# Textbook of
# Animal
# Husbandry
## Extension Education

## Fourth Edition

# Textbook of Animal Husbandry

# Extension Education

## Fourth Edition

**P Mathialagan** PhD
Professor and Head
Department of Veterinary and AH Extension Education
Madras Veterinary College (TANUVAS)
Chennai

# CBS Publishers & Distributors Pvt Ltd

Delhi • Bengaluru • Chennai • Kochi • Kolkata • Lucknow • Mumbai
Hyderabad • Jharkhand • Nagpur • Patna • Pune • Uttarakhand

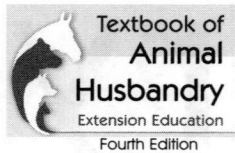

**Textbook of Animal Husbandry Extension Education**
Fourth Edition

ISBN: 978-93-88902-98-4

Fourth Edition: **2020**
Reprint: 2022

First Edition: 1997

Published by Satish Kumar Jain and produced by Varun Jain for
**CBS Publishers & Distributors** Pvt Ltd
4819/XI Prahlad Street, 24 Ansari Road, Daryaganj, New Delhi 110 002, India
Ph: 23289259, 23266861, 23266867  Website: www.cbspd.com
Fax: 011-23243014          e-mail: delhi@cbspd.com; cbspubs@airtelmail.in

*Corporate Office:* 204 FIE, Industrial Area, Patparganj, Delhi 110 092
Ph: 4934 4934      Fax: 4934 4935      e-mail: publishing@cbspd.com; publicity@cbspd.com

**Branches**

- **Bengaluru:** Seema House 2975, 17th Cross, K.R. Road,
  Banasankari 2nd Stage, Bengaluru 560 070, Karnataka, India
  Ph: +91-80-26771678/79          Fax: +91-80-26771680          e-mail: bangalore@cbspd.com
- **Chennai:** 7, Subbaraya Street, Shenoy Nagar, Chennai 600 030, Tamil Nadu, India
  Ph: +91-44-26680620, 26681266          Fax: +91-44-42032115          e-mail: chennai@cbspd.com
- **Kochi:** 42/1325, 1326, Power House Road, Opp KSEB Power House,
  Ernakulam 682 018, Kochi, Kerala, India
  Ph: +91-484-4059061-65          Fax: +91-484-4059065          e-mail: kochi@cbspd.com
- **Kolkata:** 147, Hind Ceramics Compound, 1st Floor, Nilgunj Road, Belghoria, Kolkata 700 056, West Bengal, India
  Ph: +91-9096713055, 7798394118, 9836841399          e-mail: kolkata@cbspd.com
- **Lucknow:** Basement, Khushnuma Complex, 7-Meerabai Marg (behind Jawahar Bhawan), Lucknow 226001, UP, India
  Ph: +91-522-4000032          e-mail: tiwari.lucknow@cbspd.com
- **Mumbai:** PWD Shed, Gala No. 25/26, Ramchandra Bhatt Marg, Next to JJ Hospital Gate No. 2,
  Opp. Union Bank of India, Noorbaug, Mumbai-400009, Maharashtra, India
  Ph: +91-22-24902340/41          Fax: +91-22-24902342          e-mail: mumbai@cbspd.com

**Representatives**

| • Hyderabad | 0-9885175004 | • Jharkhand | 0-9811541605 | • Nagpur | 0-9421945513 |
| • Patna | 0-9334159340 | • Pune | 0-9623451994 | • Uttarakhand | 0-9716462459 |

*Printed at:* Glorious Printers, Delhi, India

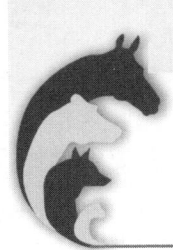

# Preface

I am happy that readers have shown a lot of interest in this book, especially undergraduate and postgraduate students of veterinary colleges across the country, teachers of extension, researchers, field extension officers, trainers, civil services aspirants and general educationists. It is true that a small number of good books have been recently written on agriculture extension but to the best of my knowledge, there is no book which deals comprehensively with all the important aspects of animal husbandry extension education and community development.

This book is intended to make a beginning in this direction by discussing in detail the principles and concepts of extension, growth and development of India's rural reconstruction and community development, the current Panchayati Raj system, animal husbandry programmes and co-operatives, rural sociology, educational psychology, extension systems, extension methods and aids, communication of innovations, programme planning, evaluation and livestock marketing extension.

A textbook remains valuable only when it is modified to take account of new developments. This edition is thoroughly revised and greatly enriched in both quality and quantity. A few new chapters have been added. Most of the examples given have been taken from Indian experience in general and my own experience in particular. It would be highly fitting, to express my sincere gratitude to the predecessors who have authored books on extension education in community development, which gave an insight into various concepts in the field of extension.

I am indebted to all the authors whose books, bulletins and articles I have consulted in the preparation of this book. The sources of information are acknowledged at the end of the references and also in the footnotes. I would also take this opportunity to thank my colleagues Dr A Manivannan, Dr P Thilakar, Dr N Vimal Rajkumar and Dr P Athilakshmy who encouraged and helped me to revise this edition and publisher who has taken keen interest in bringing out this book.

**P Mathialagan**

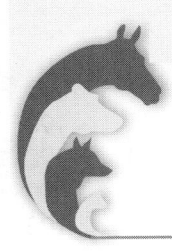

# Contents

# Chapter 1

# Principles of Extension

## GENESIS OF EXTENSION

The term was formally used for the first time in 1873 by Cambridge University to describe a particular 'Extension' of educational innovation. This was to take the educational advantages of universities to the ordinary people, where they lived and worked. The term 'extension' was first coined in England in the 1840s. James Stuart, considered to be the father of extension, was the first to deliver lectures to women's, men's clubs in 1867-68 in the north England and create the first record in the history of extension.[1]

The first Director of Extension within the United States (University of Chicago, 1892) was Moulton. He had been one of the Cambridge University's early extension workers and in 1885 had documented the first ten years of the extension movement—the world's first real treatise on extension. Agricultural extension developed much later than the other extension programmes. The Scottish Advisory Service is one of the oldest agricultural extension services in the world. It was established in its present form as a co-operative county, agricultural college and national programme. Concurrent agricultural education and advisory movement developed in England, Continental Europe, and also in Australia. Animal husbandry extension emerged in Australia as early as 1889, Queensland started a successful dairy extension programme based on the use of two 'mobile' dairy extension units (trains).[2]

Since the beginning of the 20th century the 'extension education' has been used in the United States. The university extension of England leads the isolated agricultural extension work of the US Land-Grant colleges. The farmers' institute movement originated in the north eastern United States. The Woman's Institute was adopted by US and UK from Canada.

Dr. Seaman Knapp's 'Farm and Home Demonstration' programme started in southern USA in 1902. It was sponsored by US Department of Agriculture. Later it became a co-operative extension service.

### Extension in Abroad

Extension concept is well developed in USA, Israel, China, Japan, Taiwan and Australia. In USA, the extension activity is mainly done by the co-operative extension and home economics service. In Israel extension service is given by the joint centre for agricultural extension run jointly by the Government and the settlement department of the Jewish agency. In China, the attempt was first made by the National Committee of the Chinese YMCA in 1915. National Extension Service Programme and the Republic of China made immense role of extension activity in that country.

In Japan, the extension work was started as early as 1870. In this context the approach was same as USA system with a slight change. Imperial agricultural association took part active role in Japan for extension service. In Taiwan rapid progress made since 1948. Here the extension work is undertaken by the farmer's association. In Australia, now it is very well developed. The animal husbandry extension activity is implemented by the department of primary industries (DPI). There is separate extension officer for dairy, sheep, etc. Other countries like Philippines, Republic of Korea, Nepal, Burma and Pakistan also have started their extension division.

The present pattern of American agricultural extension resulted from the merger of major national agricultural rehabilitation programmes, plus some farmer and adult education movements, with university extension. Further, agricultural extension closely integrated into a much wider programme of extension or 'community development'.

Agricultural extension, animal husbandry extension, dairy extension, home science extension, horticulture extension, agri-engineering extension and all other forms of extensions take education to people.

1. Farquhar R.N. Australian Agricultural Extension Conference: Reviews, Papers and Reports, 1962
2. United Nations Science and Technology for Development: Report of the UN Conference on the Application of Science and Techonology for the Benefit of the Less Developed Area, Vol.6, Eduction and Training, 1963.

## MEANING OF EXTENSION

The term extension has its origin in the Latin word "tensio" meaning "stretching" and "ex" meaning "out". The literal meaning of extension is "stretching out". In our context, extension is stretching out to the villages for imparting scientific information beyond the limits of universities and research stations where formal education is given. Hence extension is informal education of rural people in an out-of-school situation. The common meaning of the term is that extension involves the conscious communication of information to help people form sound opinions and make good decisions.[1]

a. **Extension is education for all people.** It is the education of all the farmers, farm women, youths and villagers as a whole.

b. **Extension is changing knowledge, skill and attitude of all the people.** Extension aims at bringing about desirable changes in the attitude, knowledge and skill.

c. **Extension is working with men and women, young and old, boys and girls to answer their needs and wants.** Working with all people irrespective of sex, age to answer their needs and wants.

d. **Extension is helping people to help themselves.** Helping people is service. But service makes people dependent. On the other hand, if we educate them they become self-reliant (independent). Education makes people self-reliant by bringing about desirable changes in what they feel (attitude), what they know (knowledge) and what they do (skill). Extension teaching aims at helping people to help themselves through education and not merely by service. "If you give fish to a man you feed him for a day (service approach) but if you teach him how to fish, you feed him for life long (educational approach)". The educational approach is desirable because it helps a person to help himself.

e. **Extension is "learning by doing and seeing is believing".** "What a man hears he may doubt, what a man sees he may possibly doubt, but what a man does he cannot doubt." About 80% of the people learn by seeing, hearing and doing. Implication for extension worker is to make the farmers work by doing themselves. The benefit of the new practice is appreciated and continued to be adopted without reverting to old method.

f. **Extension is teaching people what to want (i.e. converting unfelt needs into felt needs) as well as how to work out ways of satisfying these wants and inspiring them to achieve their desires (wants).** At present, due to lack of knowledge and convictions, many farmers adopt traditional methods and do not know that their livestock and poultry need balanced feed for optimum production. If the extension worker teaches the farmer, the benefits of balanced feed (learning by doing) becomes a want and thereafter a felt need. Then the farmer should be taught how to mix the balanced feed or where from to get it. Thus the farmer learns the new practice of feeding the balanced rations and he continues to use it in his farm. Balanced ration becomes a felt need thereafter in future.

g. **Extension is the development of individuals in their day-to-day living, development of their leaders, their society and their world as a whole.** To begin with, the extension worker influences two or three individuals to take to scientific livestock or poultry farming and eventually these individuals assume leadership to teach the rest of the people in the area to have livestock farms or to raise poultry through scientific methods. In course of time the entire village may be covered and most people would follow new methods of livestock or poultry farming and derive profits. Thus extension is the development of individuals, leaders, society as a whole, in day-to-day living.

h. **Extension is working together to expand the welfare and happiness of the people, their families, the village, the country and the world.** The research worker, extension worker and farmer together form a team for development and progress of country. Research workers (investigators) evolve new methods. The extension workers are interpreters of scientific information in the popular form so that the farmers may understand, accept and adopt the new and improved practices for increasing production, which is the basis or foundation for expanding the welfare and happiness of the people.

i. **Extension is working together in harmony with the culture of the people.** Culture means approved way of life. Improved practices recommended by the extension worker should be compatible with the approved way of life of the local people, e.g.

    1. Vegetarian—dairying, horticulture

    2. Non-vegetarian

        a. Hindu—piggery, poultry, etc.

        b. Muslim—poultry, fishery, etc.

j. **Extension is a living relationship between the village workers and village people, respect and trust for each other, sharing of joys and sorrows and results in friendship through which village extension work continues.** The extension work can be conducted through close and continuous contact between the extension worker and the farmers in the area. In proportion to the number of contacts, more and more people are influenced or changed to adopt new methods. The extension worker is a friend, philosopher and guide.

k. **Extension is a two-way channel** (Fig. 1.1). Researches bring out innovation. The extension worker carries this new scientific information and passes it onto the farmers. The farmers may have some problems and difficulties in day-to-day farming while applying the new practices and techniques. The extension worker may not have ready answer or solution for this problem faced by farmers and seeks answers. The research worker conducts experiments and passes on his results as answers.

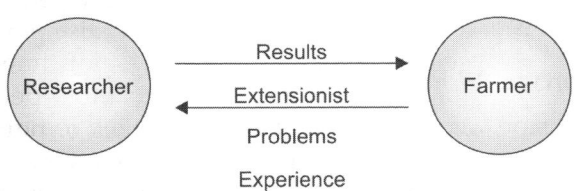

**Fig. 1.1:** Two-way channel

Therefore, the extension worker has dual responsibility of bringing the results of research to the farmers and at the same time has also the responsibility to transmit the problems faced by the farmer to the research worker for answers or solution. Thus it is a two-way channel.

l. **Extension is a continuous educational process (in which both the learner and teacher contribute and receive)**

In 1955, 7 kg of poultry feed was required for 14 weeks for a poultry to gain 1.5 kg in live weight. In 1958, 6 kg of feed was recommended for 12 weeks for a bird to gain 1.5 kg of weight. During 1970, 5 kg of feed was advised as a feed for a broiler to gain 2 kg in 10 weeks. In 1980s, 4 kg of feed was recommended per bird for 8 weeks to gain 2 kg body weight. Now (2019) it requires 3.8 kg of feed to gain 2.1 kg live weight in 5 weeks.

We can understand from this that farmers should be informed of the latest findings of research for efficient production and it is the job of the extension worker to continuously educate the farmer about the latest

scientific information relating to feeding, breeding and management of livestock for increased production.

## DEFINITION OF EXTENSION

By definition, extension and extension education are synonymous. Extension is out of school system of education in which adults and young people learn by doing.[1]

Extension is education and its purpose is to change the attitude and practices of people with whom the work is done.[2] Animal husbandry or veterinary extension is a special branch of extension education which deals with the people through educational procedures, for improving livestock farming methods and techniques, increasing the animals and bird production efficiency and income, stepping up the level of living and elevating the social and educational standards of rural life.[3]

Extension education is an applied science consisting of content derived from researchers, accumulated field experiences and relevant principles drawn from the behavioural sciences, synthesized with useful technology in a body of philosophy, principles, content and matters focused on the problems of out of school education for adults and youths.[4]

Extension education is the process of teaching rural people how to live better by learning ways that improve their farm, home and community institutions.[5]

## COMPONENTS OF EXTENSION

Over a period of time, extension has become highly specialised in nature, with status of a discipline and well-developed profession. It has now its own methodology, philosophy and principles together with systematised body of knowledge.

Extension has three broad components, viz. Extension Education, Extension Service and Extension Work. Each one has its own merits and yields, different results depending on the abilities, capabilities and potentialities of the individuals, organisation and users who practice them in the field situation.

1. Kelsey L.D. and Hearne G.C. "Co-operative Extension Work". Comstock Publishing Associates, New York, 1963.
2. Ensminger Douglas, "A Guide to Community Development", Govt. of India, New Delhi, 1962.
3. Mathialagan, P. "Principles of Extension Education-Manual" Department of Extension Education, VC & RI TANUVAS, Namakkal, 1993.
4. Leagans, J.P. "Extension Education in Community Development", Directorate of Extension, Govt of India, 1961.
5. Ibid.

## Extension Education

This is basically a need-oriented, local-resource based, problem-solution oriented system and concerned with tripod for modernisation, viz. teaching, research and extension education. Here the extension efforts are research-based, mostly concerned with development of communication media-mix, training-technology, and evolving research-based extension methodology and organizational dynamics duly charged with an efficient management of technologies, both in terms of its (i) products, viz. new breeds, medicines, vaccines and (ii) processes, viz. artificial insemination, cross breeding, feeding methods and educating people to change their attitudes towards microbes, parasites' control, etc.

In an academic parlance, "Extension Education" is a behavioural science following a continuous, persuasive and discriminating educational process. It aims at affecting the behavioural changes in people in a desirable direction through conviction, communication and diffusion by its proven methods, principles and philosophies, all cumulatives resulting in (mutual) learning involvement of both client and change agent systems.[1]

The extension education role is generally performed by higher learning institutions, viz. research institutes, universities and apex level training and extension organisations.

## Extension Service

It is an organisation and/or programme for animal husbandry, agriculture, development and rural welfare, employing the extension process as a means of programme implementation. Extension service is location-specific, input-intensive, service-oriented and field level professional activities concerned with advising the target beneficiaries on the various facts of technologies on one hand, and communicating field and user's problems to the research scientists, on the other. Thus it bridges the gap between research results and their application in the field through continuous persuasion, communication, motivation and involvement of inputs/credits as well as other supporting agencies. It serves as a catalytic agent in bringing people, problems, production processes and productivity together for achieving prosperity in an assigned influence area.

Extension service has the role and responsibility of bridging the gap between research and users of technology through transplanting, transmitting and translating research results (technology) into practice by way of establishing co-ordination and linkages with institutions of higher learning on the one hand, and people's institutions and organisations, on the other. It establishes two-way communication processes, i.e. (i) transferring technology in the field through demonstrations, delivery and direct teaching of target beneficiaries, and (ii) providing feedback, feed-in, feed-up and feed-down processes in strengthening and using national and international knowledge to make it more useful to the research from the users' point of view so as to enable reorientation of location-specific researches, duly matched with the felt needs of the people as per availability of indigenous knowledge, resources and inputs.

Extension services also work hand-in-glove with other development departments, inputs and credit institution and try to multiply their efforts (effects) through mass and local media of communication. Extension service is the mission and mandate of various development departments like animal husbandry, agriculture, health, industry, education (instructional technology, information and communication technology) etc.

## Extension Work

Extension work is to assist people engaged in farming and home-making to utilise more fully their own resources and those available to them for solving current problems and meeting changing economic and social conditions. Extension work is through educational and service approach. Rural people are stimulated to make changes that result in more efficient production and marketing of farm products, conservation of natural resources, more comfortable homes, improved health and more satisfying family and community life.

Extension work is the education of people to help themselves in decision-making in the right direction. It is a system of service and education designed to meet the needs of the people. This concept is at the lowest in hierarchy but extremely broad-based in usages as it is highly popular. It is also extremely location-specific, and usually susceptible to outside criticism. At the same time it gives best results from the altruistic motive of the users of the concept.

Extension work is actually performing task(s) in helping the people to help themselves in making them self-reliant, self-respectful, self-acting through self-help projects and activities and in inculcating self-will (obstinacy). Here, the emphasis is on development of 'self' so that in performing each task one may not require 'push' from others to start their vehicle of socioeconomic life and self-development, maturation and growth every time.

Extension work is to help farmers to solve their own problems through the application of scientific knowledge as now generally accepted. If this be true then extension must be regarded as largely educational. If extension workers devote more effort at creating of a desire for information, farmers would come and ask for it, rather than wait for it to be brought to them. Farmer motivation thus becomes a phase of extension work worthy of careful study in any area. The effectiveness of extension work is measured by its ability to change the static situation which prevails in rural areas into a dynamic one.

Many farmers will ask the local extension worker to dehorn their calves, deworm their sheep and debeak their chickens. Unless the farmer is also taught to do these things himself, it is not extension education but a service.

In the developing countries extension work is done mostly by agencies and/or individuals wedded to altruism and/or on minimum payment. This is generally the role and responsibility of individuals and agencies having mission and mandate to uplift the people. Extension work requires a fair degree of emotional commitment on the part of the extension worker to fulfil such tasks specially in educating people in the desirable direction. This agency is termed "Extension", and the personnel manning this agency or organisation are called "Extension Workers".

## SCOPE OF EXTENSION

The dictionary meaning of "scope" is "space for action", "the end before the mind". The scope of extension is unlimited, mostly dealing with the problems concerning every day life. It teaches people how to do something and to work out ways and means to satisfy their own felt need. It teaches people as to how to recognize and solve problems of life which are considered inevitable. It is an education of action–action in groups and masses, within a democratic framework of society.

It emphasises on change of mental outlook of the people and filling in them ambition of higher standards of life, the will and determination to work for such standards. This higher standard of life may be possible by directing attention to the following items:

  i. Increased employment and increased production by application of scientific methods of animal husbandry, fisheries, agriculture, etc. and the establishment of subsidiary and cottage industries.

  ii. Self-help and self-reliance and the largest possible application of the principle of co-operation.

  iii. Developing the vast unutilised resources of the country-side for the benefit of the country.

  iv. Closest co-operation with the best unofficial leadership.

So, in short, the scope of extension is to enable the people to have higher standards of life through the above-mentioned four right and self-motivated means and as this higher standard of life is a growing one without limit, the scope of extension also becomes limitless.

## CONCEPT OF EXTENSION

Concept means 'idea'. The basic concept of extension is that it is education. "Briefly we can define education as shaping of behaviour or modification of behaviour of the individual for adequate adjustment in the society".[1]

### Basic Changes in Behaviour

Change in behaviour means, change in knowledge and understanding, skill and attitude.

### Knowledge and Understanding

Knowledge is a component of behaviour which is the ability or act of knowing remembering recallecting and things learnt and experienced.

Knowledge (or things known) is the intimate acquaintance with facts. It is the information one has acquired and can use in various situations, e.g. knowing that the newborn calf should be fed with colostrum about 1/10th of its body weight.

Understanding is the comprehension of the meaning of things, the ability to interpret situations. It often includes cause and effect relationships. How and why events are related to each other, e.g. 1 kg of broiler finisher mash costs ₹ 5 and hence 4 kg costs how much? $5 \times 4 = 20$ (understanding).

### Skill

Skill is an ability in action. It is the ability to do a job. It is the competency in using knowledge effectively. Skills are two types manual and mental or technical. Manual skill or physical skill means proficiency in handling tools, machines and materials, e.g. using de-beaker, constructing brooder, etc.

---

1. Chauhan, SS.Advanced Eductional Psychology", Vikas Publishing House Pvt. Ltd., New Delhi, 1982.

Technical or mental skill means expertise in the use and application of technical knowledge, e.g. how to use flame gun for disinfection, operating incubator, preparing solution for dipping of sheep, etc.

### Attitude

Attitude is the degree of positive or negative effect associated with some psychological object[1]. Attitude is a predisposition to behave in a given manner.[2]

Attitudes (what one feels) are emotional reactions usually expressed as feelings towards something. They are likely to imply the direction of potential action, e.g. generally poultry farmers used to dispose their dead birds by simply throwing away but nowadays they have started disposing them either by burying or incinerating (change in attitude).

Extension education may combine all these changes in human behaviour in getting one job done.

### Three Concepts[3]

i. All inclusive concept: A number of countries still conceive that extension means the work that is done by the Government departments at village level, including the supplies to the rural farmers.

ii. Service concept: To gain more confidence of the farmers, more work of service nature was also added later on.

iii. Educational concept: The ultimate aim is to help people to help themselves through education to bring a change in outlook. But effective education is possible only if there is a separate agency to assume the responsibility for supplies and services enabling the extension workers to devote themselves to the task of training the farmers.

### Steps in Extension Education Process

Any effective education programme involves five essential phases. The diagram (Fig. 1.2) participatory rural appraisal/rapid rural appraisal shows the sequence of steps that result in the process from a given situation to a new or a more desirable one.[4]

1. Thurstone, LL et al. "The Measurement of Attitude", Chicago: Univ. Chicago Press, 1929. As quoted by Allen. L. Edwards, "Techniques of Attitude Scale Construction," 1969.
2. Mathialagan, P. "Attitude of Livestock Farmers", A Mimeographed Lecture Note, Department of Extension Education VC & RI, TANUVAS, Namakkal, 1994.
3. FAO Survey Report on Extension in Asia, 1975
4. Leagans, JP. "Extension Eduction in Community Development" op.cit.

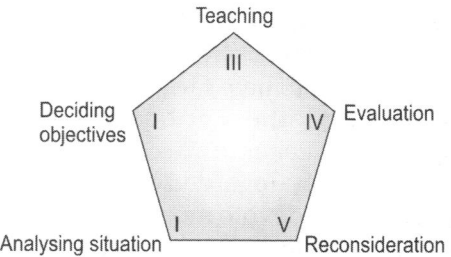

**Fig. 1.2:** Steps in extension education process

### Analysing the Situation and Identifying the Problems

This needs detailed information about a number of factors. It is very necessary to know the interests, education, social customs, habits and folkways of the people. It is also necessary to know physical factors such as soils, types of livestock and poultry farming, cropping system, markets, housing conditions, communications, etc. (Leagans, JP) These details can be acquired by conducting participatory rural appraisal/rapid rural appraisal (PRA/RRA).

All these factors are essential prerequisites and by knowing them the extension worker should be able to introduce new facts and research findings to stimulate a fresh approach to the problems of the people. A thorough analysis of situation will help to compare conditions that exist with goals that are desired.

### Objectives

The general objectives and the specific or working objectives (mainly teaching objective) should be stated separately, among different levels of objectives that are recognized. A limited number of problems should be selected and their objectives stated in simple, direct language. The solutions to be offered must give satisfaction. They should satisfy the people and the extension workers. People would take interest in planning and execution of the programme if they feel that it is "their programme".

### Teaching

Teaching must take into consideration. Selection of subject matter which will be the teaching objective. Appropriate methods and tools to convey the subject matter. The methods to be used should be consistent with the economic, social and educational levels of the people. For instance, the mass media, which are very effective in advanced countries where literacy and economic levels are high, are not yet effective in India. On the other hand, individual and group contact methods are very effective in India.

## Evaluation

Evaluation is a continuous process and must be planned for the initial stages of the programme. A few important objectives should be selected for evaluation and the process of evaluation must be as simple as possible.

## Reconsideration

As a result of the teaching programme, the situation changes and becomes different from that in the beginning. The physical, social and economic conditions of the people also undergo change. Hence, reconsideration to meet the fresh needs and interests of the people becomes imperative, as evaluation shows certain goals as being accomplished.

The extension education process is to consider each of the five steps in succession. The steps are not separate but overlap one another. Planning, teaching, evaluation and reconsideration take place continuously throughout the entire process of extension work.

## The Concept of Salesmanship[1]

Extension teaching is something compared to commercial salesmanship. It is pointed out that the extension worker is primarily engaged in the "selling" of ideas. Certainly, many of the techniques employed by a good salesman in selling physical goods are services that have direct application in extension. But while one is a commercial transaction conducted for private profit, the other is an educational process conducted by a public agency to bring about changes in the knowledge, attitude or skill of the individual.

## ▌AIMS OF EXTENSION[2]

Extension aims at: (a) Human resource development, (b) increasing production, and (c) bringing suitable changes in the cultural aspects.

## Human Resource Development

Human resource development for multiplier effect by:

i. Imparting knowledge, skills, understanding about the use of various components of technology (education/training).

ii. Bringing desirable changes in the behavioural patterns, attitudes, values, goals, and confidence as well as the practices of the people (communication skills).

---

1. Reddy, AA. "Extension Education", Sree Lakshmi Press, Bapatla, Andhra Pradesh, 1993.
2. Adopted from "Extension Management on Communication Skills–Reading Material", NIRD, Hyderabad.

iii. Firing the imagination of the people through the gateway of 'learning-by-doing' and 'seeing is believing'.

This will help people in taking their own decisions and initiatives by themselves (demonstrations).

iv. Making available fund of knowledge, wisdom and observations for perennial use and as references (publications).

v. Providing continuous flow of information and data for decision making so as to keep their (clientele) morale and motivation high for learning more and more and for the actual harvesting of resultant benefits for self-development (information and documentation).

vi. Continuously providing technological back-stoppings for recycling of their (clientele) economic gain.

## Increasing Production

Increasing production by (i) Making realistic assessment and availability of need-based inputs (knowledge and physical) for given set(s) of technology in maximisation of their outputs (training). (ii) Prepositioning of needed inputs in order to make them available at a reachable point, so as to conserve their resources, energy and efforts and thereby hasten the pace of development (grants-in-aid, subsidy, loan provision all put together). (iii) Organising interest groups, societies and markets for getting maximum economic gain and thus eliminating middlemen and exploiters (gate keeping). (iv) Developing farmers' organisations and linking them with respective farm-organisations (public, co-operative and private).

## Cultural Change

Bringing suitable changes in the cultural aspects of the people so that the changes in practices automatically bring changes in the knowledge, skills and attitudes.

All the above changes must raise higher techno-socio-psycho-cultural standards (together) with economic prosperity in the community duly linked with the national programmes and policies of overall development of the people. In achieving the above aims, the extension workers have to acquire skills in practising the philosophy, principles and methodology of extension.

## ▌OBJECTIVES OF EXTENSION

Objectives can be defined as expression of desired ends towards which our efforts are directed. According to Paul Leagans, objective means "A direction of movements". If objectives are defined as the direction of movement then a goal may be defined as the distance in any given direction during a given period of time. Some say objectives, aim, goals and purposes are "Synonyms" but it is not so.

### Classification of Objectives

There are different types of classification of objectives (Fig. 1.3). They are as follows:

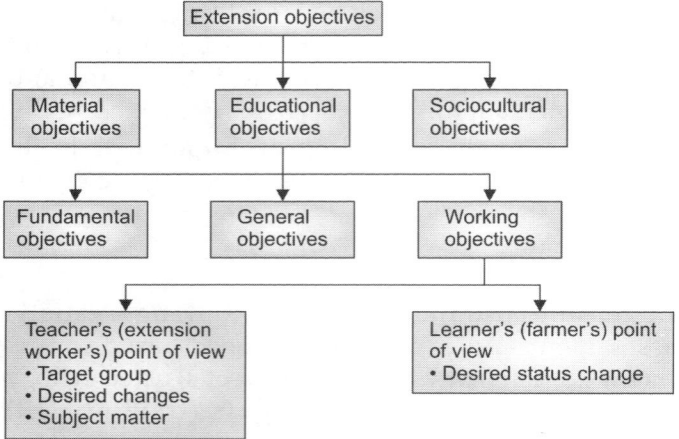

**Fig. 1.3:** Classification of objectives of extension

### General and Specific Objectives

a. General objectives are those which are broad-based and general in nature, e.g. raising the standard of living of the farming community
b. Specific objectives are those which are concerned with single item and are more particular. eg. intensive health cover to scheme animals, better sanitation in village.

### Long-term and Short-term Objectives

Long-term objectives are more permanent and are carried out for considerable period. e.g. (1) augmentation of milk production by artificial insemination and cross-breeding in cattle, (2) twelve-year perspective plan, (3) five-year plan, etc.

Short term objectives are those which are mostly temporary and immediately useful ones, e.g. programmes launched for a short period of one year or six months (one-year poultry programme).

### Material, Educational and Sociocultural Objectives

#### Material Objectives

Increase in the livestock farm income by improving production performance of the animals, e.g. European Economic Community (EEC) Sheep Development Programmes.

### Educational Objectives

To develop people through behavioural changes from traditional and static to scientific and dynamic in nature. Extension objective must be educational. Education means the production of desirable changes in human behaviour, e.g.:

1. Farm Radio School on buffalo management (objective change in knowledge).
2. Peripatetic (out campus) training about disinfection of poultry house—demonstration of fumigation, flamegun sterilization, etc. (objective change in skill).
3. By proper education convincing the vegetarian to include eggs in their daily diet (objective change attitude)

There are three levels of educational objectives, namely fundamental objectives, general objectives, and working objectives.

#### Fundamental Objectives

This includes all basic requirements of a society (food, shelter, and cloth), e.g. better life, better citizenship. It is the function of extension service to teach the people to determine accurately their own problems, to help them acquire knowledge and to drive them to action, but it must be their own action out of their own knowledge and conviction.

#### General Objectives

Though these objectives are general in nature, they are more definite, e.g. helping rural people for better amenities. Constant improvement of physical and social well-being such as wealth, health, knowledge, sociability, beauty and arts, righteousness are essential to achieve this. Efforts should be made on the following lines:

1. Improvement of the well-being of family.
2. Improvement of farm income through the application of scientific methods and farm mechanisation.
3. Encouragement of people to be wiser consumers.
4. Improvement of health through better nutritive and more adequate health facilities and services.
5. Improvement of family living through better housing, rural electrification and more adequate labour-saving equipment.
6. Improvement of educational and recreational facilities for the home and community.

7. Development of better understanding, more active participation in community, state, national and international affairs.

8. Improvement of resources so that future generations may also have good living and the general welfare safeguards.

### Working Objectives

This may be determmed in two ways. First being teacher's stand point, (a) target group, (b) desired changes and (c) subject matter, e.g. teaching rural population to have mixed farming. The next being farmer's stand point—desired status change, e.g. to make more money to educate their children up to college level.

It is important to bring harmony among rural people to make them feel what they need and extension workers to think what they ought to have. The difference between wants and needs is roughly difference between what is and what should be. It is essential to reach working objectives through full discussion.

### Sociocultural Objectives

Sociocultural objectives are: 1. Developing the community. 2. Promoting the cultural, social, recreational and intellectual life of the rural people. 3. Creating opportunity to improve the talent of rural people. 4. Developing youth as an active member.

### Objectives of Animal Husbandry Extension

1. To give knowledge to the farmer and help him perform still more efficiently to produce his own food, and increase his income.

2. To help in changing the farmer to produce his own food, set a good table and live well.

3. To help the member of the farm community in the larger appreciation of opportunities, the beauties and privileges of country and in knowing something about the environment in which they live.

4. To promote the social, the cultural, the recreational and the intellectual life of the rural people.

5. To place opportunity before the rural people to develop native talents through work, recreation, social life and leadership.

6. To make rural citizen proud of his occupation, independent in his thinking, constructive in his outlook, efficient, self-reliant with a love for home and country.

## FUNCTIONS OF EXTENSION

The function of education is to bring about desirable changes in human behaviour through education. The education may bring changes in their knowledge, skill, attitude, understanding, goals, action and confidence (Ray GL, 1996).

Change in knowledge means change in what people know. For example, through extension programmes livestock farmers who did not know about clean milk production (CMP), came to know about the technology.

Change in skill means change in the technique of doing things. The livestock farmers learnt the right method of milking which they did not know earlier.

Change in attitude involves change in the reaction towards certain things. The livestock farmers developed favorable attitude towards CMP.

Change in understanding means change in comprehension. The farmers realized the importance of clean milk production in dairy farming and its direct impact on disease prevention.

Change in goal is the distance in any given direction one is expected to go during a given period of time. The farmers directed their goal towards increased milk yield through clean milk production.

Change in action means change in the way of doing things. The farmers who did not follow the practice of CMP started practising it in their farm.

Change in confidence means change in self reliance. Livestock farmers felt that they could follow CMP and prevent mastitis in their animals. The development of confidence or self reliance is the solid foundation for making progress.

## DIMENSIONS OF EXTENSION

Extension education is a multidimensional branch of science which has lead role in sustainable development of the society. Misra (1990) and GL Ray (1996) have quoted ten dimensions of agricultural extension. Here we discuss on ten dimensions of veterinary extension.

1. Help to help them self: The main objective of extension is to help the farmers to help themselves. "Self help is the best help"—Aesop. Thus, altruistic dimension is an important dimension of extension. Altruism means concern for others. The base of the extension is the desire to help others.

2. Empowerment through education: Extension is an educational process focused towards sustainable development and empowerment of the society.

3. Communication for development: Extension is communication process meant for the development

of the society. In extension, different modes of communication, individual, group and mass communication are used in coordination with one another to disseminate information.

4. Desirable change in the behavior: Extension education by imparting knowledge, skill, attitude and action brings desirable change in the behavior of an individual.

5. Disseminating technologies: Extension education role is to disseminate scientific technologies on need basis. It also disseminates the skill to adopt the technologies. All technologies developed need not to be adopted at field level. Thus extension education also analyses the reasons and feedbacks for adoption and nonadoption of technologies.

6. Lab to land: Extension education acts as a bridge between research station and the field. The research should be done on the basis of the need of the farmer. But in many instances, the research is done independently, without analyzing the field.

7. Sustainable usage of resources: Intensive usage of natural resources is practiced to meet the growing demand for food. Extension education plays a key role in imparting skills to utilize inputs and natural resources in sustainable way.

8. Income generation: Ultimate aim to disseminate technologies among farmers is to improve their livelihood through income generation. Extension education focus on strategies to improve the income generation and livelihood of farmers

9. Curriculum development: Extension education is nonformal in nature. But it also has a formal role in imparting education to college students at university level. The students who are the future officers should have exposure on extension education, so that it will help them in their professional development and client dealing.

10. Human resource management (HRM) which is the hot topic in all fields of education has also finds its place in extension education. Framing objectives to monitoring and evaluation detailed programme planning is must for the success of any project. Thus extension education clearly defined the steps in programme planning for the successful implementation of projects.

## PRINCIPLES OF EXTENSION

Principle means guide for action, fundamental or theoretical basis. It also means law or settled rules for action. "A principle is a universal truth that has been observed and found to be true under varying conditions and circumstances. A principle is a fundamental truth and a settled rule of action".[1] In this context principles are rules of conduct for extension workers for executing their job efficiently. There is no set of rules, guides, principles that can be passed on to extension workers to follow for rural development. There is no such formula because every situation is different, every potential leader (or farmer) has a different personality, a different background and different attitude that he has acquired through his experiences.

The groups an extension worker will work with will be different in many respects, depending upon the kind of problem he will tackle, the environment in which he is in, and the money available to carry on such functions. There is no formula in the strict sense that one can find identical ways to tackle all problems and always predetermine the results. Extension worker can gain by the experiesces of others that have proved successful in eliminating the mistakes and indicate proper actions that should be adopted. Thus, we do not attempt to acquire a formula that all can follow, but strive for guides (or rules) which, within their broad scope, if we understand them, can be usefully applied.

### Principle of Existing Environment

The situation or condition that exists means, taking into account all the forces that are present and by utilising these forces, gradually building the programme and momentum necessary to arrive at the objectives. To do this, means to know what the conditions (situations) are. For this, decisions are quickly taken and opinions are hurriedly determined in trying to get on with the job. Taking time to learn about the environment is a very important part of the job.

Extension work should be related to the local situation, local leaders, and capability of the people in that social system. Every social system (village or community) has its own special characteristics, personalities and problems. Stereotyped programmes will not be workable in all areas because problems, need and current interest differ from village to village, block to block, district to district and state to state. Therefore, taking time to study the environment is very important aspect of the extension work.

### Principle of Participation and Co-operation

Participation of people in all of the activities of extension programme means involvement, co-operation of people in planning the programe, determining objectives, setting up plan of work, carrying on actions

1. Dahama, O.P. and Bhatnagar, O.P. "Educational and Communication for Development, op.cit.

and evaluating results. The extent or degree of participation will vary and cannot be predetermined. But a sincere desire to involve the recipients of the service and make efforts to permit their involvement must be accepted as necessary prerequisites to work in rural extension programmes. If people participate in programmes they develop a sense of belonging. This also develops leadership and increases the confidence of the people. This will pave way for the success of the programme and future extension programme will be easily introduced and will be readily accepted by the people.

## Principle of Developing Programme Gradually

Many problems and failures arise proceeding with the programme in haste even before all facts are present, before the people develop confidence in themselves or their extension leader or before resources are available. We could go on with this list, but let us remember the above principle. It will not guarantee success, but may help to eliminate failures. It is very important to note that no programme should be pushed through. Every programme must progress only at the pace at which the people can understand, appreciate and actively participate in it. Otherwise, we may achieve only physical development of the villages without developing the ability of the people to sustain the development. It is of paramount importance that the solutions found are within the capacity of the people of being adopted.

## Principle of Interests and Needs

This is the one feature of extension that usually stands on its own and if correctly applied, usually leads to success. People are drawn together in worldwide organisations and across many barriers, real or imaginary, when united for common interests or needs. The extension education should fulfil the needs of the people and create interest among them for extension programmes. Unfortunately many times the needs of the people and extension programmes are different as when the extension worker identifies clearly the core unfelt needs of the society but the people feel some other needs to be more important. In such situations, the extension worker should give priority to the felt needs of the people. During this period he should create an atmosphere of confidence, which would help in converting the unfelt needs of the people into the felt needs in future. In this way only can the extension agency mould the needs and interests of the people into realistic needs.

## Principle of Applied Science and Democracy

Applied animal husbandry and veterinary science is a two-way channel. The field problems are taken to the scientists to find out suitable solutions. The extension agency translates the technology of the university findings and works for their adoption by democratic teaching approaches like discussions and suggestions. All the merits are presented before the targeted groups. Ultimately, the people are free to decide their line of action, the method to be adopted in the local situation with their own resources and those available with government and non-government assistance.

## Principle of Adaptability in the Use of Teaching Methods

The selected village may consist of different groups. The level of knowledge, understanding, socio-psychological and biophysical characters of each group and its members may be different. So, no single method can carry all information to bring about desirable change in all the members of the group. Therefore, suitable selection, proper combination and skillful handling of the methods will transfer technology effectively and bring out desirable results. The extension worker can also use available resources to devise low-cost teaching aids that can be used in his teaching.

## Principle of Learning by Doing

During the extension programme the farmers should be encouraged to learn new practices by doing them. It is learning by doing, which is most effective in changing peoples' behaviour and in developing the confidence to use the innovation in future. "What a man hears he may doubt, what a man sees he may possibly doubt, but what a man does he cannot doubt.

## Principle of Using Existing Local Agencies or Grassroot Organisations

Panchayats, village co-operatives, schools, youth clubs, farmers' associations, woman's clubs and other welfare organisations are called grassroot organisations or local agencies. These organisations already have group of local people who have been brought together for special reasons. These groupings, their leaderships and the interests can be utilized to make contacts and develop programmes. The use of local groups would also make for a faster way to learn about the people and their culture and status. Learning about the agencies and their roles in a community or area also is one way for the extension education worker to be more intelligent about the area he must work in. Extension worker should fully utilize the services of local organisations and agencies in promoting the development activities.

### Principle of Cultural Differences

For effective implementation of any extension programme, the approach and procedure must be suited to the local culture. In a big country like India different extension approaches need to be used for different states, regions and localities, as people in those areas differ in their thinking, living environment and culture. A blueprint of the extension programme developed for one area may not be applicable as such in another area mainly because of the cultural differences. These differences can be perceived in the way of life of the people, their attitudes, values, loyalties, habits and customs.

### Principle of Cultural Change

The extension worker who works personally with the rural people must be aware of what they know and think. The change agent must find out and understand the limitations, the taboos and the cultural values. This can be related to each aspect of his programme, before it is introduced, so that an acceptable approach may be selected. Also, suitable programmes should be formulated and introduced to change the undesirable culture.

### Principle of Trained Specialists

Since animal husbandry, agriculture, fisheries, homes science and other sciences are rapidly growing with new innovative techniques, the extension worker should be aware of the current information to provide them to the needy. It is impossible for a village level multipurpose extension worker (e.g. RWO or Gramasevak) to keep himself abreast with all the latest findings of researches in all the branches of science he has to deal with in his day-to-day activity. Instead, the trained personnel or specialists from the developments departments concerned like extension officers of animal husbandry. Agriculture and Veterinary Assistant Surgeons should be provided with all recent advancement in their discipline which have scope for adoption in particular field through periodical in-service training in the universities.

### Principle of Satisfaction

Any successful programme results in satisfaction of the clientele. If they are satisfied with one programme the participation will be more in any future extension programmes. When the adoption of a new practice results in more production and profit they derive full satisfaction and develop confidence.

### Principle of Leadership

Local leaders are the guardians of local thought and action. So, for introducing any new practice the extension worker should identify, select and train the local leaders. It is said that there is one leader in ten person. The use of local leaders is one of the unique differences between formal education and extension education in the approaches. We can make available more number of teachers in the rural area by proper selection and training of the leaders. Extension service development and expansion depends directly upon the degree of involvement of local leaders.

### Principle of the Whole Family Approach

A rural family is an integral social unit in which all members have a part in carrying out the farming. Therefore, all the members of the family have to be developed equally by involving each of them. While introducing new practice, if the extension worker neglects one member of the family there is a possibility of the rejection of the innovation. If the farmer is alone persuaded or taught the extension worker teaches only one member of the family. If the extension worker persuades the housewife, the entire family is taught. "If woman moves, the household moves, if a household moves, the community moves, if the community moves, the village moves: if the village moves the country moves"(Nehru).

### Principle of Continuous Evaluation

Evaluation is an analysis by which one understands the merits and deficiencies of objectives, programme content, methods used in carrying out the programme and the results of the programme. The results of evaluation would help the extension workers in improving the quality of the programme.

### Principle of all Classes of Society

Since extension education is basically a programme aimed at rural people, it is for all classes in the rural areas. To improve rural welfare means to help all segments of the society. If the programme favours or ignores any segment or group, the results will be poorer by that degree.

### Principle of National Policies

No organization will be sanctioned if it is not in line with the ideas and opinions of national leaders. No programme will get necessary backing to operate if it is in conflict with national policies. We must face the fact that educational organization and programmes are a part of the nation in which they serve. It is very important to keep abreast of national policies. National policy and programme take over all view of the balanced development of country as a whole. Local programme and policies should be as far as possible in line with national policies and programmes to make the best use of the financial resources.

## PHILOSOPHY OF EXTENSION

Philosophy means the search, by logical reasoning, for understanding of the basic truths and principles of the universe, life and morals, and human perception and understanding of these. It is also a system of ideas concerning this or a particular subject, a system of principles for the conduct of life.

"Philosophy is an attempt to answer unlimited questions critically after investigating all that makes such questions puzzling and after realising the vagueness and confusion that underlie our ordinary ideas."[1]

The practical implication is that the philosophy of a particular discipline would furnish the principles or guidelines to shape or mould the programmes or activities relating to that discipline. The philosoply of extension education is based on the hypothesis that rural people are intelligent and they are interested in obtaining new information and at the same time have a keen desire to utilize this information for their individual and social welfare.

When an extension worker approaches the people to introduce a new technology, the people test the message against their philosophy of life and if that message fits in their philosophy then they act on it. The first step in this direction is to communicate the innovations. An atmosphere of natural trust and friendship between the extension worker and the people should be developed. The extension worker should gain full understanding of the problems and difficulties of the people in order to solve them.

There are two ways of solving the farmers' problems. One is by compelling people to adopt and another is by using a democratic approach, in which people are taught by educational method to solve the problems. The basic philosophy of extension is directed towards changing the outlook of man by educating him. Compulsion does not persuade the people to act in a particular way. The only way to secure the participation and co-operation of

1. "Southern Regional Extension School," held at University of Arkansas, 1949.

a person is to educate him. Education is not mere transfer of information. It is to transform the people by bringing about desirable changes in their behaviour.

The philosophy of extension education has been explained and interpreted in many ways by various authors and a clear-cut picture can be developed by trying to form a comprehensive idea by examining the views of different authors.

### Philosophical Characteristics of Extension[1]

The philosophical characteristics of extension work listed are those principles, attitudes, practices, or conceptions related to the people we serve that are commonly used by many extension workers:

1. Extension has philosophy of democracy.
2. Extension has a philosophy of education for all.
3. Extension has a philosophy of culture.
4. Extension has a philosophy of social progress.
5. Extension has a philosophy of leadership.
6. Extension has a philosophy of dignity of the individual and his profession.
7. Extension has a philosophy concerning teaching.
8. Extension has a philosophy about truth.
9. Extension has a philosophy of local responsibility.
10. Extension personnel have philosophical characteristics.

### Kelsey and Hearne (1955)

The philosophy of extension work is based on the importance of the individual in the promotion of progress for rural people and for the nation. Extension educators work with people to help them to develop themselves and achieve superior personal well-being. Together they establish specific objectives, expressed in terms of everyday life, which lead them in the direction of overall objectives. Some will make progress in one direction while others will do so in another direction, the progress varying with individual needs, interests and abilities. Through this process the whole community improves, as a result of co-operative participation and leadership development.

### Ensminger (1962)

According to Ensminger, the philosophy of extension can be expressed as follows:

• It is an educational process. Extension is changing the attitudes, knowledge and skills of the people.
• Extension is working with men and women, young people, boys and girls, to answer their needs and their wants. Extension is teaching people what to want and ways to satisfy their wants.

- Extension is "helping people to help themselves".
- Extension is "learning by doing and seeing is believing".
- Extension is development of individual, their leaders, their society and their world as a whole.
- Extension is working together to expand the welfare and happiness of people.
- Extension is working in harmony with the culture of the people.
- Extension is a living relationship, respect and trust for each other.
- Extension is a two-way channel.
- Extension is a continuous educational process.

## Dahama (1965)

According to Dahama, the following points are the "Philosophy of Extension".
- Self help.
- People are the greatest resources.
- It is a co-operative effort.
- It has its foundation in democracy.
- It involves a two-way channel of knowledge and experience.
- It is based on creating interest by seeing and doing.
- Voluntary, co-operative participation in programmes.
- Persuasion and education of the people.
- The programme is based on the attitudes and values of the people.
- It is a never-ending process.

Having all the author's idea in mind we can say extension has a philosophy of education, individual development, democratic approach, leadership development and cultural change. The basic philosophy of extension is changing the outlook of rural people by educating them.

## BASIC ELEMENTS IN EXTENSION

Basic elements in extension education are man himself (physiological and psychological man's environment (physical, economic and social) and man-created devices for improving his welfare.

### Man Himself

When we view a man, he is an individual human personality, a product of inherited traits shaped by forces in the environment in which he lives/exists. He possesses extensive mental as well as emotional powers with desire to resist many acts and conditions and to improve many things. He also possesses great potential physical skill. In short, a man must be viewed as possessing an extensive capacity for developing himself and shaping his environment.

### Man's Environment

Some of the major environmental/external forces facing a typical Indian villager are low agricultural and livestock production, low per capita income, poor housing facilities, insanitary conditions, poor health, underemployment, unemployment, poor educational opportunities, over population, unsatisfactory and insecure system, inadequate water resources, unsystematic or no credit facilities, traditional unproductive and uneconomical agricultural implements and farming practices, adherence to outmoded customs and traditions.

### Man-created Devices for Improving Welfare

Trained personnel, scientific knowledge, improved production tools, improved production methods and materials, expanded communication media, government aid for credit, inputs, guidance and for self-help along with freedom and encouragement are some of the man-created devices.

Therefore, these three basic elements lie at the use of extension education for community development. People are constantly in a state of trying to create and maintain a satisfying balance between the elements of man and his environment. The third element, man-created devices in the form of community development programme in India, is designed to help people make desirable adjustments between the elements of man and his environments.

The methods by which this adjustment must be made in a free society are by education. Only the human element is controlling the progress today. Therefore, the key to community development lies in the *mind*, *heart* and *hands* of the people and those of their professional readers.

## THREE LINKAGES IN EXTENSION

For a prosperous future, you cannot apply "yesterday's methods in today's production". In other words the rural people should constantly seek new information concerning improved livestock and latest agriculture production techniques, knowing, understanding, accepting and then adopting these modern methods in day-to-day farming to increase the productivity and income. As far as animal husbandry is concerned, the farmers are expected to produce milk, meat and eggs in more quantities.

Any research finding from the research stations of universities will be useful only when it reaches the users. Besides it should fit to the user's need and should be "user-friendly". To develop need based technologies the researcher should have contact with the farmers or users. But the researchers neither have the time to meet the rural people on a continuous basis nor they are equipped to meet the people and persuade them to adopt scientific and profitable methods and to ascertain from them the rural problem. On the other hand, it is impracticable for the millions of farmers to visit the research stations and universities to learn things for themselves.

Hence, an agency is required to bridge the gap between the researchers and the people at large and to play the dual role of interpreting the results of research to the farmers in such a way that they accept and adopt the recommendations and to convey the farmers' problems to the researchers for solutions. This agency is termed "Extension" and the personnel manning this agency or organization are called "Extension Workers".

There are three interrelated agencies which play a vital role in the process of rural development (Fig. 1.4).

## Research Agency

Manned by people highly trained in research work to evolve modern methods for more efficient, profitable livestock and poultry production and improved practices.

## Teaching Agency

Colleges of veterinary and agricultural sciences teach modern methods covering all aspects of animal

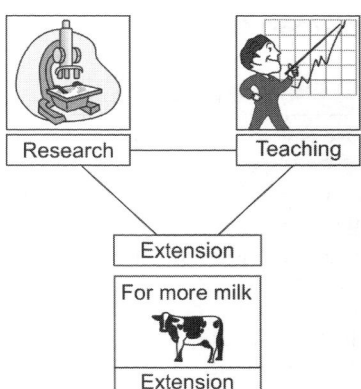

**Fig. 1.4:** Three linkages in extension

husbandry and agricultural production to the students so that they are better equipped when they take up jobs as extension workers, research workers and teachers.

## Extension Agency

The extension agency has the responsibility to communicate the results of research to the farmers in simple terms and encourage them to modern methods and improved practices in day-to-day farming to increase production. On the shoulders of extension workers lies the responsibility and functions of effectively conveying the practical and useful information to the farmers.

## Contrasts Between Formal Education and Extension Education

| Formal education | Extension education |
|---|---|
| 1. This is specialized in nature with fixed curriculum and is highly formal | This is highly informal in nature. There is no fixed curriculum |
| 2. This has organized classrooms, laboratories, prescribed books, fixed time and examinations | There are no classrooms, the extension worker does his job in actual life situation, no prescribed books, no fixed period and no examinations |
| 3. Learners adopt themselves to the syllabus offered | Here it should be flexible to meet the different needs and demands of the learners |
| 4. Pupils are requested to strictly follow the institutional norms and there is no free choice for the student | Freedom and choice of subject matter left to the learners |
| 5. The learners are homogenous with common goals | Here the learners are heterogenous and they vary in age, education level, experience and have preconceived ideas. There may also be differences in their value systems and cultural background. Their goals are diversified |
| 6. Learners go to the teacher for learning | Mostly teacher goes to the learners to teach |
| 7. Teacher alone teaches the student | The extension worker educates selected local leaders, then the local leaders are also used as teachers to teach their friends, neighbours and relatives |
| 8. Students learn from the teacher. Instructor is mostly elder than students and has more experience than the pupils | Teachers also learn from the farmers. The extension worker may be younger than the farmers and always ready to learn from the farmers' experience |
| 9. Teaching is more vertical | Teaching is highly horizontal |
| 10. Formal education is mostly deductive in approach | Extension teaching is invariably of the inductive type |

## Contrasts between animal husbandry extension and agricultural extension

| *Animal husbandry extension* | *Agricultural extension* |
|---|---|
| 1. Clientele base is very wide, ranging from landlords to the landless, from Prince to Pauper | Narrow clientele base restricted to land owning farmers |
| 2. Clientele territory ranges from village halmets to cosmopolitan cities | Clientele territory is mostly rural |
| 3. In addition to technology transfer Veterinarian as an extensive worker does the job of clinician and doctor (treatment, prevention and control of diseases of livestock) | The worker is confined to technology transfer |
| 4. In animal husbandry extension the workers are prone to many life-threatening occupational hazards, since they work with all varieties of the animal species | The actual work is done by the farmers themselves under guidance of the extension hazards, since they work workers |
| 5. Besides extracting the economic benefits from the animals, the clients are sentimentally attached with their animals. Hence, a tactful, wise and specialized approach is required while treating the animal and dealing with the clients. It is indeed an Herculean task for the animal husbandry extension worker | Since agricultural activity is purely for economic benefits, standard extension approach is sufficient |
| 6. Result demonstration takes longer time. Hence, the diffusion and adoption time may usually take months to years. This being the case the extension worker has to apply strenuous and sustained efforts to bring forth the adoption | Result demonstration can be seen in shorter period-in hours to days. The efforts of the extension worker is relatively less than that of animal husbandry extension worker |
| 7. The physical presence of the animal husbandry extension worker is essential due to risk prone complexity of technology | Once the extension worker imparts the skills to the farmer the farmer can adopt the methods learnt even in the absence of the extension worker |
| 8. Since 70% of the livestock farm labour is carried out by women, more gender specialised extension approach is needed | Equal attention is needed for both men and women |
| 9. Women do involve in decision-making process | Man has a greater say in decision making |

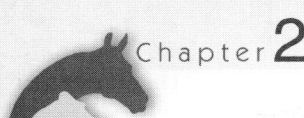

# Chapter 2

# Extension Educational Psychology

## EDUCATIONAL PSYCHOLOGY

Psychology is the science of human behaviour. "Psychology deals with response to any and every kind of situation that life presents. By response to behaviour is meant all forms of process, adjustments, activities and expressions of organisms."[1]

### Importance

Increasing use of psychology is noticed in various spheres of life and extension education is no exception to it. In extension education, the development workers deal with rural people. They teach the rural people about innovations to be adopted in their farm, home and village. In as much as the extension worker is involved in educating rural people most of the concepts discussed in this part applicable to them.

Bringing desirable changes in the knowledge, values and attitudes are one of the major concerns of extension educational psychology. Thus, the main job of the extension worker is to teach the rural people. The learning experience is given in the areas in which rural people are interested.

### Educational Psychology

It deals with the behaviour of human beings in educational situations. This means that it is concerned with the study of human behaviour or the human personality—its growth, development and guidance under the social process of education. It is a branch of general psychology which deals with various aspects of psychology, factors affecting education, teaching and learning process. It describes and explains the learning experiences of an individual from birth through old age. Its subject matter is concerned with the conditions that affect learning. Educational psychology can be regarded as an applied science in that it seeks to explain learning according to scientifically determined principles and facts concerning human behaviour.

1. Skinner, C.E. "Essentials of Educational Psychology", Printice-Hall Metra, New Delhi.

## SCOPE OF EXTENSION EDUCATIONAL PSYCHOLOGY

Its scope in Animal Husbandry Extension is as follows:

1. Educational psychology studies the limitations and qualities of individuals—physical capacity, intelligence, aptitude, interests, etc. which play a major role in one's learning.

2. It helps in improving teaching and learning. This branch helps in formulating training programmes for improving the skills of teachers and methods for organising good learning situations.

3. It helps to have better education through evolution of syllabi for different levels of education, preparation of different textbooks, development of examination patterns, etc.

4. Psychology attempts to discover the source of knowledge, belief, customs and to trace the development of thinking and reasoning so as to find the kind of environmental stimulation that produces certain type of activity.

5. It helps extension workers to find the causes of prejudices, the habit of sticking to old practices and ways of doing things, the doubts and lack of confidence and factors affecting motivation.

6. It also helps the extension workers to know the emotions and feelings of farmers, how villagers or farmers learn new practices, what type of approaches should be adopted and teaching aids that should be used.

## TEACHING AND LEARNING

### Teaching

Teaching is the process of arranging situation that stimulates and guides the learning activity in order to bring about desired changes in the behaviour of the learners. Their interest is developed desire, aroused, conviction created, action promoted and satisfaction ensured.

### Acquiring Art of Teaching

Extension teaching is an art. The art of teaching can be acquired once the science of teaching is learned and sufficient practice has taken place. Teaching can result in effective learning.

If we are to become proficient as extensionists (teachers) we must[1]

1. Be sincere in our desire to be teacher.
2. Understand the desire, needs and interest of those with whom we work.
3. Believe in education but not so strongly that we may be tempted to use force.
4. Not underrate those we wish to help.
5. Know the subject.

### Qualities of a Good Teacher[2]

A good teacher possesses the following qualities:

1. A true teacher should have burning desire to learn and to keep uptodate his subject. According to Rabindra Nath Tagore "A lamp cannot light another lamp unless it itself is also lit. A teacher cannot truly teach unless he himself is also learning".
2. He should be enthusiastic, love his profession and show a lot of potential for taking initiative. All those who have love, aptitude and flair for teaching, certainly turn out to be wonderful teachers.
3. He must have interest in his students. Good teachers are generally very fair, friendly and free with the students.
4. He should be unbiased.
5. He should have good communication skill.
6. Have a sense of humour.
7. He must be always alert and perceptive.
8. Have wide experience and broad interests.
9. Encourage and motivate his students. An effective teacher is one who takes the students along with him.
10. He is not satisfied with poor performance of his class.
11. He should not merely teach the subject matter but by his action and example inspire the students and develop and strengthen their character. A poor teacher tells, an average teacher explains, a good

teacher demonstrates and the great teacher inspires.

12. He involves himself in extracurricular activities and pursues certain hobbies. All such teachers who freely mingle and involve with students are generally well respected and accepted by students.

Unless teachers are able to acquire these qualifications they will only be teachers in name but not in deed. They will draw their salaries and may have a professional title, but they will not be educators. This applies to the extension workers. Once they accomplish this ability they can join the group of successful teachers who are the artists of their profession.

In order to bring about the desired changes in the behaviour of people, the extension worker should organize activities so that there will be repetition of the desired behaviour. This conscious attention to organization of teaching activities in a sequence greatly increases the efficiency of learning.

### Steps in Extension Teaching (Fig. 2.1)

According to Wilson and Gallup[1] (1955), the following are the steps involved in teaching–learning process:

1. Attention
2. Interest
3. Desire
4. Conviction
5. Action
6. Satisfaction

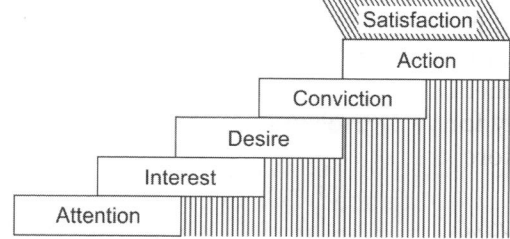

**Fig. 2.1:** Steps in extension teaching

### Attention

The first task of the extension worker is to attract attention of the learner to the new and better ideas. Farmers are to be made aware of the improvement until the individual's attention has been focussed on the change that is considered desirable. There is no recognition of a problem to be solved or want to be satisfied. Attention is the starting point to arousal of the interest.

1. Franco, Joseph Di. Agricultural Extension, A Reference Manual", FAO, Rome, 1972.
2. Mathialagan. "Extension Teaching Methods and Aids – Manual". Department of Extension, VC&RI, TANUVAS, Namakkal, 1993.

1. Meredith C.Wilson and Gladys Gallup. "Extension Teaching Methods". Federal Extension Service, U.S. Department of Agriculture, Washington, D.C., 1955.

## Interest

Once attention has been captured it becomes possible for the teacher to appeal to the basic needs or urges of the individual and arouse his interest in further consideration of the idea. Extension worker reveals how new practice will contribute to the farmer's welfare. The message should be presented attractively.

## Desire

The desire is concerned with the continuation of learner's interest in the idea or better practice until that interest becomes a desire or motivating force. The extension worker explains to the farmer that the information applies directly to the farmer's situation and that the doing of this would satisfy his needs.

## Conviction

Action follows desire, conviction of the people and prospect of satisfaction. In this step the learner knows what action is necessary and just how to take that action. The extension worker also makes sure that the learner visualizes the action in terms of his own peculiar situation and has acquired confidence in his own ability to do the thing.

## Action

Unless conviction is converted into action, the efforts are fruitless. It is the job of extension worker to make it easy for the farmers to act. If new control measure is the action needed the recommended chemical should be available within the farmers' reach. Necessary equipment should also be available. If action does not quickly follow the desire the new idea will fade away. Therefore, this phase should never be neglected.

## Satisfaction

This is the end product of the teaching process. Follow-up by the extension worker helps the farmers to learn to evaluate their progress and strengthens satisfaction. Satisfaction helps to continue his action with increased satisfaction. It is the motivating force to further learning. The saying that "A satisfied customer is the best advertisement" will also apply to the extension worker.

The teacher has to arrange the learning situations in all the six teaching steps with the help of the extension teaching methods. Various teaching methods are not equally suited to advance each of the different steps in teaching, each method under certain circumstances makes a contribution to each step. It depends on the teacher how he handles the situation. The above six steps often blend with each other and lose their clear-cut identity. Of course, these steps are based on motivation.

### Principles of Teaching

1. The learner should understand the purpose of the course.
2. The student should want to learn.
3. The teacher should keep friendly and informal relationship with learner.
4. The physical condition should be favourable and appropriate for learning.
5. The teacher should involve the learners so that they participate and accept some responsibility for the learning process.
6. The teacher should make use of the learner's experience.
7. The teacher should prepare, keep his teaching aids handy and be enthusiastic about teaching it.
8. The method of instruction should be varied and appropriate.
9. The teacher should update his notes with the availability of new knowledge on the topic of subject.

### Factors Contributing to Teaching

1. **Need based teaching:** Teaching should be related to actual problems and needs of the learners. The learner should be made to understand how this knowledge or skill acquired will fulfil his needs.
2. **Suitable teaching aids:** Audio-visual aids related to the subject should be prepared well, arranged sequentially and should be presented impressively so as to attract the learner's attention and facilitate learning.
3. **Physical facilities:** All the minimum physical requirements like seating, lighting, ventilation, etc. should be provided to make teaching and learning comfortable.
4. **Learner-centre:** The teaching programme should be so organized that it is based on the learners standpoint.
5. **Teacher's personality:** Teacher should have pleasing personality. An extension teacher should have patience, cheerfulness, sincerity, helpfulness, clarity, firmness and a sense of humour.
6. **Practical-oriented:** Field-oriented, practical-oriented teaching will help more in problem solving than theoretical way of teaching.

## Learning

Learning is a process by which a person becomes changed in his behaviour through self activity.[1] "Learning is a process of progressive behaviour adaptation."[2]

Any change of behaviour which takes place as a result of experience may be called learning. Teaching and learning are not two separate processes. They are actually one process or they are the reverse of the same coin. The interaction can be symbolized as

Teaching ⟷ Learning.

### Learning Situation

A learning situation is a condition or environment in which all the elements necessary for promoting learning are present. These elements are teacher, learner, subject matter, physical facilities, and teaching methods and aids. These five elements react with each other. The symbolic representation of the learner's reaction to the other elements are given in Fig. 2.2.

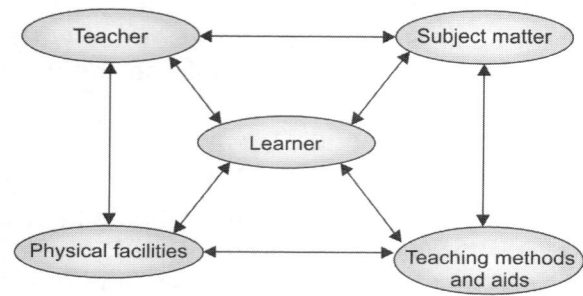

**Fig. 2.2:** The elements of a learning situtation

The above five elements should have the following conditions for an effective learning situation.

### Teacher

The quality of learning will depend upon the quality of conditions created by the teacher. A successful extension worker is one who takes into account the following important considerations:

1. He should select those experiences which suit to the abilities and needs of the learners and to the needs of the society at large. Be skillful in the use of extension methods and aids.
2. Understand the learners, their needs and ability.
3. React appropriately to the feelings, emotions and attitudes of learners.

---

1. JP Leagans, "Extension Education in Community Development", op. cit.
2. CE Skinner, "Essentials of Educational Psychology" op. cit.

4. Is well convinced with the worth of the job.
5. Is well composed, even in the event of irritating situations.
6. Has better human relations.
7. Has clear objectives.
8. Is a good communicator.
9. Is democratic in his leadership.
10. Knows the subject matter.
11. Is sincere in his desire to be a teacher.

### Learner

Learner is the key figure in learning and teaching. If he is unwilling and gives negative response, desirable change is hardly achieved. The learner must obtain and retain the knowledge. This obtaining and retention of the knowledge by the learner depends upon the following:

1. Needs for information.
2. Interest.
3. Level of aspiration.
4. Nature and level of understanding.
5. Capability to attach desired meanings.
6. Use the information gained.

Most of the adult learners think that they are too old to learn. But this is not correct, people always learn irrespective of their age.

### Subject Matter (Contents)

Subject matter is the content of any teaching and learning process. Selecting the subject matter is the most important work and requires skill and careful study. Transfer of subject matter will be easy and effective if it fulfils the following qualifications:

1. Valid and correct, based on facts.
2. Applicable in practical life situations.
3. Well organized.
4. According to needs, interests and level of understanding of the learner.
5. Timely and appropriate.
6. Vital, important and related to the particular specific teaching objective.

### Teaching Methods and Aids

Subject matter cannot effectively be transferred without the help of suitable teaching methods and aids. Proper selection and skillful handling of teaching aids facilitate in creating the desirable learning situation. The teaching methods and aids should be:

1. Simple and easy to handle.
2. Suitable to subject matter.

3. Readily available.
4. In working condition.
5. Diversified, flexible and suited to the environment and needs of the clients.

### Physical Facilities

If the physical settings like place, light, ventilation, seating arrangements, etc. are not properly provided, effective teaching and learning cannot take place. Physical facilities must be satisfying both to the teacher as well as to the learner. It is one of the most important responsibility of the teacher to ensure that the desirable physical facilities are made available for creating good learning situation. Presence of proper physical facilities become rather more important in informal settings, because learners are not bound by the formal classroom regulations.

### Principles of Learning

The main aim of extension education is to provide effective learning experience to the farming community. Therefore, the extension worker should know the basic principles of learning. Many principles, however, are well established and have useful application in extension education.

1. **Learning is growth-like and continuous (*principle of association*):** Extension teacher must know the state of the learner's mind and capacity and begin teaching at learner's level for better learning. New ideas must be related to those already known to the farmer. A new idea must be repeated intermittently to emphasise its importance.

2. **Learning should be purposeful (*principles of clarity*):** Seeing is believing. So farmer will realize the importance or value of a practice only when he sees the result in practice. Teach the farmer when there is a need of the knowledge and then retention will be more. Practice must be continuously evaluated and redirected. Objective must be clear to the learner and to the teacher.

3. **Learning engages a maximum number of senses (*principle of self activity*):** Any information is read by our brain only through five senses. Broadly speaking, seeing, hearing and doing are the most important way in which maximum messages are to be learnt and retained for long time. Good teaching tries to teach any learner through as many avenues to the human mind as can be employed. The ability of learning also differs according to the learner's power of imagination and creativity. One aspect of learning is creating an imaginary picture of the desired results. Demonstration, visuals and other symbols help in making this picture of a new idea more vivid in order to facilitate effective learning.

4. **Learning must be challenging and satisfying (*principle of rewards*):** Not only the student's interest, also the teacher's skill in arranging effective situation and timely appreciation to student's achievements will motivate the learning process and lead to satisfaction. A favourable attitude accelerates learning; a bad attitude retards learning. Motivation makes the student more challenging. Standards demanded by learners should be suitable to their ability. Farmer can have satisfaction by learning new things taught by a challenging and efficient way of extension teaching. A friendly atmosphere will boost the level of satisfaction.

5. **Learning must result in functional understanding (*principle of practice*):** Effective learning means not only acquiring knowledge but thorough understanding of the practice. Useful learning requires that students not only acquire new ideas, but also understand how to apply them in realistic situations. Memorising is one way of gaining knowledge but unless what is learnt is applied it will be forgotten and the learning will be of no use in reaching the desired objectives. For development of functional understanding it is essential that the farmer understands the whole subject as well as different topics and their inter-relationship. If a farmer is interested in delicing his calf then he should understand the dose, dilution time and method of administration as well as the inter-relationship and after effects so that he can apply the medicine successfully.

To gain a workable understanding of technology requires knowledge of the whole, recognition of the parts and ability to see distinction among the parts of related knowledge. To attain this the extension worker should divide the entire teaching programme in meaningful units and decide the methods to be used in making the learning effective.

6. **Learning is affected by the physical and social environment:** The physical and social environment creates a favourable background for successful learning. The physical environment includes seating, lighting, temperature, ventilation and quiet atmosphere. The learners should be required to spend least energy in adjusting to the environment. Social environment and the mental make-up of the

student are closely associated. The instructor should create a suitable environment.

7. **Learning ability varies widely among individuals:** Some may be slow learners and some fast learners, hence the level of communication of the extension worker should be according to the level of understanding of the farmer/group. Similarly, the subject matter also should suit the farmer's ability.

8. **Learning is a gradual process, and needs multiple exposures for change:** Ultimate objective of technical teaching is to encourage the farmer to adopt improved practices. No single attempt or method can carry information to all the people. So, by using combination of teaching methods one can have a cumulative effect on the learners' mind that results in adoption. For example, a new idea may be introduced to a village people through AIR or TV and then to village leaders through contact by extension functionaries. This might be followed up by a village meeting, followed by demonstration and supplemented with reading materials. The percentage of adoption will be more when the farmers are exposed four to eight times over a period of time.

9. **Normal adult life has significant learning capacity:** Adult education programmes are based on the assumption that adults have the capacity to learn. Learning ability, starting about the age of six, rapidly grows until the age of 20, then it begins to level off until around 50. The rate of learning declines about 1% a year after the age of 35. The main reason for this decline among the adults is their less acute vision, less acute learning, low external motivation, habits and impact of a particular ideology.

   Some of the methods that create suitable physical situation are the use of visual aids, speaking clearly, distinctly and at an appropriate speed, presenting topic step by step; repetition and providing rewards and encouraging. It is necessary to avoid ridicule and punishment.

10. **Learning is an active process:** To learn new skill, the learner must practice the acquired facts and relate them to each other and to a problem. He should change his attitude. Extension worker can create an atmosphere for learning but the farmer will have to learn by himself. Hence, learning is an individual or personal matter.

11. **Learning requires effective communication:** A teacher should have good communication skill to share his knowledge with the learner and to bring about desirable change in him. Anyone can acquire this skill provided he is really interested in teaching. Better communication can be achieved by integrating suitable visuals in a teaching process. A visual is equivalent to thousand words. Especially in the case of rural farmers, visuals communicate very well to them, but they should be appropriate to the subject matter.

12. **Theory and practice must be related in learning:** Theory explains the why and how of an idea. Many times even though a farmer understands theory he cannot use it in practice. Sometimes, he knows how to do it but does not know the theory behind it. There should be a balance between these two and for acquiring high professional competency it is necessary to know both theory and practice.

## Process of Learning

Learning takes place at different levels depending on prior experience of the learner, his intellectual ability and presentation of materials. The process can be categorized as:

1. **Association:** All initial learning consists of information of association, includes Pavlov's condition learning as well as operant conditioning of Skinner. Most of the S-R learning come under association. Most of the knowledge and attitude come through association. This type of learning is comparatively easy to evaluate.

2. **Conceptualisation:** It is the process of grasping the commonalities or relationships. It is the process of abstracting the commonality in association, meaning that the relevant relationship is grasped. If the process of association learning is considered to be a linking of neurons in chains, the conceptualisation process may be thought of as a grid which short circuits some of the chains. Most of the higher learning in cognitive as well as effective domains takes place by conceptualisation.

3. **Creative self direction:** This is the highest level of learning and under favourable conditions people are able to progress from association formation through a process of conceptualisation to a kind of learning that characterizes the creative artist. This motive power comes from the emotional or affective dimension of learning. When the learner has reached this level of learning he can work independently on his own initiative.

## INTELLIGENCE

Individual farmers differ in their ability to learn, to adjust to new situations, manage things, persons and ideas. This difference is due to the intelligence level of the individuals.

## Definitions

The dictionary says that intelligence is "the capacity to acquire and apply knowledge".

1. As quoted by Supe, "It is the capacity of solving problems and by using past experience, adjusting with new things and understanding abstract things by using symbols".[1]
2. "According to Vernon, intelligence is the capacity to adopt relatively in new situation of life. C. Burt, an English psychologist defined, intelligence as invoking general cognitive ability.[2]
3. As per Alfred Binet, intelligence is the ability to think in terms of abstract ideas.[3]

## Types of Intelligence

a. **Concrete intelligence:** It means intelligence in relation to concrete materials. It is the ability of an individual to comprehend actual situations and react to them adequately.
b. **Abstract intelligence:** It is the ability to respond to words, numbers, and letters, etc. It is required in the process of reading and writing.
c. **Social intelligence:** It is the ability of an individual to react to social situations of daily life. High social intelligence is possessed by those who are able to handle people well. Adequate adjustment in social situation is the index of social intelligence.

Factors affecting intelligence:

1. Inheritance of intellectual capacity.
2. Influence of environmental factors.

## Development of Intelligence

It is generally agreed upon by almost all psychologists that intelligence increases up to adolescence and declines in old age. The extent to which intelligence in old age declines is still an open question. Many studies have shown that a decline begins in the middle or late teens.

## Difference in Mental Growth Among Groups

1. Sex difference—boys and girls tend to show, if any, little difference in intelligence as measured by tests of mental ability.

---

1. S.V. Supe. "An Introduction to Extension Education". Oxford & IBH Publishing Co. Pvt. Ltd., New Delhi, 1994.
2. Adopted from S.S. Chauhan, "Advanced Educational Psychology", op. cit.
3. Adopted from Lester D. Crow and Alice Crow, 'Educational Psychology", Urasia Publishing House (P) Ltd., Ram Nagar. New Delhi, 1979.

2. Racial differences—findings about racial difference is no longer accepted. The difference may be due to environmental influences. The 'bright' and 'dull' can be found in any group.

## Measurement of Intelligence

Intelligence can be measured by mental ability tests. Types of mental ability tests:

1. Individual or group tests.
2. Language or verbal tests.
   • Non-language or non-verbal tests.
   • Performance test.
3. Simple or more difficult tests.

## BINET TEST

Alfred Binet evolved intelligence tests to discriminate intelligent learner from lazy ones. He made a set of questions for learners of different age groups. By asking questions to each age group he evolved a concept of mental age (MA) which is indicative of the intellectual development of the individual.

This mental age was related with chronological age (CA) to obtain the intelligence quotient (IQ) of the individual.

The ratio between mental age and chronological age can be called intelligence quotient.

$$IQ = MA/CA \times 100$$

e.g. if a boy of 6 years can do all the tests meant for a 9-year-old, then his mental age is 9 and his IQ may be ...

$$IQ = 9/6 \times 100 = 150$$

## Importance of Measurement

It is a measure of prediction of growing youth's future. The intelligence quotient as a means of estimating the degree of mental development has great value if it is interpreted wisely as one indication of a learner's probable future success in learning.

## Application in Animal Husbandry Extension

The results of intelligence tests combined with other techniques available for the evaluation of learning success can help a teacher to discover what the livestock farmer or youth can learn and how quickly he can learn, as well as the teaching methods that should be applied and learning content that should be utilised to guide the learner to use his mental potentialities to their utmost.

A farm youth or farmer in any group may range from "bright" to "dull" in intelligence. The extension teaching should begin from the level of intelligence of the farmers. The farmers of various mental abilities will be frustrated, if they are taught by any one method and similar material. The intelligent farmer who is fast learner will be bored and the poor minded will not be able to understand. It will be better if the farmers are categorized on the basis of their intellectual level and training programmes and syllabus are planned according to their capacities.

# MOTIVATION

Motivation is what moves or activates an individual. In psychology it refers to some internal activator within an individual. The motives are the directing tendencies inside the individual to follow a particular course of action.

## Definition

The goal-directed, need-satisfying behaviour is called motivation. It is a process of initiating a conscious and purposeful action. Motive means an urge or combination of urges to induce conscious or purposeful action.

Motives, arise out of natural urges or acquired interests, or dynamic forces that affect thoughts, emotions and behaviour, e.g. motive for earning more money by poultry farming (economic motivation).

## Needs which Motivate Human Beings

i. **Organic needs or physiological motives:** Man is so built that he requires certain things in order to keep living. He is also constituted that these needs initiate activity that will eventually satisfy him. These are all basic organic needs which demand periodic or continued satisfaction. These needs are called appetites, e.g. breathing air, appetite for thirst, appetite for sleep or rest, etc.

ii. **Wants:** People have unique personal wants, e.g. likes and dislikes for specific food, play, etc.

iii. **Emotions as motives:** Under the influence of fear, anger, etc., people may do many things that they would not do normally, e.g. parents use fear to direct the behaviour of children. Organisations use fear to produce a desired form of behaviour.

iv. **Feelings and attitudes as motives:** An experience by an individual is evaluated by him as pleasant or unpleasant. When the experience is pleasant, individual has an attitude of approaching that experience and if it is unpleasant, his attitude is of withdrawal.

v. **Social motives:** Most people have a strong desire to achieve social approval. For this, they try to improve their personality through clothes, possession of things, knowledge, skills, etc.

vi. **Others**

**Habit:** It is a person's settled practice, especially something that cannot easily be given up. Established habit becomes almost automatic and requires only a stimulus to set it in action.

**Objective environment:** People act differently in different situations. The objective environment produce a 'set' or 'readiness' to respond in a particular way.

## Functions of Motivation

i. Motives encourage a learner in his learning activities, e.g. extrinsic motives like prizes, medals, etc. motivate.

ii. Motives act as selectors of the type of activity in which the person desires to engage, e.g. selection of courses.

iii. Motives direct and regulate behaviour, e.g. discipline in school, etc.

## Significance of Motivation

The motivation will depend on the needs of the learner. The order of needs of human beings is from lower (basic) to higher level. The basic needs are more dominant in the first instance in the life of an individual. Once he is satisfied he tries to seek satisfaction of the higher order of needs.

Motivation is concerned with the arousal of interest in learning. This forms the basis for learning. So, the teacher has to find the right type of stimuli in the individuals that will produce satisfaction in order that the interest of the learner shall be maintained long enough to master definite ideas or subject matter. The students will not be interested in learning if there is no proper motivation.

## Value Aspects of Motivation

a. **Intrinsic values:** These are what a learner does for the sake of engaging in the activity itself. This is to be desired in learning and is more immediate.

b. **Extrinsic values:** These are when incentives and goals are artificially introduced into a situation to cause it to accelerate activity.

## Techniques of Motivation

1. **Need-based approach:** The approach should be need-based so that it could satisfy five categories of

needs by knowing the level of motivation and patterns of motivation among them. The six categories of needs are:
 i. Safety need, e.g. security.
 ii. Desire for recognition, eg. promotion.
 iii. Organic needs, e.g. thirst.
 iv. Physiological need, e.g. hunger.
 v. Sense of belonging need, e.g. affection.
 vi. Esteem need, e.g. prestige.

2. **Training to set a realistic level of aspirations:** Any attempt to revise the expectations of farmer should be done with full understanding of their socio-economic status, e.g. (i) Creating an aspiration in a farmer who does not have any cattle of his own for possession of one or two cattle. (ii) A person who attains a yield of 1000 litres milk/cow could be made to aspire for 3000 litres/cow. Such a realistic level of aspiration would ensure slow and steady progress.

3. **Participation:** The involvement of farmers in the programmes of agricultural change acts as boost of motivation not only for the immediate participants but also for others.

4. **Use of audio-visuals:** The proper selection, combination and use of various audio-visuals for the appropriate purpose will act as lubricants of motivation.

## Classification of Needs

Dealt in detail in Chapter 10.

## Importance of Motivation in Extension

1. Mobilizing the villagers and extension workers.
2. Knowledge of biological drive/need helps the extension worker to realize the problems of the people. It helps in sympathetic handling.
3. Knowledge of psychological and social drives helps the extension worker to formulate programmes and make effective approaches in changing their attitude.
4. Knowledge of other motivating forces helps in avoiding conflicts or tensions.
5. Motivation helps in the better involvement of farmers in development programmes.
6. The role of audio-visuals in motivating farmers needs no emphasis. The proper selection, combination and use of various audio-visuals for the appropriate purpose will act as lubricants for motivation.
7. Various studies conducted in India indicate that economic motivation is much predominant followed by innovativeness. Among the economic motives also providing better food, clothing and education for ones children seem to be the dominant motives.

## ATTITUDE

Attitude is the intensity of positive or negative feeling associated with some psychological object. Attitudes are important determinants of behaviour. If we are to change them we must change the emotional components. It is a mental and neutral state of readiness organized through experience, exerting a directive or dynamic influence upon the individual's response to all object with which he is related.

A farmer may buy a particular company's medicine for his poultry farm because he has been brought up to believe that it is the "right" organization. In the course of experience he may learn something about the products of that company. In that case his attitude will probably change. As a result, he may be expected to buy a different product. Knowledge, attitudes and behaviour are then very closely linked.

### Measuring Attitudes

1. **Direct questioning:** If we want to know how individuals feel about some particular psychological object, the best procedure would be to ask them some questions. Direct questioning may, indeed, be satisfactory for some purposes, e.g. opinion poll.

   A large number of people are asked only a question or two because they do not have much time to respond to many items. There are two major problems in public opinion poll: (i) Wording or questions, and (ii) sampling.

   For the poll to be accurate, the sample must be representative. For this we have to use stratified sampling. In stratified sampling, the polling agencies set quotas for certain categories of people based on census data. The most common categories are age, sex, socioeconomic status and geographical region, all of which are known to influence opinions. By seeing to it that the quotas in the sample are in proportion to the categories in the general population, the sample is made more representative.

2. **Direct observation:** By direct questioning sometimes we may not be able to measure the attitude accurately. Instead of asking questions we can measure the attitudes by direct observation There are limitations to this approach also. An

extension worker interested in the attitudes of a large number of individuals towards some object may not have the opportunity to observe in detail the attitude of all the individuals with whom he is working.

3. **Attitude scales:** It is a highly scientific method of measuring attitudes. A well constructed attitude scale consists of a number of items that have been just as carefully edited and selected in accordance with certain criteria as the item. Many scales have been developed for measuring the attitudes. Each scale consists of a group of statements related to a particular attitude. Some scales ask the person to respond by indicating whether he agrees or disagrees with each statement. Other scales ask the person to specify the degree of his agreement with a statement. The degree of agreement or disagreement is given predetermined values.

## Attitude Change

Well established attitudes tend to be resistant to change, but others may be more amenable to change. Attitudes can be changed by a variety of ways. Some of the ways are as follows:

1. By obtaining new information from other people and mass media, resulting in changes in cognitive component of a person's attitudes.
2. Attitudes may change through direct experience.
3. Attitudes may change through legislation.
4. Since people's attitudes are anchored in their membership group and reference groups, one way to change the attitude is to modify one or the other.
5. Attitude change differs with reference to the situation also.

## Factors Influencing the Development of Attitudes

1. **Maturity:** The young child has only a very limited capacity for understanding the world about him and he is consequently incapable of forming attitudes about remote, or complex, or abstract things or problems. At about a mental age of twelve years the child begins to understand abstract terms. As a result of this growth in capacity, he is able to understand and react to more abstract and more generalized propositions, ideas and ideals.
2. **Physical factors:** Clinical psychologists have generally recognized that physical health and vitality are important factors in determining adjustment, and frequently it has been found that

malnutrition or disease or accidents have interfered so seriously with normal development that serious behaviour disturbances have followed.

3. **Home influences:** It is generally accepted that attitudes are determined largely by social environment and that home influences are especially important.
4. **The social environment:** The home environment is of primary importance in the formation of early attitudes, but friends, associates, and the general social environment come to have an increasing influence as the child grows older and has wider social contacts.
5. **Government:** The form of the government seems to be an important factor in determining attitudes both towards government itself and towards other things.
6. **Movie pictures:** Movies influence the people much and change their attitude.
7. **The teacher:** Personalities of the teachers bring about significant change in the attitudes of the learners.
8. **The curriculum:** Literature and the social sciences have more influence than other subjects on the determination of attitudes.
9. **Teaching methods:** The "manner of presentation" of subject matter has a favourable effect on attitudinal change.

## Development of Attitude

Attitude is developed in three phases, first towards the object, then the effect connected with the object, and finally the action that can be undertaken with respect to that object. Attitudes are not innate but formed as a result of the individual's contact with the object and the environment. Attitudes are not mere accidents of individual experience. They result from day-to-day living in the home, in the school, and in the community. Whatever attitude children have is the result of teacher's precept and example. The challenge to teacher is that of helping the learner retain his identity, develop his individuality and absorb a background of democratic culture.

Attitudes are formed without direction and also by direction as the result of careful planning by a person or persons who desire to encourage the development of certain attitudes in others. It is through initiation, emotional experience and deliberate efforts on the part of the individual himself, teacher, and others that the new attitudes arise.

Child is a great initiator and builds most of its attitudes in that way. Adolescent develops attitude by his enlarging experience. Adjustment to the situation to which the adolescent is exposed influences the attitude either desirable or undesirable. Radio, television, film and printed matter also contribute to the development of attitude. Thus, there are so many factors that influence the adults to develop attitudes.

## Social Incentives

1. **Motives and incentives:** Motives are a set of internal conditions which give rise to action in an organism. Incentives are conditions set up in order to alter behaviour of other individuals. Thus, incentives may be positive or negative. A positive incentive reinforces action while a negative incentive inhibits action. The modification of the individual by the society is based upon the operation of these incentives. This is how social learning takes place.

2. **Incentives modify behaviour:** Incentives top the motives and change the attitudes of the individuals in the group. When appropriate incentives are given the efficiency of performance improves considerably. On the other hand, inappropriate incentive may lead to decrease in efficiency. Material rewards are positive incentives which release drives and thus influence the speed and accuracy of performance. Similarly, punishment or the removal of a reward is a negative incentive which inhibits certain drives, apart from rewards and punishments, praise and reproof of or scolding are also very powerful incentives affecting behaviour.

3. **Rewards and punishments:** A combination of rewards for right responses, and punishments for wrong responses will lead to more efficient learning.

4. **Praise and reproof:** These incentives help children as well as adults to conform to social norms. Consequently conformity leads to rewards or approval and satisfaction while non-conformity leads to punishment or disapproval and self-dissatisfaction. Socialization is achieved by these methods in all grades of human society in the tribal as well as in the most highly civilized groups.

5. **Competition and co-operation:** Competition may be based on a motive when it is spurred by the desire for recognition and improvement in status or it may be due to an incentive when the desire is to win a competition or to earn more money.

   Competition means striving to equal or surpass the speed and quality of another person's performance, or it may be to improve on one's own past performance.

6. **Competition and rivalry:** Rivalry is a drive to equal or surpass the skill of another person. Many times brothers and sisters become rivals and try to excel each other. In the same way in the old Indian society, there was a great deal of rivalry among the different wives of a single individual.

## Difference between Competition and Rivalry

| Competition | Rivalry |
| --- | --- |
| The term competition may be restricted to the attempt by an individual or group to improve the level of performance so that one is superior to the other. | The term rivalry may be limited to those situations where the persons or group try to crush the rival. An attempt is made to become superior to the other not by improving one's performance but by dislodging the other. |
| It is much more impersonal. | It is related to face to face relationship. |
| It does not lead to jealousy and hatred. | It may inevitably lead to both of them. |

The attitude affects an individual's course of action. Due to unfavourable attitudes towards artificial insemination in cows, an individual is not likely to participate and follow the recommendation of the practice. In such a situation the first duty of the extension worker is to make efforts to change the attitude of the person. The change in attitude may lead action.

# Chapter 3

# Rural Development

## GROWTH AND DEVELOPMENT OF INDIA'S EXTENSION ORGANISATION

India is primarily a rural country and her prosperity means the prosperity of the rural areas. The present age has often been described as age of common man. Throughout the world there is a widespread desire to improve the lot of the rural folk.

"India lives in villages" is a familiar saying. More than 80% of the population is ruralite. Rural areas are the nursing grounds in so many respects in any country and more so in India. Nobel laureate and renowned poet Rabindra Nath Tagore says, "Villages are like women. In their keeping is the cradle of the race. It is the function of the village like that of women to provide people with their elementary needs, with food and joy, with the simple poetry of life, and with those ceremonies of beauty which the village spontaneously produces and in which she finds delight. But when constant strain is put upon her through the extortionate claims of ambition; when her resources are exploited through the excessive stimulus of temptation, then she becomes poor in life and her mind becomes dull and uncreative. From the time-honoured position of the wedded partner of the city, she is degraded to that of maidservant while in its turn, the city in its intense egotism and pride remains unconscious of the devastation constantly worked upon the very source of its life, health and joy".

Village development was not a big need in earlier days, since the village in the past functioned as a self-contained and self-sufficient unit. A balanced system of society was capable of looking after the needs and wants. But this situation was disturbed by invaders and the Mogul rule and for a long time no people felt the need for rural reconstruction work.

### British Administration's Attempts in Extension

When it is remembered that the British administration was primarily motivated by commercial considerations, there is hardly any need to search as to why it did not devote adequate attention to the improvement of the rural areas, If, however, now and then the Britishers attempted something in a sporadic manner, it was done either under the stress of particular situations or to sidetrack the political issue.

Apparently they did not realise that their responsibility was particularly great because the Village Panchayats, which had hitherto looked after village welfare, were liquidated with no other agency set up in their place. It has been said that the British administrative system was negative in its outlook, its main business being to maintain law and order. Rabindra Nath Tagore said that his country's government had become something like patent food untouched by hand. W.S. Blunt stated that we have given the right security from death by violence, but we have probably increased danger of death by starvation.

British Government never seriously attempted to uplift the villages. They woke up only under some compelling situations, such as famines or similar widespread economic distress. As for famines these occurred more or less regularly.

Between 1800 and 1825 it was reported that there were five famines; between 1825 and 1850 two famines: between 1850 and 1875 six famines; and between 1875 and 1900 eighteen famines in different parts of the country.

Famines spurred the government into action, The Famine Commission of 1880, 1898, 1901, the Irrigation Committee of 1903, the Commission on Co-operation of 1915 and the Royal Commission on Indian Agriculture were among the efforts of the government to improve the economic lot of the common man; but seldom were the reports of the commissions translated into action in a through-going fashion. 'If you want to shelve a problem, "said Disreli, once, appoint a Royal Commission". The various commissions appointed during the British period only shelved the economic problem of the country.

However, Department of Revenue, Agriculture and Commerce as one department commenced (1871) due to representation made by the Manchester Cotton Supply Association. This department could not exercise any influence on the problem of agricultural development except the collection of simple agricultural statistics.

Based on the Famine Commission's (1880) recommendation, Agricultural Department in most of the states started functioning. As a result of the report of the Famine Commission of 1901, the Imperial Agricultural Research Institute and Agricultural College at Pune: District level agricultural and livestock farms and experimental stations were started. The Indian Agricultural Service was constituted at the Centre. Later, the other development departments like Animal Husbandry, Irrigation, Rural Development were started. The Government of India Act of 1919 empowered the transfer of all the development departments closely connected with Rural Development to the major provinces and Agricultural Development became a state subject.

The Royal Commission (1928) suggested the government (1) to establish a body for agricultural research at the national level for promotion, guidance and co-ordination of agricultural and animal husbandry research; (2) to develop linkages between administration, research and teaching.

The activities drawn up by various departments were such that they did not involve the people concerned. Further, the developmental work taken up by the departments were not based on detailed studies.

## Individual/Group/Community Initiatives for Extension

The 20th century extension work owes its beginning to a few outstanding individuals of philosophic and philanthropic bent of mind. But they worked in most part in isolation from one another and without government assistance, their interest being aroused through their official contact with the villagers. In others, their imagination and sympathy enabled them to visualise a better way of life for the villagers. But the work of most of them confined to relatively small areas. Sometimes, it appears that compassion and fellow feeling were the considerations for a few attempts to uplift villages.

A study of some of the isolated but concerted efforts in extension under individual initiatives, that served as precursor and pace-setter for extension management is relevant.

1. **Scheme of rural reconstruction (1903):** Daniel Hamilton formulated a scheme for creating model village in an area of 'Sunderban' near West Bengal on co-operative principles. One village of this type and co-operative credit society were organised. In 1934, a Rural Reconstruction Institute was also established. It provided training facilities in cottage industries.

**Limitations**
1. The scheme was organised by an individual without the financial and moral support of the government.
2. The area of operation was small and activities were also limited.
3. Involvement of people was also not adequate.
4. The staff employed was untrained.

2. **Servants of India Society (1905):** This was founded by Gopala Krishna Kokale as a political society at Pune. It laid strong emphasis on socioeconomic and educational activities. Later Kokale started training centres in Madras state (Chennai), United Province and Central Province (Madhya Pradesh) and published booklets on basic education, labour problems, etc.

**Limitations**
This scheme did not get much success due to:
1. Lack of finance and government support.
2. Lack of involvement of people.
3. Untrained staff of the organisation.

3. **Economic Conference of Mysore (1914–18):** This was launched by Dr M.S. Visweswarya as the Diwan of Mysore state. It was a purposeful and methodical plan for achieving improvements over a wide range of subjects. Agriculture was one of the main points in this scheme. It comprised District and Taluk committees with their respective Revenue Officer as Chairman, the officers of Development Departments and selected non-officials. These committees surveyed the needs and possibilities, examined them carefully, arranged priorities, fixed targets and designed ways and means of achieving them. Things possible immediately and in the long range were tested out and noted.

**Limitations**
1. The scheme was wound up due to immense load of the programme.
2. The involvement of people in the programme was also limited.

4. **The Gurgaon experiment (1920):** The Gurgaon experiment was a landmark in the history of rural reconstruction in this country. It was a pioneer effort in the field and was marked by several novel methods which had not been previously tried anywhere on a considerable scale especially under

government auspices. The scene of the experiment was Gurgaon, a district of the old Punjab situated halfway between Delhi and Mathura.

F.L. Brayne took charge of this district as Deputy Commissioner towards the end of 1920. He was struck by the miserable condition of the people by their lack of health, primitive methods of agriculture and animal husbandry, ignorance and squalor, wastefulness of their social customs and the depressed state of their women and took more than an 'official view' of the situation. He lost no time in initiating an uplift campaign and this was generally known as the Gurgaon experiment.

The objective of the campaign, as defined by the Brayne himself, was "to jerk the villager out of his old groove, convince that improvement is possible and kill his fatalism by demonstrating that climate, disease and pest can be successfully fought; further to laugh him out of his unhealthy and uneconomic customs and teach him better ways of living and farming".

Brayne in the first place wanted to create in the villager a desire for improvement and then launch his innovations. For this, propaganda was carried out through a variety of media and these included broadcast, magic lanterns, cinemas, cartoons, dramas, songs, and glees, gramophone records, newspapers, coloured pictures, and posters, books, leaflets, pamphlets, models, exhibitions, shows, and melas, competition, public meeting, demonstration, etc.

The machinery employed to carry out the programme was manned mainly by voluntary organisation and paid village guides. The main burden of the work fell on the guides and they constituted the main spring of the uplift campaign. The central idea behind the appointment of guides was to provide a single agency to whom the villager could turn for advice. These guides resided within their respective villages and propagated the whole gospel of village regeneration. They attended to a variety of jobs, such as agriculture, public health, education propaganda, etc. There were 65 guides and some of them maintained notebooks for each village separately in which a page was devoted to each family.

Brayne also started a school for rural economics. There was also a school of domestic economy for women. The Gurgaon experiment aimed at the more scientific collection and use of manure, improved method of cultivation and irrigation, a better system of dry farming, the re-division of

holdings into a large and better shaped blocks the more economical use of money, improvements in methods of keeping village cattle and preventing of breeding by immature bulls and heifers, development of communication and encouragement of co-operation.

But after the transfer of Brayne, there was lack of interest and hence the scheme did not make any headway. Again this programme gathered momentum after 1933 when Brayne was appointed as the Commissioner of Rural Reconstruction in Punjab. This work was subsequently transferred to co-operative department.

**Limitations**

1. The village guides were not technical men. They were inexperienced and untrained.
2. The scheme was taken up by the orders of one superior office. So very little permanent improvement was made.
3. The work lost its momentum as soon as the central figure was transferred from the place.
4. Attempts were limited to a few villages.
5. **Marthandam attempt (1921):** This project was started in 1921, by Dr Spencer Hatch, an American Agricultural expert, who had special training in rural reconstruction work in different parts of the world. He selected Marthandam (place near Kanyakumari in Tamil Nadu) as a centre for rural reconstruction work and it was run by YMCA. The main objectives of this project were five-fold, namely mental, spiritual, physical, economical and social development. Figure 3.1 shows the emblem of the centre.

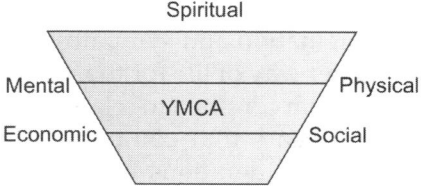

**Fig. 3.1:** Marthandam project emblem

The motto of this centre was "self-help and intimate expert counsel". Self-help comes into play only if the villagers are given a share of responsibility in the conduct of the various ameliorative activities. Keeping this in mind, village associations were formed. Each association had its Honorary Secretary who constituted its leading spirit. The association assisted the implementation of various innovations. Above these associations there was the

Regional Development Association which concerned itself with the developmental activities of the entire region.

The chief powerhouse in the whole system was the demonstration centre at Marthandam. The actual field work commenced with a rural survey of the particular locality selected for work. The data were studied and findings framed. Then action plans were drawn. Suppose in any particular locality, the survey disclosed the need for improved cattle, a plan of action was thereupon drawn up. The first part of the plan consisted of a publicity campaign to educate the people on the necessity for improved dairy farming. All possible media of propaganda were utilized. After creating awareness, co-operative bull clubs and breeding associations were formed and these assisted the villagers financially and otherwise in securing improvement in the breed. The same process was repeated with or without variation in other fields of village welfare.

Similarly, under the guidance of this centre, egg selling club, honey club, weavers' club, etc. were organized in the villages. The egg selling and honey clubs did well and were very successful. At the centre (Marthandam) prized bulls and goats, model beehives, demonstration plots for improving grain and vegetable seeds, poultry run with prized laying hens, weaving shed, equipment like honey extractors were maintained for the purpose of imparting knowledge on these to the villagers.

Propaganda proved a major contributory factor in the success of the campaign there. The chief media of propaganda used by the centre were: (1) Rural dramas, (2) rural exhibitions, (3) inter-village competitions, and (4) demonstrations.

### Limitations

1. There was neither adequate funds nor government backing for the work.
2. There was no continuous contact with the villagers since workers were required to return to the centre in the evening.
3. The programme was sponsored by a religious institution and hence co-operation of the village was partial.

6. **Shriniketan attempt (1921):** This was established by the Poet Rabindra Nath Tagore in collaboration with L.K. Elmhirst for a village reconstruction. The Institute of Reconstruction was inaugurated in 1921.

### Objectives

The objectives of the institute were briefly as follows:

1. To take a real interest in village welfare.
2. To study rural problems and translate the conclusion to action.
3. To help the villagers to develop their resources by teaching them better methods of cultivation, improvement of livestock, encouragement of cottage industries and inculcation of the benefits of co-operation.
4. To improve village sanitation and to make villagers sanitary conscious.
5. To work out practically an all-round system of elementary education in the villages based on the scout ideal (*Brati Balika*).
6. To encourage a spirit of service.
7. To train students and leaders in rural matters. The institute conducted demonstrations on farmers holding on improved agricultural practices, established a dairy and poultry to supply milk, eggs, better animals and birds to the farmers for breeding. The villagers were given training in weaving. Co-operatives were organized and provided facilities for giving training in tanning, pottery, embroidery, tailoring, etc. to students and workers of the institute. Night school, mobile library, film shows, meetings were also organized with villages.

### Limitations

1. The institute did not get much help from the government and no research work could be conducted.
2. The work was confined to eight villages only.
3. The programme was also organized by a single person.

7. **Sevagram attempt (1923):** This was started under the guidance of Mahatma Gandhi in 1923 but it had really began in 1920 as All India Spinners' Association. The objectives of the project were to provide service to the underprivileged for achieving self-dependency and basic education to the people. The main activities of the project were, organisation of training centres for cottage industries, prohibition, removal of untouchability, stressing women's education and basic education and preaching and practising communal unity.

### Limitations

1. No well-defined methods.
2. Gandhiji set very high personal standards, which were difficult for the common man to reach and therefore the project could not provide the expected results.

8. **Firka Development Scheme of Madras State (1947):** This scheme was launched in the last quarter of 1947 in 34 firkas throughout the state and on 1st April 1950, it was extended to another 50 additional firkas at the rate of 2 for each district. The selection of firkas was based on the consideration of general backwardness of the area and the possibilities of indentifying the production of handloom cloth, Khadi and other cottage industries. The scheme consisted of short-term plans for the development of rural communications, water supply, formation of Panchayat, organisation of co-operatives and programmes for sanitation, The long-term plans were for making the area self-sufficient through agriculture, irrigation and livestock improvement and development of Khadi and other cottage industries. The plan thus involved the close co-ordination of the various government services such as agriculture, veterinary, irrigation industries, medical, public health and communications.

The programme was directed in each firka by Firka Development Committee consisting of officials and non-officials. A Firka Development Officer was selected from among the social workers and appointed for 2 to 3 firkas. Each firka was divided into 5 to 10 groups of villages which were put in charge of gramsevak in the rank of Revenue Inspectors. Each firka or group of firkas was provided with special stall-like agricultural fieldman, PWD supervisor and minor irrigation overseers. The Collector was in charge of the scheme in the District. It was planned that after giving the initial impulse, the programme would grow out in their own experience and momentum.

At the state level, State Rural Welfare Board was formed comprising the heads of the department and influential constructive social workers and this board drew up the comprehensive plan for firka development. The development schemes were entrusted to non-official agencies engaged in doing constructive work by the government and these agencies were paid grants also.

### Limitations

1. These efforts were found restricted in scope and lacked co-ordination.

2. The scheme was also found ineffective owing largely to lack of direction, support and encouragement from the central authority.

9. **India Village Service:** This service was established in 1945 by its founder-author A.T. Mosher of New York and B.W. Gupta. It was directed by Dr W.H. Wiser as a mission project in United Province in 1948. The object of this organisation was to assist the village people to realise the best in their own villages by developing individuals, voluntary leaders and local agencies to enable them to become capable of helping themselves and others.

India Village "Colleagues" were appointed and were provided with good facilities. Co-operation of government and other agencies was sought. Stress was laid in informal discussions, use of books, songs, exhibitions and other visual aids, tours, trips and dramas. Residents of the adopted villages were the beneficiaries of this organisation. The colleagues lived 3 to 5 years at a allocation. The work was very slow but with definite results.

10. **Etawah Pilot Project (1948):** The idea of this project was conceived in 1948. The project was put into action with headquarters at Mehewa village, about 11 miles from Etawah in United Province, in September 1948.

Lt. Col. Albert Mayer of USA was the originator of the project. Initially, 64 villages were selected and later their number was increased to 97. The Government of United Province helped Mayer in setting up a machinery at district level and extra appointing staff for the project. The 4-point programme of America also provided finance.

In 1951, 125 more villages were covered, and in 1956 another group of 122 villages was included.

### Objectives

i. To see what degree of production and social improvement, initiative and co-operation could be obtained from a compact area;

ii. To see how quickly results could be achieved; and

iii. To see whether results achieved could be permanent and reproducible in other areas.

The project was started on a pilot scale to study the above objectives. The rural problems tackled by the project:

a. **Concerned with the broadening of the mental horizon of the villager, to ensure he not only accepted new and tested ideas but that those ideas became self-generating and self-perpetuating.**

**b. Dealt with the villager's land, his tools and his surroundings, the approach being educative and persuasive rather than coercive.**

In this project the village level workers were trained and appointed, co-operation of other departments and agencies was enlisted and demonstrations were conducted. The activities included increasing farm yields, soil conservation, animal husbandry, village sanitation and social education. In short, a general awakening in respect of all-round village uplift was aimed at.

The project was found to be successful and the pattern was accepted for the community projects. Villagers' participation was a strong point in this. There was thorough planning and an integrated approach to village life. Finally this project was merged with National Extension Service (NES).

11. **Nilokheri Project (1948):** This was originally started in 1948 to rehabilitate 1000 persons displaced from Pakistan. This scheme was started in an area of 1100 acres of swampy land. Nilokheri was a swamp, midway between Karnal and Piph along the grand trunk road in East Punjab. The swamp was reclaimed as the nucleus of an agro-industrial township. A township with a population of five to six thousand was developed without any difficulty, to house essential services like health, education, public works and power supply and provide facilities for marketing, shopping, recreation, etc.

The township (Nilokheri) also offered extension service in agriculture, animal husbandry village and small industries, besides being a supply and service centre. A training centre for village artisans, craftsmen, and young farmers was also established there. The township also served the villages around and in turn received the surplus of food and other commodities for the urban population. Thus, there was a reciprocal economy between the village and the town and neither could be said to have exploited the other. The development phase was more or less completed by the end of 1951. The scheme was also called "Muzdoor Manzil" aimed at self-sufficiency for rural-cum-urban township in all and essential requirements of life. The programme was conducted under the supervision of the Ministry of Rehabilitation at the Centre. The central figure of this project was S.K. Dey, the then Union Minister of Community Development and Panchayati Raj.

A committee appointed under the chairmanship of Sri P.A. Narielwala strongly recommended the adoption of agro-industrial economy for the future pattern of development of rural area.

12. **Paul Hoffman—15 Pilot Projects (1951):** In 1951, Paul Hoffman, President of the American Ford Foundation, came to India with the object of exploring how Ford Foundation could help India in her basic development.

The Ford Foundation started 15 pilot projects, more or less on the pattern of Etawah, in various states about the middle of 1951. A centre for training extension personnel was also opened. The idea was to produce a multipurpose worker who would know how to offer first aid in the various facets of the programme of agriculture. Five training centres, attached to five agriculture colleges in India, were started with financial aid from Ford Foundation. The pilot projects provided extension staff in Agriculture and Animal Husbandry. These were besides the specially trained multipurpose village level workers.

13. **Chester Bowles (1951):** After reading about Etawah and Nilokheri and holding discussions with the Government of India, Chester Bowles came to India and promised 50 million dollar US aid for India's reconstruction. It was decided that a new programme of village development would be undertaken as a pilot project in all the then states of India Part A, B and C. The US Government promised to provide the necessary technical personnel and other things required in the programme. Under this programme 15 pilot projects started earlier under the Ford Foundation were absorbed. Hence, it was decided by the central governments in consultation with the state governments in May 1952, to launch the Community Development Programme in India.

## Constraints

Reasons for the failure of past efforts in community development work in India:

i. The attempts were mostly based on individual initiative, inspired by humanitarian considerations.

ii. Government backing and financial support were lacking.

iii. Attempts were sporadic.

iv. Staff employed was inadequate, inexperienced and untrained.

v. Objectives were ill-defined and lopsided in their development.

vi. Plans, programmes and organisations involved were weak and were unbalanced.

vii. Parallel programmes of supply and service, guidance, and supervision were not developed.

viii. Need for proper methods and skills of approach to the task were not fully realised.

ix. Association and co-operation with other development departments was very limited.

x. Research and evaluation were lacking.

xi. Involvement of village population in thinking, planning and executing village development was not properly achieved.

## Community

The term "Community" popularly has been loosely used to refer to groups such as community of nations, a community of teachers, community of musicians, Hindu community, Muslim community, Christian community or world community or international community or UNO. These usages do not communicate the sociological meaning of the word.

Sociologists have defined several components essential to the concepts of community. "Community may be defined as a group of people living in a continuous geographic area, having common centres of interest and activities and functioning together in the chief concerns of life."

The community is an organized group of associated individuals. The people are geographically oriented. They reside in a given local area and carry among themselves economic, political, educational, religious and recreating activities. A community is a social group with degree of "we feeling and living in a given area".

## Development

Development means gradual and step by step progress. MacIver used the word development to signify an upward course in a process "that is of increasing differentiation". When it is used in conjunction with community it refers to bringing the potential abilities of the people who live together in a community.

## Community Development

The 1948 Cambridge conference defined community development as a movement designed to promote better living for the whole community with the active participation and if possible on the initiative of the community but if this initiative is not forthcoming spontaneously, then by use of techniques for arousing and stimulating it in order to secure its active and enthusiastic response to the movement.

According to United Nations, Community Development can be defined as a process designed to create conditions of economic and social progress of the whole community with its active participation and the fullest possible reliance upon the community initiation.

Community Development is a balanced programme for stimulating the local potential for growth in every direction. It promises reciprocal advances in both wealth and welfare, not on the basis of outside charity but by building on the latent vitality of the beneficiaries themselves with the minimum of outside aid.

### Community development (CD) has been described

- As a **process of change** from the traditional way of living of rural communities to progressive ways of living;
- As a **method** by which people can be assisted to develop themselves by their own capacity and resources;
- As a **programme** for accomplishing certain activities in fields concerning the welfare of the rural people; and
- As a **movement** for progress with a certain ideological content.

### Principles of CD

In order to promote the systematic study and practice of CD, people have drawn up a series of what they have termed 'principles'. The United Nations, in a report of concepts and principles of CD, set forth ten such principles. These principles are applicable to most parts of the world and were not formulated to deal with any particular community.

### *Principles Stated in UN Report*

1. Activities undertaken must correspond to the basic needs of the community; the first project should be initiated in response to the expressed needs of people.

2. Local improvements may be achieved through unrelated efforts in each substantive field. However, full and balanced programme requires concerted action and establishment of multipurpose programmes.

3. Changed attitudes in people are as important as material achievements of community projects during the initial stages of development. The people should be changed educationally to bring a change in their farming, home making and health.

4. CD aims at better participation of people.

5. The identification, encouragement and training of local leadership should be the basic objective in any programme.

6. Much thought has been given to participation of women and youth in CD programme.

7. To be fully effective, self-help projects for communities require both intensive and extensive assistance from the government.

8. Implementation of CD programme on national scale requires adoption of consistent policies, specific administrative arrangements, recruitment and training of personnel mobilization of local and national resources.

9. The resources of voluntary organisations should be fully utilized in CD programmes at local and national level. This is another universally applicable principle in CD programme. The voluntary organisation can promote a spirit of service in people.

10. Economic and social progress at the local level necessitates parallel development on a wider national scale.

The rate of progress that can be achieved by the process of CD is slow to raise the awakening in underdeveloped countries, CD methods do not produce quick results, and process of change is slow and difficult. The rate of progress will get faster as success is achieved and human development takes place. The best guarantee of success is the successful follow-up of it.

## Community Development Programmes

Three-fourths of India's population live in rural areas. Seventy percent of India's population gets employment through agriculture and animal husbandry. Bulk of raw materials for industries comes from agriculture and rural sector. Increase in industrial production can be justified only in rural population's motivation and purchasing power to buy goods can be increased. Stable and developing agricultural economy can help in stability of prices of industrial goods. Growing disparity between the urban elite and the rural poor can lead to political instability. After independence, it had become essential to change the outlook of the Indian rural people. Their thinking and behaviour required to be shaped according to the growing modern age. Hence, a strategy was developed to promote the social life of village people in general and in particular to extend the economic and social benefits to the rural poor. Therefore policy makers developed and launched the community development programmes for the uplift of rural community.

## Objectives of CD Programmes

1. Development of material and human resources in the area and thereby raise the rural community to higher levels of living.

2. Achievement of increased production by the application of scientific know-how to the rural occupation of animal husbandry, agriculture, cottage industries, etc.

3. Provision of opportunities for full employment to the under and unemployed rural population by developing agricultural programmes livestock programmes, cottage and small-scale industries.

4. Training of agriculturists, artisans and extension workers of various kinds for proper implementation of the programme.

5. Creation of more living activities mainly through the efforts of the concerned communities, by making them to devote their unutilized energies and spare time.

6. Improvement of health and sanitation, provision of housing facilities and promotion of educational and other social activities.

7. Provision of proper communication facilities.

8. Changing mental outlook, creation of ambition for higher standard and will to live better life.

9. Development of self-reliant and harmonious village communities.

10. The fundamental or basic objective of community development in India is the development of people or "Destination man": Reddy (1993). Its broad objectives are economic development, social justice and democratic growth (Mukerji, 1961).

### Organised Efforts in CD

In March 1950, the Government of India set up a Planning Commission to formulate the First Five-Year Plan. CD is an integral part of the plan. It was the first organized effort for community development. The programme emphasized the importance of working through people's rural institutions (e.g. Panchayats). It was to ensure their involvement in planning and to secure the fullest possible public participation.

From the conception behind the pilot projects of 1952 to the emergence today of a community development ideology, there has been a big development. The following are the various stages of evolution of the organisation and its set-up.

1. **Community Development Project (CDP):** The pilot programme was started on October 2, 1952. It aimed at finding out how people reacted to it and what constraints were encountered in this movement. Each of the 55 community projects covered about 300 villages with an area of about 450 to 500 square miles and with a population of about 2 lakhs. Each project area was divided into three development blocks. A development block consisted of about 100 villages and a population of 60,000 to 70,000. Each block in turn was divided into groups of 5 to 10 villages each. Each group formed the field of operation for a village level worker (VLW) now known as "Rural Welfare Officer". To begin with, only areas with assured rainfall and facilities for irrigation and soil suitable for giving quick returns were selected. The project suffered from several handicaps which retarded the pace of progress. As a result of this three-year project was extended on the recommendation of the third Development Commissioners' Conference by one year and continued to operate up to September 30, 1956.

2. **National Extension Service (NES) Programme:** This programme was formulated in April 1953 and was inaugurated on October 2, 1953. The National Extension Service Programme and Community Development (CD) had the same idea and the two were integrated under one agency at the centre as well as in the states. Both the programmes were complementary and interwoven and ran concurrently. The idea behind the programmes was to cover the entire country within a period of about 10 years.

The movements had identical aims. The NES was a permanent organisation and covered the whole country. It provided the basic organisation, official, non-official and a minimum financial provision for development. Further funds were allotted from the centre and states under different heads. National Extension Service blocks, in which successful results had been achieved with the maximum popular co-operation, were selected for intensive development for a period of three years. These were called 'community projects'. The number of community projects taken up by NES blocks depended on the available financial resources and local support and enthusiasm (Sri V.T. Krishnamachari).

1. **CD and NES blocks:** Both NES and CD programmes have uniform unit of operation called development block, representing 100 villages with a population of 60,000 to 70,000. But out of NES block, selection was made periodically for intensive development work under CD Programme and the selected block was called CD block.

2. **Post-intensive block:** Community Development blocks after completion the scheduled period of operation were called post-intensive blocks. The intensive phase of the programme financed by specific provisions in the block budget ceased at this stage. The programme, continued by inclusion in the various departmental budgets for implementation as part of the Second Five-Year Plan with regard to various subjects such as education, health, agriculture, communication, cottage industries, housing, etc. was applied to those areas and implemented through the staff provided by the blocks. It was at the post-intensive stage that all the loose ends had to be skillfully interwoven to produce the finished tapestry.

3. **Stage I and Stage II CD blocks:** Sri B. Mehta, as Chairman of a study team, expressed the view that the division of Community Development Programme into three, viz. the extensive, intensive and the post-intensive development stages, was unnecessary or inconvenient. He suggested the implementation of the programme in two stages of six years each and extension of the period of the coverage of the entire country by this programme by at least three years, since it was a continuing programme and needed continuous efforts.

These recommendations were accepted by the Central Committee and the National Development Council with some modification in April and May 1958, respectively. Accordingly, the new plan came into force with effect from April 1, 1958. There was no distinction between NES and CD blocks and there was no phase like post-intensive phase. The programme was implemented in two stages of five years each. The complete coverage was to be achieved by October 1963.

4. **Reorganised Panchayat Samiti blocks:** Community Development Programme was implemented through panchayat and advisory bodies, viz. the block planning and development committee with the assistance of voluntary organisations and workers. The Balwantrai Mehta Team's report resulted in Community Development becoming the main activity of the peoples' democratic institutions at the village, block and district levels. The whole process was known as the Panchayati Raj and the three-tier institutions are the Panchayat, the Panchayat Samiti and Zila Parishad.

Administration of the CD Programme (prior to Panchayati Raj) (Fig. 3.2).

1. **National level:** The Central Committee headed by the Prime Minister and comprising members of the Planning Commission, Ministers of Community Development and Food and Agriculture implemented the Community Development Programme from the top. The committee laid down the broad policies and provided general supervision. They were also responsible for holding consultation with appropriate authorities in various states regarding economic development. The committee was assisted by an Advisory Board consisting of the Secretaries of Central Ministries of Food and Agriculture, Finance, Health, Education, the Additional Secretary of the Ministry of the Natural Resources and Scientific Research, etc. The Central Committee was informed of the progress of work from time to time through periodical reports prepared by the Community Projects Administration (CPA). The Ministry of Community Development had the overall charge of the programme. Earlier, the administration was under the CPA till 1956. Then it was upgraded to the Ministry of Community Development. Later this ministry was called Ministry of Community Development, Panchayati Raj and Co-operation.

2. **State level:** The State Development Committee presided over by the Chief Minister was entrusted with the execution of both the CD and NES programmes. The members included the Ministers of all development departments. The Development Commissioner was the secretary and was responsible for directing CD blocks in the state. The Development Commissioner had the following functions:

   i. He maintained a two-way relationship with the Centre for receiving National Programme guidance and reporting suggestions and modifications to the centre.

   ii. He performed at the State level the role performed by the Ministry of CD at the Centre.

   iii. He maintained an administrative relationship with the District Collector, who in turn was responsible for planning, co-ordinating, executing and evaluating the work of each block in his district.

3. **District level:** The Collector was the Chairman of the District Planning or Development Committee. He was assisted by the Block Development Officers (BDOs). The Committee consisted of all the heads of the development departments in the district and the Chairman and Vice-Chairman of district board, MLAs and other non-officials.

4. **Block level:** The Block Development Officer was assisted by a team of technical experts in agriculture, co-operation, animal husbandry, cottage industries, etc. The Block Development Committee consisted of representatives of panchayats, co-operatives, progressive farmers, social workers, MPs and MLAs of the area.

5. **Village level:** The Village Level Worker (VLW) or the Gram Sevak acted as a multipurpose man. Each Gram Sevak was in charge of about 7 or 10 villages. He was guided and assisted by various technical specialists and was the last official administrative person in the chain.

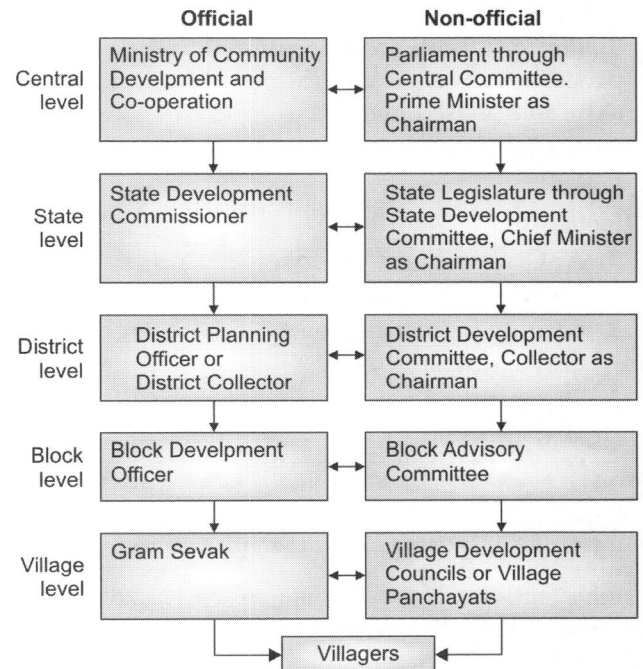

**Fig. 3.2:** CD/NES organisation prior to Panchayati Raj

## Extension Education *vs* Community Development

The inter-relationship between Community Development and Extension is detailed in accordance with objectives, processes and form.

1. **Objectives**

   *Similarities:*

   i. Basically an educational approach.

   ii. Designed to extend knowledge to rural people.

   iii. Aims to bring about change.

   iv. Tackles the problem at people's level.

v. To improve social and economic development.

vi. Recognises that people need help if they are to help themselves.

| Extension Education | Community Development |
|---|---|
| 1. Emphasis on the individual | Emphasis on co-operation |
| 2. Education aimed at individual development to attain economic prosperity | Education aimed at groups of individuals to work collectively to attain social improvement |
| 3. Its main focus is on individual needs | Its main focus is on community needs |
| 4. Emphasis on decision making for change by individual and families | Emphasis on decision making by group and representation of groups. |

2. **Process**

   *Similarities*: Both are educational and democratic processes involving rural people relatively in a slow and phased manner.

   *Dissimilarities*: No dissimilarity seems to exist.

3. **Form**

   *Similarities*:

   1. A Government sponsored and supported organisation to do the job.
   2. Permits a great flexibility in types of organisation to do the job.
   3. Organization emphasizing co-operation.

   *Dissimilarities*:

| Extension Education | Community Development |
|---|---|
| 1. Emphasizes on organization that either carries out transmits technologies from other sources to the farmers | Emphasizes the co-ordination of service agencies by a working team made up of representatives of different services |
| 2. Usually represents a transfer of responsibility from administering Government Organization to another 'Educational group' | Usually a rigid control held by a Government administering agency to cut across participating Government Department—to recognize and include the various departments that must provide service—to eliminate departmental reluctance to participate |
| 3. Permits co-operation between departments, agencies | Forces departments and agencies to participate |
| 4. Essentially a branch of the Department of Agriculture/ Animal Husbandry | Essentially a branch of Government serving department |
| 5. Not directly involved in promotion of local units of Government | Tied into promotion of local units of Government |

## Comparison of US Co-operative Extension Service and Community Development Programme of India

| Co-operative Extension Service of USA | Community Development Programme in India |
|---|---|
| 1. An integral part of Land Grant College and university | A department of Government. Away from college and universities |
| 2. Administered and manned by educationists and professional teachers | Administered by professional administrators |
| 3. Emphasizes the educational process of bringing about desirable changes in knowledge, attitude and practices | Emphasizes achievement of physical targets |
| 4. Emphasizes formulation, implementation and evaluation of educational objectives | Emphasizes formulation of physical targets and their achievement |
| 5. Teaching, research and extension are fully integrated at one place under one head | Teaching, research and extension are separate, integration and co-ordination inadequate |
| 6. Extension workers are responsible for mainly education | Extension workers are mostly engaged in service activities |
| 7. Rural people are fully involved in implementing rural development programmes | Limited involvement and participation of rural people in implementing rural development programmes |

## PANCHAYATI RAJ

The earlier Panchayati Raj institutions at the grassroot level were "grass without a root and caricature of local government".

### History of Panchayati Raj in India

Panchayati Raj system is not new to India. In fact it was developed earliest and preserved longest in India among all countries of the earth. There are two kinds of panchayats in traditional Indian villages. Village panchayat and caste panchayat. Caste panchayats dealt with their internal matters. All castes were represented in the village panchayat by their elders. The village headman held office on a hereditary basis and was elected by consensus when necessary. He was responsible for village administration.

The village has its own traditional methods of conflict resolution, enforcement and social mobilization. The village has an identity, fixed revenue and forest limits, common property like grazing land and shared resources like wells and tanks and have places for meeting and worship.

The Indian village community has been recognized as a unique entity quite different from the settlements in China, Russia and Germany. The villages have been a constituent of large political units and subjected to various officials. A *Gramik* was responsible for village administration. The next higher official (*Dashi*) was in charge of ten villages. There were others at higher level covering twenty, hundred and thousand villages. Though responsible to the state for collecting dues, looking after village defence in co-operation with the body of elders, and administration of justice was primarily the task of bodies at the village level.

There were democratic bodies or panchayats in the villages of Tamil Nadu. The members of the council were chosen by lot drawn from names picked from the pots. This was prevalent during Chola era as per the Uttramerur stone inscription (AD 10). Available inscriptions and records highlight that the institutions in south had acquired their distinctive characteristics and had established order by tenth century AD. There existed several communities for village administration. Annual committee, garden committee, tank committee, gold committee and committee of justice. The list of officials and public servants, quoted by Methyl from 1812 select committee report of the House of Commons, included the headman, accountant, watchman, boundary man, tank and water resources super-intendent and teacher.

Under the British rule, the Indian village community was subjected to several changes. There was an all round decay in local self govertment agencies. The state judiciary took over the powers of the village panchayat and village officials were to appointed to look after the interests of the ruled and collect taxes. Private property pervaded and intermediaries like *zamindars* emerged in the rural structure. Later *zamindari* abolition led to soaring aspirations followed by rising frustration. The new panchayat system was interjected into the village power structure with civil status, national democracy and greater interlinkages at the block, district and state levels.

In his book "Discovery of India", Jawaharlal Nehru mentions a 10th century book, "Neetisara", written by Shukracharya in which he observed that the village panchayat or elected council had large powers, both executive and judicial, and its members were treated with the greatest respect by the King's officers. Panchayati Raj institutions in India refer to a statutory multi-tier administrative structure entrusted with development work, duties and responsibilities by the state legislatures. This form of local self-government has its origin in Lord Ripon's famous resolution of 1882 in which he recommended "the smallest administrative unit", the sub-division or *taluka* shall ordinarily be placed under a local board, which would further be controlled by the district boards.

The legislation was enacted as early as in 1947, known as the Panchayati Raj Act, 1947. A real push to the revitalization of the panchayats was given after independence when a specific role was assigned to them in administration. This was as per the Constitution in which mandated that the state shall take steps to organize village panchayats and endow them with such powers and authority as may be necessary to enable them to function as units of self-government.

## Committee on Plan Projects (COPP)

It is usually referred to as study team on plan projects or Mehta Committee since it was headed by Balwantrai Mehta in 1957. The study team was appointed by the Planning Commission to identify the drawbacks and the weaknesses of Community Development Programmes and NES and to suggest remedial measures. The Mehta Committee recommended the setting up of elected bodies at village and block and district levels. It was called the institution of democratic decentralisation. The committee suggested that these bodies should be entrusted with the task of planning and development. "Development cannot progress without responsibility and power". "CD can be real only when the community understands its problems; realises its responsibilities; exercises the necessary powers through its chosen representatives and maintains a constant and intelligent vigilance on local administration."

The committee suggested introduction of three-tier structure of local self-government bodies from the village to district and said these bodies should be organically linked up.

- The agency of government at each level was to be made subject to the control and guidance by elected representatives of the people thus providing for the growth of democratic administration from below, called democratic decentralisation, i.e. transfer of power and responsibilities to these bodies.

- The block should as far as possible be treated as the administrative unit of all the development departments, so that there is one unified set-up without duplication and overlapping of jurisdiction of the responsibilities.

- The block (Panchayat Union, Panchayat Samiti), the middle-tier of this system was the new innovation and the district level, new body district development council (Zilla Parishad) was to replace the district boards.

- Adequate resources should be transferred to the new bodies to enable them to discharge their responsibilities.
- The system evolved should facilitate further devolution and distribution of power and responsibilities in future.

## Panchayati Raj

The recommendations of the Balwantrai Mehta Committee came as a fresh breeze and gave a new lease of life to CD and extension service projects. It paved the way for new era of Panchayati Raj institution which was inaugurated by Jawaharlal Nehru on 2nd October, 1959 at a national rally at Negaur. This introduction of the three-tier system of democratic decentralisation was later known as Panchayati Raj. In Tamil Nadu state this was inaugurated on 2nd October, 1960 Rajasthan and Andhra Pradesh were the first states to implement the Panchayat Raj on 2nd October, 1959, and November, 1959 respectively. The District Boards and other institutions below the State Legislature except village panchayats were abolished. Pandit Jawaharlal Nehru described the new beginning as "the most revolutionary and historical step in the context of new India". In a sense, it was an act of faith in republican democracy and was as important event as the establishment of the parliamentary system itself for the people of India and by the people of India.

### Definition

Panchayati Raj is a system of governance, horizontally it is a network of panchayats and vertically it is an organic growth of panchayat.

### Revitalisation of the Panchayati Raj

Initially democracy and development seemed to march hand in hand. There was a climate of optimism and resurgence, but within a few years of the inauguration of the new era, the Panchayati Raj institution began to sag, stagnate and decline.

At the end of three decades from the inauguration of the Panchayati Raj movement, it was felt appropriate to focus attention and reflect on the process of democratic decentralisation, review the growth, status and functions of Panchayati Raj institutions and consider the measures required to revitalise these institutions and make them truly effective instruments in the constructive task of rural development and nation building. In order to draft this concept paper, the

Department of Rural Development constituted a committee with Dr. L.M. Singhvi as chairman in 1986.

### Committee's Report

1. **Cause of decline**
   - The potential of Panchayati Raj institutions centres on people's power, aroused apprehensions and jealous hostility all around.
   - Elected representatives in Parliament and State Legislatures were not quite willing to share power.
   - There was chronic insufficiency of resources at the disposal of these institutions.
   - The bureaucracy was becoming alienated after the initial face and programme after programme was launched without involving Panchayati Raj institution (Chairman) and Panchas (President) and other Panchayati Raj functionaries were suspended and Panchayati Raj institutions were superseded frequently and indiscriminately.
   - Facilities for training were meager. Research and reform inputs were negligible. Political factionalism and certain public disenchantment with these institutions weakened them further. Corruption began to creep in.
   - What is worse, Election to Panchayati Raj institutions were not held for years together.
   - Elected Sarpanchas (Panchayat Union Chairman) and Panchas (President) and other Panchayati Raj functionaries were suspended and Panchayati Raj institutions were superseded frequently and indiscriminatively.
   - The state governments, which were primarily responsible for nurturing these institutions, began to look askance at them.
   - These institutions also suffered from being neglected at the national level, although occasional expressions of concern were not lacking.
   - Panchayati Raj declined because of lack of conceptual clarity, absence of political will and denial of national priority, lack of continuous process of research, evaluation, feedback and correction at these institutions in a blind alley.

April 24th, 1993 is a landmark day in the history of Panchayati Raj in India as on this day the constitution (73rd Amendment) Act, 1993 came with force to provide constitutional status to the Pahchayati Raj (Fig. 3.3). The 73rd Constitutional Amendment brought in 30 lakh elected members all over the country into Panchayats and Municipalities. The constitution of

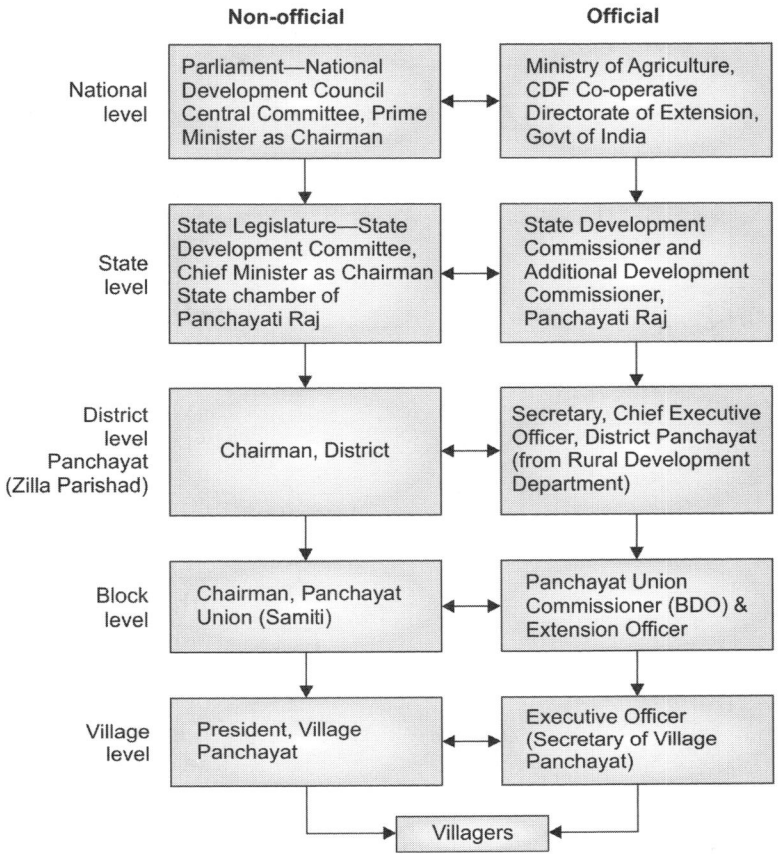

**Fig. 3.3:** Organisation of Panchayati Raj in India

Gram Sabha consisting of all adult members of a Village Panchayat will give 'voice' to 'voiceless' people living in 6,00,000 villages of India.

### Salient Features of the Panchayati Raj Law

The 73rd Constitution Amendment defines Panchayats as units of "Self-Government" for the rural areas.

1. **Three-tier structure:** A three-tier structure has been provided thereby bringing some amount of uniformity in the Panchayati Raj system through-out the country. Thus, Panchayati Raj institutions are to be established at the village, intermediate and district levels. Smaller states with a population of 20 lakhs or less are given option of not forming the middle-tier. Panchayats vary in their population ranging from 500 to 10,000.

2. **Exemption of certain areas:** While the application of the 73rd Constitution Amendment is to be uniform in the entire country, the scheduled and tribal areas as defined under Article 244, viz., the North Eastern States of Nagaland, Meghalaya and Mizoram and certain hill areas of the district of Darjeeling, have however been exempted.

3. **Population size of villages in India:** The Government of India publication, "Panchayati Raj in India, 1991" gives the distribution of average population per Gram Panchayat. It shows that with the exception of Meghalaya, Lakshadweep and Puducherry, about 7% of Gram Panchayats have a population below 1,000, about 28% between 1,000 and 2,000, about 14% between 2,000 and 3,000, 21% between 3,000 and 4,000 and about 31% 5,000 and above. This means that about 70% of Gram Panchayats have the viable demographic size of below 5,000.

Between 1983 and 1991, the average size of the Gram Panchayats in 50% of the cases reduced, in 19% it increased and in the rest there had been no change. The size of Gram Sabha in no case should increase more than 1,000 to ensure face-to-face dialogue.

4. **Election to Panchayati Raj institutions (PRIs):** Elections to the Panchayats are to be conducted regularly under the overall supervision of separate Panchayati Raj Election Commission of the state.

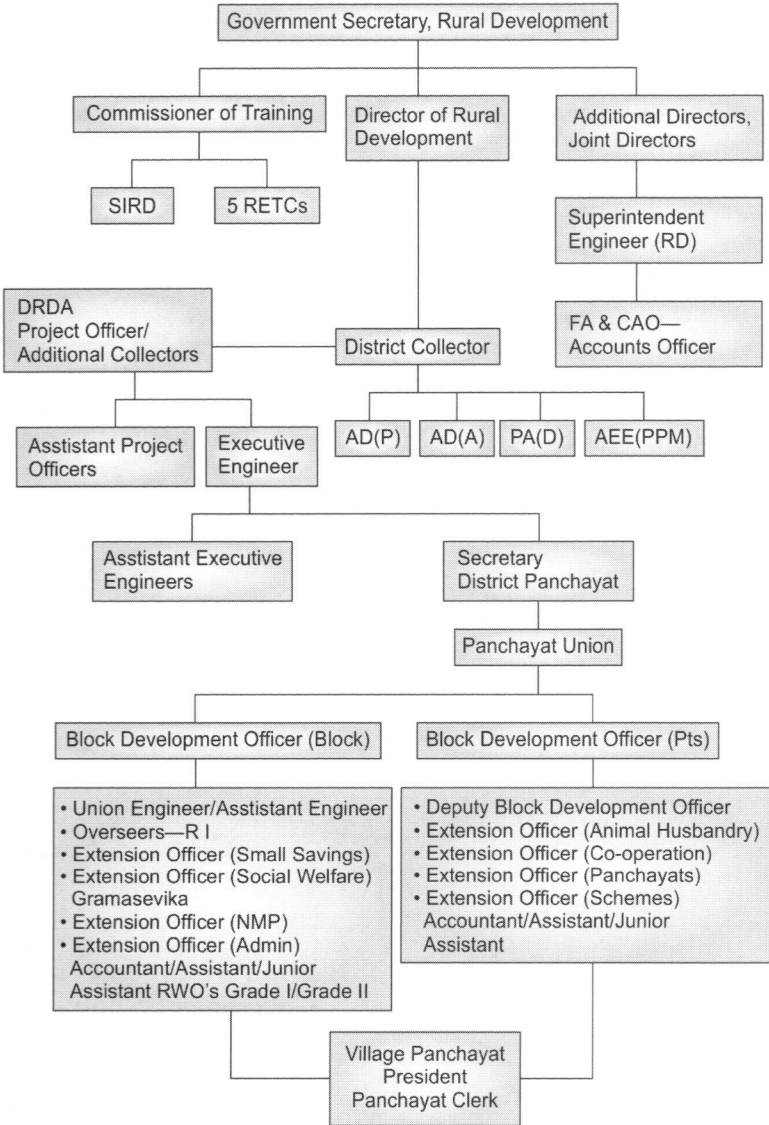

**Fig. 3.4:** Organisation of Panchayati Raj in state (Tamil Nadu)

The elections of members of Panchayats at the village, intermediate and district levels are compulsorily direct. The Chairpersons at the intermediate and district levels have to be compulsorily elected indirectly by and from amongst the elected members. However, the Chairman of Village Panchayat is elected directly.

5. **Reservation of seats**
   1. Reservation for the candidates belonging to weaker sections, namely the Scheduled Castes and Scheduled Tribes, at all levels in proportion to their population and in proportion to the area has been provided for in order to ensure participation of these groups in the decision-making processes.
   2. One-third of the total number of seats has been reserved for women (including the number of seats reserved for women belonging to SC and ST).
   3. Not less than one-third of the total number of Chairpersons' post in Panchayats at each level have been reserved for women. Similarly, reservation for the offices of Chairpersons belonging to SC and ST categories has also been made.
6. **Tenure:** A term of five years has been provided for every Panchayat unless it is dissolved earlier on specific grounds. In the event of dissolution, election will be compulsorily held within six months. The reconstituted Panchayat will serve for the remaining period of the five-year term.

### Village Panchayat

There are 2,18,116 Panchayats against 5.8 lakhs villages. A Gram Sabha (village assembly) consisting of all adult members registered as voters in the area of a Panchayat is to be constituted. It was intended to provide effective peoples' participation in various programmes at local level. As Gram Sabha is considered as the only means of "direct democracy" where all important decisions have to be arrived at and it may serve the purpose of training ground for all the people especially the younger generation.

The Gram Sabha has to meet at least four times in a year. The quorum for its meeting has been fixed at one-tenth of the total number of members of the Gram Sabha. The meetings of the Gram Sabha are presided over by the Chairman of the Panchayat and in his absence, by the Vice-Chairman and in the absence of both, a member chosen by the members present at the meeting.

Panchayat means an institution of self-government constituted for local administrations of the village/town. A revenue village with a population of not less than five hundred is treated as one village panchayat. For each panchayat 5–15 members are elected directly by the people.

**Wards:** Village Panchayat is divided into wards and the number of persons to be elected from each ward has been determined.

**President :** Directly elected. In some states indirectly elected. Some states are encouraging election by consensus to avoid the influence of political parties.

**Vice-President:** Among the elected members Vice-Chairman is indirectly elected.

**Reservation:** For SC, ST, men and women belonging to SC, ST community based on their population seats are allotted by rotation.

**Term:** Five years

**Meetings:** For every village panchayat at least three meetings in a year should be conducted and six months shall not intervene between two meetings. In some states minimum two meetings.

**Items discussed:** 1. Approval of the village plan, 2. Approval of the village budget for the year, 3. Review the progress of the implementation of all schemes.

**Quorum:** One-third of the total members of panchayat. It varies from state to state. The Chairman presides over the meeting and in his absence the Vice-Chairman chairs it. In the absence of both any member chosen by from the quorum presides over the meeting. However, no minimum quorum for Gram Panchayat was fixed by the Union Government.

**Functions:** 1. Provision of water supply, sanitation and lighting. 2. Formation and maintenance of roads, land management and collection of statistics. 3. Welfare of backward classes. 4. Act as an agent of the panchayat union in executing the schemes entrusted to it. 5. Opening and maintenance of burial and cremation grounds. 6. Sinking and repairing of wells, repair and maintenance of ponds, tanks, construction and maintenance of water works.

### Powers

1. Planting and preservation of trees.
2. Lighting of public roads, places other than built-up areas.
3. Opening and maintenance of public market other than those classified as public markets.
4. Control of fairs and festivals.
5. Opening and maintenance of cart stands, public landing and halting places, public cattle sheds.
6. Opening and maintenance of public slaughter house.
7. Opening and maintenance of reading rooms.
8. Establishment and maintenance of radio/TV sets, playgrounds, parks and sport's clubs.
9. Opening and maintenance of literacy centres for imparting social education.
10. Construction of works of public utility, provision of facilities for safety, health, comfort, conveyance, culture or recreation of the inhabitants of the village.

**Revenue:** House tax, vehicle tax, duty on transport of property (exchange of immovable property, gift of immovable property, mortgage of possession of immovable property, perpetual lease of immovable property).

The Panchayats have been authorized to levy, collect, and appropriate suitable local taxes. A state can also provide grants-in-aid to Panchayats from its consolidated fund. In each state, a Finance Commission was established within one year of the 73rd constitutional amendment and thereafter every five years. This State Finance Commission reviews and assesses financial position of the Panchayats and recommend to the state the pattern of distribution of funds between the state and PRIs.

**Committees:** One or more joint committee may be constituted at the Panchayat level.

**Administration:** The executive authority is appointed by the Government at the village panchayat level. He is the Secretary of the village.

### Panchayat Union Council (Panchayat Samiti)

The Panchayat Union Council is the intermediate-tier, i.e. block. Panchayat Union Council means the body constituted for the administration of a Panchayat Union. The nomenclature of a Panchayat Union Council in different states is as follows:

| State | Nomenclatures |
|---|---|
| Tamil Nadu | Panchayat Union Council |
| Andhra Pradesh | Panchayat Samiti |
| Karnataka | Taluka Development Board |
| Gujarat | Taluka Panchayat |
| Assam | Anclialik Paiicilayat |
| UP | Kshetra Samiti |

### Composition

According to previous Panchayati Raj Act (1958) of Tamil Nadu state, all the village and town panchayat presidents are the members of the Panchayat Union Council. Now, according to the present law:

i. Persons elected from the wards at the rate of one member for every five thousand population.

ii. Members of Lok Sabha and Rajya Sabha and MLAs.

iii. One-fifth of the presidents of the village panchayat, are the members of the Panchayat Union Council and have the right to vote.

**Reservation:** As per the scale.

**Chairpersons:** Chairman and Vice-Chairman— indirectly elected.

**Term:** Five years.

### Revenue

1. Local Cess Surcharge.
2. Local Education Grant.
3. Local Cess Surcharge Matching Grant.
4. Local Roads Grant.
5. Village House Tax Matching Grant.
6. Fees for licence and permissions given.
7. Fees levied in the public markets after deducting the consolation, if any, paid by the Panchayat Union Council to the Village Panchayat on the scale fixed by the government.
8. Contributions paid by the Village Panchayat in respects of markets classified as Village Panchayat markets.
9. Fees for the use of public rest house.
10. Income from endowments and trusts.
11. The proportional share of proceeds of the entertainment tax.
12. Sale proceeds of tools and plants.
13. Income from Panchayat Union ferries and fisheries.
14. Interest on loans and securities.
15. Income from lease and sale proceeds of buildings, lands, and other property belonging to the Panchayat Union.

### Committees

a. *Appointment Committee*: Composed of the Chairman of Panchayat Union Council is the Chairman of Appointment Committee. This committee looks after all posts under Panchayat Union Council and the pay which is debitable to the funds of the Panchayat Union Council.

b. *Agricultural Production Committee*: Composed of the Chairman of Panchayat Union Council the Commissioner and three persons nominated by the Panchayat Union Council who possess adequate knowledge and experience in the field of agriculture and animal husbandry.

c. *Education Committee*: Elected persons from among Panchayat Union Council members specified by the council as ex-officio members.

d. *General Purpose Committee*: Elected persons from among themselves. Chairman as the ex-officio member.

### Administration

A Commissioner (BDO) is appointed by the Government for each Panchayat Union Council. The Commissioner is generally the Development Officer.

### Functions of Panchayat Union Council

1. Construction, repair and maintenance of public roads.
2. Maintenance of dispensaries.
3. Maintenance of maternity and child welfare centres.
4. Construction and maintenance of poor house, orphanages, shops and stalls.
5. Construction and maintenance of elementary schools.
6. Preventive and remedial measures against epidemics or malaria.
7. Control of notified fairs and festivals.
8. Veterinary relief.

9. Regulation of buildings.
10. Opening and maintenance of public market.
11. Maintenance of statistics of births and deaths.
12. Maintenance of choultries.
13. Promotion of agriculture.
14. Promotion of cottage industries.
15. Other duties as specified by the Government.

## Discretionary Function

Public utility calculated to promote safety, health, convenience and comfort of inhabitants covered by Panchayat Union Council.

Execution of community development programmes, including all matters relating to the development of agriculture, animal husbandry and village industries and others such as:

i. Construction, repairs and maintenance of all the public roads.
ii. Maintenance of statistics.
iii. Public markets' opening/closure.
iv. Control of fairs and festivals.
v. Granting permission for the construction of factories, installation of machineries, etc. in the Village Panchayats.
vi. Preparation of annual plans based on the needs of the people.

## District Panchayat (Zilla Parishad)

Constituted for each revenue district excluding townships, municipal corporations, municipalities and industrial townships.

### Composition

1. Elected members of the District Panchayat determined on the basis of the population of the district as ascertained from the last census list. One member for every fifty thousand population.
2. Members of Lok Sabha, Rajya Sabha and MLAs.
3. One-fifth of the Panchayat Union Councils' Chairmen.

### Chairperson

Chairman and Vice-Chairman are indirectly elected. (Under the previous law, District Collector was the Chairman of the District Panchayat).

### Administration

At the district level, the administration is headed by an officer not below the rank of Joint Director of Rural Development. He is the Chief Executive Officer (CEO).

### Functions

1. Preparation of District plan.
2. Advise on all matters of development undertaken by Panchayat and Panchayat Unions to Government.
3. Monitor and review progress of development.

### Committees

There are five standing committees:

1. Food and agricultural committee;
2. Industries and labour committee;
3. Public works committee; and
4. Election committee;
5. Health and welfare including prohibition.

Additional standing committees may be formed. It requires all standing committees consist of persons not exceeding five members, including the Chairman. The Chairman of the District Panchayat is the ex-officio member of the committee. Members of the standing committees elect a chairman separately for its own. No person is allowed to be a member of more than two standing committees. The CEO appoints one of his officers as ex-officio secretary for each Standing Committee. The CEO is entitled to attend the meetings of all the standing committees.

### General Fund

1. The amount transferred to the District Panchayat. Fund by appropriation from the consolidated fund of the state.
2. All grants, assignments, loans and contributions made by the Government.
3. All rents from lands or other properties of the District Panchayat.
4. All interest, profits and other money acquired by Government grants, assignments or transfer from private, individuals or institutions.
5. All proceeds of land, security and other properties sold by the District Panchayat.
6. All fees and penalties paid to or levied under this Act.
7. All sums received by or on behalf of the District Panchayat by virtue of this Act.
8. Government grant made to every District Panchayat fund to cover the expenses of establishment at a scale as may by determined.

## Dissolution of Panchayats

In the opinion of the Government, any Panchayat body is not competent in its performance, the Government has power to direct that a particular Panchayat body be dissolved with effect from a specified date which shall be within 6 months from the date of decision to dissolve the Panchayat. Before notification, the government communicates to the Panchayat body on which ground it has decided to dissolve it so that the Panchayat is able to challenge the proposal. The government consider its objection and explanation on the fixed date and if it is not satisfied the Panchayat body stands dissolved.

### Removal of the Chairperson

For removal of the Chairperson, a representation signed by not less than two-thirds of the members and containing the charges against him/her is presented to the Officer in the case of Village Panchayat or to the Government in the case of PUC/DP by two members who have signed it. If the Officer/Government is satisfied that the Chairperson is willfully neglecting the duties, an explanation is sought. If the explanation is not received within the date or it is not satisfactory, the Officer/Government forwards a copy of the notice along with the explanation to the Tehsildar/RDO who convenes a meeting after issuing notice to all members, including the Chairperson, at least seven days before. The Tehsildar/RDO only presides over the meeting but does not speak or vote in it. The charges along with the explanation is read before the quorum by the Tehsildar/RDO and he records the views of the Panchayat. The minutes of the meeting are duly recorded and copy is sent to the Officer/Government. The Officer/Government, considering the views by notification, removes/drops the proposal for the removal. In the case of Vice-President/Vice-Chairman the same procedure is applicable.

### No Confidence Motion

In the case of the Vice-President/Vice-Chairman of PUC/DP, no confidence motion is made by not less than one-half of the members after signing a written notice that is delivered to Tehsildar/RDO by two of the members who have signed it. The Tehsildar/RDO convenes the meeting giving notice at least 15 days earlier to all members to ascertain their views. Other procedures are the same as it is in the case to removal of the Chairperson.

### *Analysis*

a. **Motivating the bureaucracy:** Bureaucrats must understand that democratic decentralizations are much different from administrative decentralization. The latter is not new. However, democratic decentralisation means delegation of authority to elected representatives. This will mean that bureaucrats will lose power and work as subordinates to these representatives. In other words, they will have to consider themselves servants of the people and to masters as they used to be so far. Motivating the bureaucrats to participate in Panchayati Raj should be emphasized and the role of bureaucracy vis-à-vis the elected officials clarified. A motivated bureaucracy is a necessary condition for making Panchayati Raj a success.

b. **Silent revolution:** In India, woman is considered inferior to man. The reservation of one-third seats in Panchayat for women has ushered in a silent revolution to improve their status. So, is the case with Scheduled Castes and Tribes, who have seats reserved in proportion to their population in village.

Gangrade (1995) observed that women's involvement and participation in the third tier democratic institutions was totally absent. This was even in the village where the leaders had claimed cent per cent participation. They had a feeling that the women had no role in management and governance of village affairs. It is necessary to convince women about the importance of their active involvement in village affairs in the interest of total development of the villages.

The women will remain mere spectators and listeners unless they are made to articulate and participate in Panchayats at each level. They need to be trained and given regular intensive orientation courses, as a majority of them are illiterate.

c. **Formation of Mahila Sabha:** All adult women are members of Gram Sabha but a very few of them attend and very rarely participate in the meetings. Their Broad-based participation is limited due to traditional factors like caste, feudal approach and family status. Besides reservation of seats, not less than one-third of the total number of offices of Chairperson in Panchayats at each level have been reserved for women. The objective behind this reservation in executive bodies is to give women an effective 'say' in development and political processes of rural India. Women folk in villages generally remain at periphery.

For active involvement of women in the affairs of village, a separate Mahila Sabha may be constituted as a distinct statutory outfit of the Gram Sabha with definite rules, rights and access to funds. The forum of such sabha as sub-unit provides opportunity for 'woman to woman' contact, which will enlighten them for their meaningful participation in Gram Sabha, the general body of the village Panchayat. The Mahila Sabha may also establish contact with various voluntary women's organisations for their wider participation, emancipation and empowerment.

d. **Reservation for SCs and STs:** In order to give adequate representation to SCs and STs in the decision-making process, the law contemplates that the office of the Chairperson at all levels shall be reserved in favour of SCs and STs based on their population in the states. Women belonging to SCs and STs may not lag behind as a provision has been made to reserve one-third seats from among the seats reserved for this group. State legislature has been empowered to provide reservation of seats and offices of Chairpersons in Panchayats in favour of other backward classes also. The number of reserved seats shall be allotted by rotation to different Panchayats at each level. These reserved seats will be filled by direct election.

Following the enactment of the Constitution (73rd Amendment) Act, 1992, the states were expected to amend their Panchayat Raj Acts to bring them in conformity with the Constitutional Amendment Act, before 24th April, 1994.

Extension programmes in India had its beginning with few individuals. Their aim was to promote all-round development of the communities, economically, socially and culturally through co-operation of people in the community. Extension education concentrated on the individual in particular and community as a whole. Evolution of extension organisation took place through various programmes via Community Projects, National Extension Service Programme, Stage I and Stage II CD Block and reorganized Panchayat Samiti to the present day Panchayati Raj. The present day Panchayati Raj would help to bring about proper representation among its members. In this system a Gram Sabha, which is constituted, has to take all important decisions. A three-tier structure provides for uniformity in the Panchayati Raj system throughout the country, with the establishment of Village Panchayat (at village level), Panchayat Union (at intermediate/block level) and District Panchayat (at district level). Educating the rural masses about the efficacy of Panchayati Raj is essential. The success of the new phase of decentralisation will,

therefore, depend much on the commitment of the people. Unless a certain degree of financial autonomy is guaranted to Village Panchayat. No development worth the name can take place in Panchayati Raj system. However, democracy offers a promise to the poor and backward people, if they use their votes properly to win power and help in the well being of the community.

## ANIMAL HUSBANDRY DEVELOPMENT PROGRAMMES

Animal husbandry (AH) plays an important role in Indian economy. Agriculture contributes to the GDP to an extent of 25% of which one-fourth is through lievestock products. Livestock provides round the year income from its produce with increase in standard of living. Demand for animal protein and other products have increased several fold in this densely populated nation. To meet the demand, animal husbandry practices have been geared up all over the country. But due to intensification and extension of farming, it is competing with cereals for a key place in human consumption. To provide food to the whole nation, our pattern of food production has to be "land saving crop husbandry, and grain saving animal husbandry", so that animals do not compete with humans for grains.

Since independence many animal husbandry development programmes have been launched by both central and state governments from time to time. There have been drifts and shifts in these development strategies as well as extension systems for quicker but uniform and sustainable development. All these development programmes are implemented through and by the animal husbandry departments, rural development departments and various Non-Governmental Organisations (NGOs). The present chapter deals with animal husbandry administration and different animal husbandry development programmes.

### Animal Husbandry Administration

The management of public affairs of the animal husbandry department and related institutions is called animal husbandry administration. It can also be defined as the guidance, leadership and control of the efforts of the group of individuals in the animal husbandry department towards some common goal.

### Scope

The scope of administration of animal husbandry can be viewed to be the sum total of several activities, namely planning, organisation staffing, directing, co-ordination, reporting and budgeting. Staffing means appointing suitable persons to various posts under the organisation. Reporting means that the staff are being kept well informed of what is going on in the organisation. The other terms carry their normal literal meanings.

### Basic Principles of Animal Husbandry Administration

For increased effectiveness of animal husbandry administration, some basic principles need to be followed:

i. **Principle of hierarchy:** The members of the organisation are placed in a definite hierarchy wherein lines of positional authority and responsibility run upward and downward through several levels with a broadbase at the bottom and a single head at the top with whom is entrusted the authority of making vital decisions.

ii. **Principle of authority:** There can be efficient administration only when the authority vested with the individuals concerned is sufficient, clearly defined and is understood by all persons in the organisation.

iii. **Principle of responsibility with matching authority:** The individual should not only be burdened with responsibility but should also be delegated with matching authority, more so in an ideally decentralised form of administration.

iv. **Principle of span of control**: Span of control is the number of subordinates one has to supervise so as to permit as much decentralisation of decision-making as is needed to attain quality, decisions, increased effectiveness and efficiency. Some of the factors influencing the span of control include the intensity and frequency of the need to see the chief, the magnitude of their problems, the professional competence of the staff, the degree of control that must be exercised, etc.

v. **Principle of communication:** There should be a two-way channel of communication, both vertical and horizontal, in the organisation. It ensures common understanding of organisational values and objectives.

vi. **Principle of organisational structure:** The organisational structure should be subject to continuous adaptations as conditions warrant. Changes in basic objectives, in size of staff, in professional competence, adjustments in programme emphasis and in the nature of institutional relationships within which the organisation must operate will have to be made.

### Increasing Efficiency in Animal Husbandry Administration

Proper organisation of the administrative staff, acumen of personnel to recruit candidates with the required intellectual, moral and physical qualities and proper relations with the public increase the efficiency. In addition to these, if irregularity and unpunctuality with regard to fixed hours of work, red tapism, delay in work, overdose of formalism, obscurities in orders and abuse of power are avoided, then these may also lead to increased efficiency of the AH administration.

### Extension Organisation

Organisations are the assemblages of both human and non-human resources in addition to help in organising resources in order to attain certain common goals. Normally the administration is run from the office of the organisation. In the office there is generally a horizontal division of labour so that the head can have the supervision and attend to proper division of labours. The office is divided into different sections and sub-sections, such as Registry and Recording section, Subject section, General section, Finance and Account section, Establishment section, Intelligence section, etc.

The work of the office involves writing. This facilitates in keeping evidence, searching precedents and deliberations within/outside the organisations. This is done mostly in the form of letters, notings, orders, rules and regulations. Common and relevant papers related to a particular issue are kept together in a file.

### Technical Problems in the Building of an Organisation

The following six factors appear to contribute to the building of an extension organisation:

i. **Increase in size of staff:** With the increase in staff, there will be greater need for delegating responsibility and authority for improving the skills in dealing with people and for better co-ordination among members of the organisation.

ii. **Changes in personnel:** Changes in the organisation often bring men with varied skills and expertise into the administration. These changes may lead to increasing desire by individuals to participate in organisational decisions and problem-solving, increasing interest in being identified more closely with the parent organisation, with research and increasing degree of occupational mobility.

iii. **Changes in clientele:** Farm families are undergoing change and there has been an equally important development in terms of the type of assistance they need.

iv. **Changes in the predominant bases of organisation:** The three bases of organisational behaviour, namely function, geographic area and clientele undergo changes which may affect the administrative accountability of the staff towards the basic supervisors.

v. **Changes in objectives of the organisation:** As the organisation grows it undergoes changes in terms of its objectives which calls for modification of its structure in turn.

vi. **Changes in bases of authority available to members of organisation:** Authority is the process of influencing the behaviour of other people. It can be based on the administrative rules and regulations, on knowledge, on position, and on the situation. By recruitment policy and training, the members, who choose to belong to an organisation, can adapt themselves to any one of these forms of authority which will develop their intensive commitment to the organisation.

In addition to the foregoing factors, others like staffing, training, morale, programme co-ordination, budgets and reports are also important in building an organisation.

## Rural Development Programmes as Under Different Plans

| S. No. Programme | Year of introduction |
|---|---|
| I. **First Five-Year Plan** | |
| 1. Community Development Programme | 1952 |
| 2. National Extension Service | 1953 |
| II. **Second Five-Year Plan** | |
| 3. Multi-purpose Tribal Development | 1959 |
| 4. Intensive Agriculture Area Programme | 1960 |
| III. **Third Five-Year Plan** | |
| 5. Intensive Agricultural Area Programme | 1964 |
| 6. High Yielding Variety Programme | 1966 |
| **Annual Plan 1966** | |
| 7. Farmers' Training and Education Programme | 1966 |
| 8. Tribal Development Block | 1968 |
| IV. **Fourth Five-Year Plan** | |
| 9. Drought-Prone Area Programme | 1970 |
| 10. Crash Scheme for Rural Development | 1971 |
| 11. Small Farmers' Development Agency | 1971 |
| 12. Tribal Area Development Programme | 1972 |
| 13. Pilot Project for Tribal Development | 1972 |
| 14. Pilot Intensive Rural Employment Programme | 1972 |
| 15. Minimum Needs Programme | 1972 |
| 16. Command Area Development Programme | 1974 |
| V. **Fifth Five-Year Plan** | |
| 17. Hill Area Development Programme | 1975 |
| 18. Special Livestock Production Programme | 1975 |
| 19. Desert Development Programme | 1977 |
| 20. Whole Village Development Programme | 1979 |

*Contd...*

| S. No. Programme | Year of introduction |
|---|---|
| 21. Training Rural Youth for Self-Employment | 1979 |
| 22. National Rural Employment Programme | 1980 |
| 23. Development of Women and Children in Rural Areas | 1983 |
| 24. Rural Landless Employment Guarantee Programme | 1983 |
| VII. **Seventh Five-Year Plan** | |
| 25. New Twenty-Point Economic Programme | 1986 |
| VIII. **Eight Five-Year Plan** | |
| 26. Milk and Milk Products Order | 1992 |
| 27. National project on Rinderpest Eradication | 1992 |
| 28. Integrated Dairy Development Project | 1993 |
| IX. **Ninth Five-Year Plan** | |
| 29. Swarnajayanthi Gram Swarozgar Yojana | 1999 |
| 30. National Project on Cattle & Buffalo Breeding Programme | 2000 |
| X. **Tenth Five-Year Plan** | |
| 31. Conservation and Improvement of Native Animal Genetic Resources | 2002 |
| XI. **Eleventh Five-Year Plan** | |
| 32. National Agriculture Development Programme | 2007 |
| 33. Livestock Health and Disease Control | 2007 |
| 34. Assistance to State Poultry/Duck Farms | 2009 |
| XII. **Twelth Five-Year Plan** | |
| 35. National Dairy Plan (NDP) | 2012 |
| 36. National Livestock Mission | 2012 |

With the starting of community development project in 1952, as part of the First Five-Year Plan, various rural development programmes have been implemented. Some of these rural development programmes have animal husbandry as an important component within them. These include Intensive Agriculture Programme (IAP), Small Farmers' Development Agency (SFDA), Marginal Farmers and Agricultural Labourers (MFAL) Programme, Drought-Prone Area Programme (DPAP), Hill Area Development Programme (HADP), Integrated Rural Development Programme (IRDP), Training of Rural Youth for Self-Employment (TRYSEM), Development of Women and Children in Rural Areas (DWCRA), etc.

Intensive Agricultural District Programme (IADP) was started in restricted areas in 1960 for development of agriculture and to initiate the process of development in related areas. Due to the beneficial impact of this programme, the government extended it to other districts with slight modifications under the name of Intensive Agricultural Area Programme (IAAP) in 1964.

The gains of intensive development efforts, (including institutional credit) flow more towards large and resourceful farmers at the neglect of small farmers, landless labourers, tenants and artisans. Hence, a shift in rural development strategy was necessitated. Deliberate efforts were made for the flow of development benefits to the poorer sections and backward areas. Accordingly SFDA, MFAL, DPAP, HADP, etc. were implemented with modified emphasis.

**Small Farmers' Development Agency (SFDA):** During the Fourth Five-Year Plan the government set up two separate agencies of SFDA and MFAL. Later MFAL was amalgamated with SFDA to form a unified corporate body known as SFDA. The basic objective of this agency was to enable selected target groups of marginal/small farmers and agricultural labourers to increase their income through production activities.

**Drought-Prone Area Programme (DPAP):** It was launched in 1970. It aimed at mitigating the scarcity conditions by executing rural works to generate employment. The main thrust is to restore the proper ecological balance in the drought-prone areas. Some of the important elements envisaged in this integrated approach are changes in agronomical practices, restructuring of the farming pattern and pasture development through proper management of small and marginal farmers and agricultural labourers. Financial assistance and subsidy were given for purchasing milch animals, sheep, poultry and pigs.

**Hill Area Development Programme (HADP):** This was started for the development of agriculture, animal husbandry, etc. to improve the living condition of the farmers in the hill areas.

**Integrated Rural Development Programme (IRDP):** The Beneficiary Oriented Programme as well as Area Development Programme could not make much dent into the problem of poverty and unemployment. Considering the magnitude and dimensions of rural poverty, IRDP was launched to mitigate them. The apparent failure of Community Development Programme was the main reason for the evolution of IRDP.

IRDP was launched in 1978–79. It envisages the integration of methodology and approach of both Beneficiary Oriented Programme as well as Area Development Programme. This was done to intensify development efforts for the purpose of poverty alleviation as well as increasing productivity. The objective of the programme is to assist selected families of target groups in rural areas to cross the poverty line and to minimise inequality.

The programme aims to achieve the stated objective by providing income generating assets, including working capital where necessary, to target group families through a package of assistance including subsidy and institutional credit. The target group of the programme consists of small farmers, marginal farmers, agricultural labourers, rural artisans and others whose annual family incomes are below the poverty line.

Since the families belonging to SC and ST constitute the bulk of the poverty group, at least 30% of the assisted families should be drawn from SC and ST. At least 30% of the total beneficiaries should be women. Priority should be given to women-headed households.

The assistance to beneficiaries under the IRDP comprises two components, viz. loan and subsidy. The major part of the investment comprising the loan portion has to come through institutional credit. The unit cost of milch animals, goat unit, sheep unit and bullocks are periodically raised and fixed by the Directorate of Rural Development Agency. A subsidy of 50% is provided to SC/ST, 25% to small farmers and 33.33% to marginal farmers, agricultural labourers and others.

The assets are purchased by a purchase committee comprising of bank staff, veterinarian (Extension Officer of Animal Husbandry), etc. Insurance coverage and health coverage of animals are arranged by the veterinarian. The price fixed by the purchase committee is treated as the sum insured for the settlement of claims.

### Training of Rural Youth for Self-Employment (TRYSEM)

TRYSEM is a Central Government-sponsored scheme. It was launched by Government of India as a subsidiary scheme from 1991. It particularly concentrates on the welfare of rural youth who are partially educated, unskilled, and unemployed for want of guidance and financial assistance. Major objectives of this programme include imparting technical skill to rural youth in the age group of 18–35 from families below poverty line to enable them to take up self-employment and to an extent, wage employment in any of the economic sectors.

The training is need-based and of flexible duration. TRYSEM trainees are provided with financial assistance under IRDP on completion of the training programme. Thus, every TRYSEM trainee is a potential IRDP beneficiary. At least 30% of the trainees should belong to SC/ST and a minimum of one-third should be women. While under training, trainees are paid stipends ranging from ₹ 200–500 per month. Tuition fees of ₹ 200 per month per candidate is paid to the institution by the Project Officer of DRDA.

### Development of Women and Children in Rural Areas (DWCRA)

DWCRA was formulated as a sub-scheme of IRDP in 1982, to improve the quality of life of rural families below poverty line and to provide assistance to women as post-IRDP strategy. It is partly supported by UNICEF and jointly financed by the Union and State Governments. It operates in conjunction with IRDP and TRYSEM. Major objectives of the scheme include providing facilities for income generating activities to women of families below the poverty line which will have a positive impact on the economic and nutritional status of the family. It also provides an organisational support—to make the rural women more aware of problems they face and service they can make use of to organise production enhancing progammes in rural areas to care for the children of the working women by providing an improved environment. Various income generating activities of the scheme are poultry, dairy, sheep, goat and pig farming, mushroom production, fruit and vegetable processing, bee keeping, basket making, pickle making, embroidery, soap making, agarbatti making, etc.

### Swarnajayanthi Gram Swarozgar Yojana (SGSY)

SGSY scheme evolved from the Erstwhile Rural Development Programmes, viz. Integrated Rural Development Programme (IRDP), Training of Rural Youth for Self-Employment (TRYSEM), Supply of Improved Tool Kits to Rural Artisans (SITRA), Development of Women and Children in Rural Areas (DWCRA), Ganga Kalyan Yojana (GRY) and Million Wells Scheme (MWS). This programme came into effect from 1st April, 1999 and is funded by the centre and the state in the ratio of 75:25.

It is a holistic programme of micro-enterprises covering all aspects of self-employment, viz. organisation of rural poor into self-help groups (SHGs) and their capacity building, planning of activities clusters, infrastructure buildup, technology, credit and marketing. Emphasis is laid on group approaches involving the organisation of poor into SHGs and their capacity building.

SGSY aims at establishing a large number of micro-enterprises in the rural areas with an emphasis on the "cluster approach". For this 4–5 key activities are to be identified in each block based on the resource endowments, occupational skills of the people and availability of markets, with the approval of Panchayat Union/Samiti at block level and DRDA/District Panchayat at the district level. For identified key activities project reports are to be prepared encompassing training, credit, technology, infrastructure and marketing with the involvement of banks and financial institutions.

The objective of SGSY is to bring the assisted poor families (Swarozgaris) above the poverty line within three years by providing them income-generating assets through a unit of bank credit and subsidy. It lays emphasis on group approach and 75% of the allocation is channelised through groups with subsidy at the rate of 50% of the project cost subject to a maximum of ₹ 1.25 lakh per group. For SC/ST, subsidy is 50% of the project cost and maximum of ₹ 10,000 per individual and 30% for others, (maximum of ₹ 7,500 per individual). DRDA provides revolving fund (RF) at the rate of ₹ 10,000 per group and banks are required to sanction RF loan up to ₹ 25,000 in the form of cash credit. There are safeguards for the weaker section similar to IRDP, i.e. SC/ST 50%, women 40% and disabled 3%.

The scheme is implemented by the DRDAs through the Panchayat Unions/Samitis in the blocks, commercial banks, regional rural banks and co-operative banks. Grading has to be carried out at two stages. Every SHG that is in existence at least for a period of 6 months is subjected to grading. When the group qualifies after first grading, RF is provided. At the end of six months from the date of receipt of revolving fund, the SHG is subjected to another grading test to see if it has been functioning effectively and is capable of taking up an economic activity through higher level of investment. Basic orientation programme for all the selected groups is organised for a period of not more than two days. Training would be organised through government institutions, ITI, polytechnics, university, NGO, etc.

## Animal Husbandry Development Programmes

### Dairy Development Programmes

Cattle rearing is one among the first organised activities of civilisation. Cattle provided all the basic requirements of human being and have been man's mute companions. Several efforts have been made by governmental and non-governmental organisations for the development of dairy sector. A growth rate of 4.5% has been achieved by the dairy sector during the past decade as compared to the 2% growth recorded by the agricultural sector as a whole.

### Review of Dairying

- 1886—Department of Defenses established dairy farms for supply of milk to British troops at Allahabad as advised by Board of Agriculture.
- 1914—A preliminary study concerning the composition of milk produced by indigenous cows and buffaloes was conducted.

- 1916—Imperial Dairy Expert appointed.
- 1919—First livestock census was carried out for planned development.
- 1920—Mr. William Smith, the dairying expert recommended the following. Scientific breeding, feeding and management practices to be followed in Military Dairy Farms. Establishment of a training centre to train the personnel to manage the farms on scientific lines.
- 1923—The Military Farms at Bangalore, Wellington (Nilgiris) and Karnal transferred to Agriculture Department. The farm at Karnal was developed as cattle breeding farm and Bangalore Farm as imperial institute of Animal Husbandry.
- 1929—Imperial Council of Agricultural Research (now Indian Council of Agricultural Research) established.
- Sri Pestonji Edulji Polson established Polson model dairy at Anand. He started producing Polson butter.
- 1931—The Institute at Bangalore renamed as Imperial Dairy Institute.
- 1936—Dr N.C.Wright, Director, Dairy Research Institute, Scotland, reviewed in India, made important recommendations which formed the basis of development of dairy industry.
- 1941—The Bangalore Institute—renamed as Imperial Dairy Research Institute. subsequently, Indian Dairy Research Institute.
1. **Goushalas:** The Goushalas and 'Pinjirapoles' are charitable institutions established by the co-operation of the people. Cows, calves and bulls are kept in goushalas and other animals in pinjirapoles. These institutions are mostly concentrated in the northern north-winter parts of the country. A goushala possesses 151 acres of grazing area and about 63 acres of cultivable land. Goushalas are in existence for the last two centuries. These are being maintained on account for religio-economic considerations. The reorganisation and development of goushalas as centres for cattle breeding and milk production started with the setting up of a Central Goushala Development Board by the Government of India in 1949.

The Central Council of Gosamvardhana (CCG) was established in 1952 by the Government of India to act as the central co-ordinating and advisory body on cattle development throughout the country. In 1960, the Government of India reconstituted structure and functions of the council.

The council is actively engaged in arousing public interest in the development of cattle by organising Gosamvardhana Week and other extension work. The council also conducts a training course of one year duration at its Goushala Managers' Training Centre in Karnal where trainees are taught the most modern methods of cattle management, processing and marketing of milk and milk products.

A comprehensive goushala development scheme, sponsored by the Ministry of Agriculture was included under the Second Five-Year Plan. Financial assistance was also provided for construction of sheds, water supply and maintenance of animals. The goushalas were required to send their unproductive and unserviceable animals to the nearest Gosadans. The scheme was continued under the Third Plan but from the Fourth Plan it was transferred to the state sector and this programme received very low priority in the allocation of funds as the impact made by these institutions on cattle development and milk production was not considered significant.

Some of the Goushalas at Nasik, Urikanchan, Amritsar, Indore, etc. are providing quality indigenous and crossbred heifers and bulls. One Goushala at Mumbai has completed 100 years in 1986 and has established two institutes for fodder research and grassland development. The Sabarmati Ashram Gaushala founded in 1915 by Mahatma Gandhi near Ahmedabad is one being managed by the NDDB and has a training centre for AI service including embryo transfer.

2. **Five-Year Plan and Dairy Development**

*First Five-Year Plan (1950–55):* All the activities of rural life were initiated through community development programmes. With regard to animal husbandry the goals were to increase milk production and supply to urban areas and improve the quality of indigenous breeds so as to provide draught power. Official cattle breeding policy was laid down, emphasizing the development of dual purpose breeds. Buffaloes were included in Key Village Scheme (KVS). "Gosadans" were set up for surplus cattle. The plan recommended for setting up public milk supply schemes with provision to set up a milk board for each urban area.

*Gosadan:* The Gosadan scheme was launched during the First Five-Year Plan with the aim to segregate the old, infirm, unproductive and useless cattle from the good ones so as to control promiscuous breeding and also to relieve pressure on the limited resources of feed and fodder available for the productive stock. During this first plan period 25 Gosadans were established. Gosadans are generally located in remote forest area and waste lands. In these Gosadans, the segregated cattle, are housed in proper shelters or sheds and maintained on natural pastures and hay. Thus, the Gosadan scheme was launched to solve the problem of degraded cattle.

*Second Five-Year Plan (1955–60):* The plan provides for pedigree bull rearing farms and for pregnancy testing in KVS areas. Establishment of 196 key village blocks and expansion of existing 114 blocks with 670 AI centres. 34 new Gosadans and 248 Goshalas, 1900 veterinary dispensaries were started. Delhi milk supply scheme was established in 1960. Private entrepreneurs like Glaxo, Lever, Nestle, etc. were started there milk product factories.

*Third Five-Year Plan (1960–65):* It encouraged crossbreeding with exotic breeds, setting up of fodder banks, factories to prepare feed using agriculture wastes and byproducts, manufacture of dairy machines and equipment in private sector within the country. About 143 urban milk board and milk plants have been started. Private entrepreneurs like Gosadans, Levers, Nestler, etc. were started there milk product factories.

*Fourth Five-Year Plan (1969–74):* The fourth plan enlisted selective breeding programme and emphasized crossbreeding with exotic breeds. Second important innovation made was the international linkage of the development strategies through dairy commodity aid under the World Food Programme. The world bank's assistance to Dairy Development was started with the coverage of Karnataka, Madhya Pradesh and Rajasthan. It also envisaged an All India Co-ordinated Research Project (AICRP) for improvement of production potential of buffaloes. Operation Flood Project (OFP) was also introduced.

*Fifth Five-Year Plan (1974–79):* The plan envisaged 'agressive crossbreeding' for increasing milk production and proposed import of foreign semen doses, bulls and heifers of exotic breeds and increase in the number of exotic cattle breeding farms. Large-scale Integrated Dairy Development Projects were proposed and were later funded by the World Bank.

*Sixth Five-Year Plan (1980–85):* This plan proposed to contain the increase in the population of cows and buffaloes by replacing non-descript local stock by high yielding cows of indigenous breeds, crossbred cows and improved buffaloes. Further, 500 key village blocks and 122 ICD projects were established. Institute of buffalo research was started. Froze semen stations were established in different states.

*Seventh Five-Year Plan (1986–90):* This plan proposed to bring almost 50% of the cows under crossbreeding programme and set a target of 5.6% annual growth in milk production. Embryo transfer technology and Operation Flood II projects were introduced. Importance was given to fodder development. PTS was implemented.

*Eighth Five-Year Plan (1992–97):* Milk and Milk Production Order (MMPO) was issued.

*Ninth Five-Year Plan (1996–2001):* The realities of the post-GATT world was reflected in this plan. Importance was given for effective animal health management to reduce the economic loss and to enlarge export of livestock products. The sanitary and phyto-sanitary (SPS) measures have been introduced in the new World Trade Agreement (WTA). Milk production reached 84.6 million tones (mt) in 2001-2002. The per capita availability of milk increased from 112 gm per day in 1973-74 to about 226 gm per day. Restriction on establishing new milk processing capacity under Milk and Milk Products Order (MMPO) has now been removed.

*Tenth Five-Year Plan (2002–2007):* The tenth plan target for milk production is set at 108.4 mt envisaging an annual growth rate of 6%. Introduction of National Project on Cattle and Buffalo Improvement Programme. Major thrust will be given to genetic upgradation of indigenous cattle and buffaloes using proven semen and high quality pedigree bulls and by expanding the artificial insemination and natural service network. Improved bulls for natural breeding will be made available to private breeders, Gaushalas, NGOs and Panchayats in remote and hilly areas. A holistic approach will be taken to address the issue of clean milk production, which is imperative for marketing and promoting export of dairy products.

Enrichment of straw/stovel preparation of hay/silage to overcome fodder scarcities, conversion of fodder into feed block to facilitate transport of fodder from surplus areas, establishment of fodder banks and promotion of chaff cutters and increase the fodder productivity through promotion of intensive fodder production techniques. Completed eradication of Rinderpest and adopt a National Immunization Programme against the most prevalent diseases. All India Control of Animal Disease (ASCAD) is being implemented.

3. **Efforts through specific programmes**

*Community Development Programme (CDP):* In the CDP inaugurated on 2nd October, 1952, there were provisions for establishment of animal breeding centres. The block animal husbandry officers posted in the Community Development Blocks look after the animal husbandry programmes along with other activities. Each block has a network of artificial insemination centres.

*Key Village Scheme (KVS):* This scheme was taken up in August 1952. The scheme envisages a multifaceted approach to cattle development by giving simultaneous attention to better breeding, improved feeding, effective disease control measures, management practice and organised market facilities. Artificial insemination (AI) technique was also introduced.

*Intensive Cattle Development Programme (ICDP):* It is a comprehensive project started in the year 1964-65 covering all aspects of cattle development. The target was to operate 114 projects in 20 states, in the milk shed areas of the large dairy plants.

*Special group and area-specific programmes:* Several special group and area-specific programmes like SFDA, MFAL, DPAP, HADP, ITDP and IRDP for weaker and economically backward communities were formed with animal husbandry as an integeral part as these could increase their income and help in employment generation.

*Fodder Development Programme (FDP):* Government established seven regional stations for forage production with the objective of achieving quick transfer of technology on all aspects of fodder production.

*Special Livestock Breeding Programme (SLBP):* This programme was launched in some selected districts of the country involving small/marginal farmers and agricultural labourers in livestock production and generation of additional employment and income.

*National Project on Cattle and Buffalo Breeding Programme (NPCBB):* The National Project on Cattle and Buffalo Breeding (NPCBB) is the flagship scheme of DAHDF. Initiated in October 2000 for a period of 10 years, this envisages genetic upgradation of indigenous cattle and buffaloes, development and conservation of important indigenous breeds, and to evolve sustainable breeding policy. The project is being implemented by State Implementing Agencies (SIAs) in 28 States and one UT. NPCBB will have two main components, namely National Programme for Bovine Breeding (NPBB) and Dairy Development.

*National Dairy Plan (NDP):* It has been launched (2012) as a central sector scheme with credit support from the International Development Association (IDA) and implemented by the National Dairy Development Board (NDDB) through a network of End Implementing Agencies (EIAs), mainly dairy cooperatives and producer companies, this aims to (i) increase productivity of milch animals and thereby increase milk production and (ii) provide rural milk producers with greater access to the organised milk-processing sector. These objectives would be pursued through adoption of focused scientific and systematic processes in provision of technical inputs, supported by appropriate policy and regulatory measures.

4. **Operation Flood:** This is a major dairy project which provides for reliable source of income to the rural poor. Dr Verghese Kurien is called the "father of the white revolution" in India. He is credited with architecting Operation Flood.

*Operation Flood I 1970–81:* It was launched in 1970 following an agreement with the World Food Programme (WFP) with an attempt towards development of the dairy industry in India on the 'Anand pattern' so as to meet the country's need for milk products. To increase the capacity of milk-processing facilities. To change the urban milk markets from traditional milk suppliers to modern dairy supplies. To develop milk transport and storage facilities. To improve dairy farming standard.

*Operation Flood II 1981–85:* Success of Operation Flood formed the basis for Operation Flood II. This programme was approved by the Government of India for implementation with financial assistance from World Bank and commodity assistance from the European Economic Community (EEC). To create a viable dairy industry to meet India's need.

*Operation Flood III 1985–90:* This programme aimed at achieving financial viability of the milk unions/state federations by adopting the salient institutional characteristics of the 'Anand Pattern' Co-operatives. To establish an additional 15,500 village level milk co-operatives and to strengthen national milk grid. The Operation Flood III was funded by World Bank credit loan, food aid by EEC and NDDB's own resources.

## Strategies Adopted

Operation Flood was designed on some simple assumptions, viz. (1). Dairying is complementary to agriculture and provides supplementary income to a large number of people. (2) Millions of farmers living far off from market are involved in production. (3) Market and price incentives are essential to increase production.

## Interventions Based on Assumptions

1. **Strategic:** Traditionally, development activities in the developing countries are supported by assistance from the developed countries in the form of capital, technology and food. In the case of Operation Flood we received food aid from the UN and European Economic Community (EEC). Food assistance may be used to meet short-term food shortages due to natural calamities or it may be used to generate employment under the food for work programme or for generating resources. Had the assistance been used just for meeting the food shortage alone it would have damaged the dairy industry in the country.

2. **Institutional intervention:** In replicating the Anand pattern, Operation Flood attempted to promote a grassroot level democracy with the participation of producer members irrespective of the size of land holding or social stratification. These co-operatives must operate viably to ensure payment of remunerative prices to the members. Another important element in the strategy is its special focus on professional management.

3. **Technological intervention:** Operation Flood provided adequate price incentives to encourage farmers to make major input purchase decisions. Technology is also made use of in testing the milk, and transporting and processing it. It has been proved that once the farmers are convinced of an assured price and regular payment linked with a guaranteed marketing channel they are more responsive for better technology.

**National Dairy Development Board (NDDB):** An institution of national importance, the NDDB was formed by merging the erstwhile Indian Dairy Corporation (IDC) and it started functioning with effect from 1987, with the major objective to promote, plan and organise programmes for development of dairy and other agriculture-based or agricultural and allied industrial and biological projects on an intensive and nation-wide basis and to render assistance in the implementation of such programmes.

**Breed improvement programme:** NDDB launched the Dairy Herd Improvement Programme Action (DHIPA) to achieve genetic changes in selected cattle and buffalo populations. The Open Nucleus Breeding System (ONBS) of NDDB, which evaluates the quality of bulls and technology for the commercial production of Urea Molasses Block (UMB), was successfully transferred to various milk unions.

**National Milk Grid (NMG):** NMG was started in 1970, to provide national market for milk and milk products.

**National Milch Herd (NMH):** This scheme was to improve Indian dairy cattle (cattle and buffalo) and to develop crossbreeding technology.

**Technology Mission on Dairy Development:** The government has launched a technology mission on dairy development in association with NDDB to raise overall dairy productivity and increase rural employment and income. It also co-ordinates various research institutions in the country.

5. **Intervention by other national agencies**

   *National Bank of Agriculture and Rural Development (NABARD):* NABARD plays a vital role in the development of dairy in the country. It finances various dairy projects through state-level institutions, nationalised banks, co-operative banks and rural banks.

   *National level dairy association:* Indian Dairy Association facilitates Indian farmers and other technical people to discuss through seminars, conferences and symposia on various topics of dairy industry. Besides this many other associations do exist.

   *National Co-operative Development Corporation (NCDC):* This was established in 1972 for augmenting white revolution. It offers free technical advice to dairy co-operatives, and financial assistance to milk producers. It has seven regional offices with its head office in New Delhi.

   *National Co-operative Dairy Federation of India (NCDFI):* The NCDFI was set up in 1970 with the objectives to help and advise, offer consultancy service, help preparation of project report, and recurring financial assistance for government and institutional recruitment of personnel for dairy industry and participation in the development activities.

*All India co-ordinated research projects:* The aim of this project is to evolve a breed of dairy cattle that would adapt itself to the local environment with high breeding efficiency. A Central Frozen Semen Bank was set up at Hassaragatta (Karnataka) with four more frozen semen stations. The All India co-ordinated research projects on buffaloes, sheep and goats were also started by ICAR at different centres.

*Constraints:* 1. Improper selection of beneficiaries. 2. Poor quality animals. 3. Lack of technical know-how, technical inputs, trained personnel, transport, storage facilities, fodder and grazing lands. 4. Non-availability of locally suitable high yielding dairy cattles.

*Suggestions:* 1. Proper selection of beneficiaries. 2. Careful monitoring. 3. Training of farmers and technical personnel. 4. Fodder development. 5. Measures to reduce the feeding cost by utilising various unconventional feed and feed stuffs. 6. Improving the transport and storage facilities of milk and other inputs. 7. Extending all the technical inputs and institutional supports. 8. Inculcating the real value of dairy co-operative. 9. Research and developments. 10. Inculcating equality consciousness. 11. Consumers education about dairy products. 12. Establishing milk colonies.

## Sheep Development Programmes

Sheep rearing plays a major role in the rural economy and in the uplift of people below poverty line.

### Objectives of Sheep Development Programmes

1. To improve the socioeconomic condition of the rural population in the area of operation through sheep husbandry practices.
2. To provide adequate employment for under-employed people in villages through development of small-scale cottage industries based on sheep production.
3. Provision of adequate infrastructure support (including pasture/fodder development) for the improvement of sheep, import of exotic breeds of sheep and establishment of exotic breeding farm and ram multiplication farms.

4. To bring about improvement in the economic traits of sheep by effective genetic improvement through scientific breeding for more mutton and carpet wool production.
5. Distribution of improved rams to selected breeders for breed improvement.
6. Provision of in-service training to farmers and project staff, to improve the scientific methods of sheep management practices.
7. To augment quality mutton production through improvement in the sheep population.
8. Improvement of facilities in respect of health cover, field veterinary extension services and research.
9. Improvement of marketing system of sheep.
10. Improvement of selected slaughter houses for hygienic mutton production.
11. Insuring an effective supervised credit programme for small holders to promote breed improvement, sheep production and marketing through viable farmers, co-operative societies and their federation.

### Five-Year Plan and Sheep Development

During the Second Five-Year Plan period, a breeding policy for sheep was evolved which included, (1) definition of selective breeding, (2) upgrading of non-descriptive breeds with superior breeds, (3) cross-breeding with foreign breeds in selected hilly areas. In the Third Plan period, new sheep breeding farms were established. Old farms were expanded and quality rams were supplied to the farmers. Further, during the Fourth Plan period, Sheep and Woolly Extension Centres and Wool Grading-cum-Marketing Centres were established. In the Fifth Plan period, cross-breeding with woolly type sheep was encouraged. Various programmes were launched during the other plan periods also. During the Ninth Plan period, the production of wool was increased from 43.3 million kg in 1996–97 to 49 million kg in 2001-2002. The fine wool production in the country is around 4 million kg.

During the ninth plan focus was given to wool production. The wool production has increased from 43.3 million kg in 1996–97 to 49 million kg in 2001–02 as against the target of 54 million kg. The fine wool production in the country is around 4 million kg against the demand of around 35 to 40 million kg. In the tenth plan period the programme of providing exotic males for improvement of sheep in the Northern temperate region will continue.

Eleventh Plan initiative is entrepreneurial development for commercial rearing of small ruminants and pig. During The Twelfth Plan period NLM Programme has an additional mini mission relating to development of small ruminants.

### Other programmes

The government is implementing sheep development programmes through state Animal Husbandry Departments, Rural Development Departments and other Social Welfare Departments. The sheep development programmes like (1) Special Animal Husbandry Programme, (2) Special Assistance Programme, (3) Special Central Livestock Breeding Programme, (4) Intensive Health Cover for Sheep and (5) European Economic Community (EEC) assisted sheep development project were financed by Central and State Governments.

Apart from this assistance was given through other programmes like SFDA, DPAP, HADP, ITDP, IRDP, etc.

### Constraints

Most of the beneficiaries are selected wrongly and the unit cost is found to be inadequate. Exploitation by middlemen in the purchase of sheep. Untimely assistance and diversion of the loan amount. Absence of sufficient fodder banks to meet the demand during drought and also reduction in grazing lands. Inadequate infrastructure in production and marketing of sheep and their byproducts. Lack of modernisation of abattoirs or slaughterhouses and carcass utilisation plants.

### Suggestions

1. Beneficiaries should be selected without any deviation from the norms prescribed by the financing agency. Political and bureaucratic influences should be ended in selecting a beneficiary.
2. Before availing the assistance, the beneficiaries should be taught about the objectives and the outcome of the programmes.
3. Persons monitoring the various developmental programmes should be given adequate training to monitor the programmes effectively.
4. Unit cost should be reviewed and revised once in six months based on the prevailing market price.
5. Frequent inspections by the officials may prevent the misuse of the assistance.
6. By developing an organised marketing system, the return from sheep enterprise can be maximized.
7. The increasing demand of fodder can be met by converting the waste lands into pasture lands.

### Goat Development Programmes

Despite various adverse comments about the impact of goat rearing on the flora, the number of goats in fact has gone up in recent years. Considerable size of the rural community, especially women farmers and landless agricultural labourers are rearing one or two goats. This traditional mini goat husbandry practice is still seen or has taken roots throughout rural India because the goats are the 'poor man's cow'. They give milk and also meet the farmer's timely needs through sale of kids. They are a sort of money spinners for the poorest of the poor people. Rural poor below the poverty line are given assistance for purchase of goat, insurance, and also fodder development to promote goat rearing under the various rural development programmes like, Integrated Rural Development Programme (IRDP), National Watershed Development Programme-Rural Area (NWDPRA), Ambedkar Vishesh Rojgar Yojna, Swarnajayanthi Gram Swarozgar Yojana (SGSY) and DANIDA project. During the Ninth Plan period, instead of increasing the goat population, emphasis was made on productivity per animal, organized marketing and prevention of emergence of new diseases like Peste des Petits ruminants (PPR) which has led to higher mortality and miscarriages in goats.

During the Ninth Plan period emphasis was given on productivity per animal, creation of organised market and prevention of emergence of new diseases like PPR.

### Piggery Development Programmes

Piggery development programmes helped the weaker sections of rural community. India has a population of about one crore pigs which is less than 1% of the world population. China is the highest pig producer in the world. Before the introduction of Five-Year Plan, except for some sporadic import of a few superior quality pigs of exotic breeds by a few missionary organisations, no organised measures were taken to improve pig production in the country. But it is the most important activity and animal husbandry sector in the north-eastern region inhabited by tribal people. This region also has a substantial pig population, which constitutes around 25% of the country's pig population. The major difficulty in pig development is the acute shortage of breeding males.

### Five-Year Plan and Piggery Development

In the First Five-Year Plan, no attention was given to pig development. During the Second Five-Year Plan, a Co-ordinated Pig Development Programme was launched in 1959-60. Under this programme, schemes were drawn up for establishment of bacon factories, regional pig breeding stations, pig breeding farms/units and piggery development blocks. The selected blocks for implementation of piggery development were called 'piggery blocks'. Each piggery block was linked to a district livestock farm for supplying the foundation stock to the identified pig growers. The beneficiaries were selected from below poverty line groups of Scheduled Castes and Scheduled Tribes. They were given 50% subsidy, free health coverage and 3-4 days' peripatetic training.

These schemes were further extended during the subsequent Plan periods. The Piggery Development Scheme was strengthened by a special development programme taken up at the end of the Third Five-Year Plan. During this plan period 2 regional breeding-cum-Bacon factories, 12 Piggery Units and 140 Piggery Development Blocks were started. In preparing a model scheme for this programme, the central government rightly took the decision to attach the regional pig breeding stations to the bacon factories. The pig breeding station-cum-bacon factoreis are composite projects with a large pig breeding station and a bacon factory. These composit projects are being implemented in Andhra Pradesh, Bihar, Kerala, Maharashtra, Rajasthan, Chhatisgarh and West Bengal. Veterinary colleges and agricultural universities had started research farms and those farms were utilised for giving training to the pig farmers. The regional pig breeding stations supply pure breeding stocks of exotic pigs to the farmers for further multiplication and surplus stock for slaughter in bacon factories and local sales.

During the Fourth Plan period 4 piggery processing plants were established. In the Fifth Plan period, 23 pig breeding farms were established with the assistance provided by the North-Eastern Council. A pig breeding station for maintaining a genetic pool of high quality imported stock has also emerged. Special efforts are being made to take up piggery programmes in the North-Eastern states. Financial assistance and subsidy were given to the rural poors for establishing piggery units under several development programmes like IRDP, ITDP, HADP, SLBP and DPAP. The programme of providing exotic males for improvement of pigs in the North-Eastern region was extended during the ninth and tenth plan periods. The general approach followed in piggery development work is to use the improved breeds of pigs like Yorkshire and Landrace for grading up the indigenous population. Twelfth Plan NLM has a focus on development of non-descript pig populations, concentrated in NE region and Eastern region.

### Constraints

1. Absence of animal health cover and scientific know-how.
2. Lack of supply of balanced pig feed at economical price.
3. Wrong selection of beneficiaries and location.
4. Lack of proper system of purchase of pigs.
5. Lack of credit facilities and market outlets.
6. Absence of training programme.
7. Lack of remunerative market.
8. Religious taboos and social bias.

### Suggestions

1. Educating the people about the objectives of piggery development programmes.
2. Providing training, all the inputs and market facilities.

### Poultry Development Programmes

Poultry keeping is one of the best tools available for an integrated rural development and to bring about socio-economic transformation of small entrepreneurs. It provides round the year employment and income. It closes the mimal protein gap because the natural resources for raising cattle, sheep and goat are shrinking, hence poultry is the best alternative. No other branch of agriculture/animal husbandry has made such a big impact on their development, as the poultry husbandry. Now from a subsidiary enterprise, poultry farming has turned to be a main occupation. " The author observed that farmers engaged in poultry farming out of their total annual income more than 80% comes from poultry. Even those farmers having agriculture as a main occupation, the income from subsidiary enterprise poultry was more than 50%".

### Past efforts

Commercial poultry development in India started only in 1970s, although poultry raising in India dates back to pre-historic times. The first major step towards poultry development in modern India was taken during 1939 with the establishment of poultry research division at the Indian Veterinary Research Institute, Izatnagar in Uttar Pradesh, which developed an effective vaccine against the Ranikhet disease. Intensive poultry development made its beginning in the early sixties after the government poultry farms, particularly in Odisha, demonstrated the efficacy of modern poultry rearing. It gained wide popularity with extension activities of the then newly set up veterinary colleges under agricultural universities, state animal husbandry departments and the American Peace Corps volunteers who also helped to popularise modern poultry production in Indian villages.

### Five-Year Plan and Poultry Development

Even in the First Five-Year Plan recognition was given to poultry as a vital tool for the socioeconomic uplift of the large majority in rural areas. A pilot project approved in early 1956 had the provision to establish 56 extension centres. The scheme was assisted under the Indo-US Technical Co-operation Programme. In the Second Plan, five regional farms, equipped with superior stock, were started along with 269 poultry extension centres. Training programmes were conducted for private poultry breeders in modern methods of poultry rearing.

During the Third Plan, poultry farms emerged as vital commercial enterprise. ₹ 45 million was allotted. Development of deep litter system, multiplication of exotic breeds and organisation of inter-state poultry development projects, occurred during this period. Expansion of 60 state poultry farms, 3 regional farms and 50 extension-cum-development centres and commercial hatcheries were set up in different states. In the Fourth Plan, ₹ 110 million was alloted and much emphasis was placed on breeding better stocks and popularising the latest scientific practices in new area. The Central Government implemented a support programme with tax concessions income from poultry, special credit lines and insurance of poultry against losses through epidemic diseases. Egg and poultry production-cum-marketing centres were established. Old farms were expanded and new farms started. For supplying of high quality chicks, the government intended to encourage the establishment of a national breeding programme by a scheduled prohibition of imports of hybrid chicks first and of parent stocks and grandparents at a later stage.

During the Fifth Plan, with a tune of ₹ 355 million attempts were made to improve the quality of inputs needed for poultry farming and to establish proper marketing facilities. During this plan period, 3 central regional poultry breeding farms, 3 random sample laying test units, 61 intensive poultry producing-cum-marketing centres were established. In the Sixth and Seventh Plan periods, all aspects of poultry industry had developed. It can aptly be called the 'Decade of poultry'. Broiler farming emerged as a new wing and it now occupies the pride of place. National Egg Co-ordination Committee (NECC) was established. The

Seventh Plan (₹ 602 million) envisaged improvement in infrastructures available for taking up scientific breeding in egg and broiler strains and also the proposed development on new lines of broilers. National Agricultural Federation for Export Development (NAFED) assisted in the marketing of poultry products.

In the Eighth Plan attempts were made for establishment of poultry co-operatives on the pattern of Anand co-operative processing marketing and storage infrastructural facilities were strengthened. State level poultry training centres were started. A task force was set up to work out details of establishment and operation of National Poultry Development Board. Eleventh Plan initiative is a separate poultry capital venture fund to promote establishment of poultry estates, retail poultry outlets, and other poultry activities. Twelfth Plan of the NLM has an additional mini mission relating to development of poultry.

### Poultry

In the Ninth Five-Year Plan it was estimated that the egg production in the country was about 33.6 billion numbers (2001–02) against the Ninth Plan target of 39 billion. The most notable growth among the livestock products has been recorded in eggs and poultry meat. Since 1970–71, their output has grown at 0.87% per annum.

In the Tenth Five-Year Plan, to give a boost to export of Poultry Products, measures will be undertaken for the development of infrastructure like cold storage, pressured air cargo capacity and reference laboratory for certification of health and products. Programmes will be formulated to improve indigenous birds and promotion of backyard poultry farming.

### Other efforts

Some efforts were made to make the unorganised sector more attractive through a number of central and state sector schemes, notable among them being Intensive Poultry Development Project (IPDP). Mass Poultry Production Programme involving small/marginal farmers and agricultural labourers. These emanated from the recommendation of National Commission on Agriculture (NCA) as a result of which 60 districts were identified in 1975 for introducing poultry production as a component of special scheme called SLBP. Poultry development was also given due to consideration under the area development programme like Drought-Prone Area Programme (DPAP), Desert Development Programme (DDP), IRDP, ITDP, etc.

Various poultry development institutions like Central Poultry Breeding Farm, Central Poultry Training Institute, Central Duck Breeding Farm, Random Sample Poultry Performance Testing Centre (RSPPTC), regional feed analytical laboratories, etc. were established in various parts of India. The Government of India had increased the total outlay for the development of poultry from Rs 28 million during the Second Plan to Rs 602 million during the Seventh Plan period. The Eighth Five-Year Plan poultry development strategy includes provision of quality chicks, establishment of poultry co-operatives, processing, marketing, storage infrastructural facilities, state level poultry training centres and National Poultry Development Board.

In general, the poultry industry in India has proved to be sustainable during the last 3–4 decades. This was mainly due to a long-term strategy with clear objectives by the Government and the private sector, government support through incentives, adequate institutional framework and finally the flexible regulations for the import of essential inputs. All the inputs like chicks, feeds, vaccines, etc. were produced and supplied by the private entrepreneurs.

At present the poultry industry is well developed in the states of Andhra Pradesh, Tamil Nadu, Punjab and Karnataka. There is development to some extent in Maharashtra and Gujarat. This is due to the integrating efforts of hatcheries, and leading feeds manufacture.

## Constraints

The major constraints limiting growth of poultry development in India are:

1. Regional imbalances due to lack of entrepreneurship.

2. High concentration of poultry in certain pockets with inadequate biosecurity measures.

3. Inadequate infrastructural facilities such as disease diagnostic laboratories, specialised training centres, trained technical manpower and quality control measures for rural poultry development.

4. Lack of availability of reliable data on poultry production and market intelligence for proper planning.

5. High investment cost with decreasing profit margin.

6. High cost of insurance and inordinate delay in settling the claims.

7. Unorganised market network and lack of efforts to develop rural markets.

8. Lack of incentives and processing facilities for developing export markets.

9. Lack of corporate participation in developing the integrated poultry production and processing units.

10. Limited research and development efforts for cost effective poultry production.

11. Lack of public incineration facilities, declining financial support from government institutions, price fluctuation, lack of remunerative price, etc.

12. The status of poultry sector as to whether it falls under agriculture or industry is somewhat ambiguous and, therefore, it has deprived the sector of various benefits available to it.

## Suggestions

The following suggestions are given to overcome the constraints:

1. Planned reduction in regional imbalances.

2. Government intervention, by way of various support mechanisms, is now needed for the promotion of poultry in rural areas. Developing regional centres to provide diagnostic and feed testing facilities, manpower training, promoting the consumption of poultry products and quality consciousness.

3. Enhancement of support for research and development of cost effective housing and poultry feeds.

4. Building up of a sound database on poultry population, production and marketing intelligence and improving the monitoring and supervision system in financial institutions.

5. Encouragement for establishing integrated poultry complexes having facilities for rearing, feed production, health and marketing.

6. Developing effective biosafety measures, adequate processing storage and marketing facilities. Industry-friendly insurance cover, awareness on exports and price support mechanism.

7. Poultry farming should be declared as an agricultural activity.

8. Indigenous poultry breeds, including the improved strains that can survive with low quality raw feed and have better resistance against diseases, can be reared under free range conditions by rural unemployed youth and women for some additional income and employment.

## Rabbit Development Programmes

In India, the rabbit production is only in its infancy. Only here and there in a few states the rabbit farming has been taken up with government assistance through rural development programmes. It is estimated that the rabbit fur skins constitute more than 50% of fur trade in international market. India imports about half a million rabbit fur skins annually from France and other countries to meet the demand of fur industry in Jammu and Kashmir. The rabbit fur skins obtained as byproduct from the rabbit enterprise for meat production can serve as import substitute. This can also be adopted as a cottage industry in the area to generate employment income for rural masses.

Rabbit production is a boon for the hilly regions of our country. The task force on sheep, goats and rabbit production has recommended that Angora rabbit rearing should be encouraged in temperate regions all over the country. Maintenance of breeding lines on scientific grounds for generating highly adaptable and high wool producing breeding stocks at a central location, strengthening of extension programme to demonstrate and work hand in hand with the private breeders in implementing the managemental norms for improvement in rabbit production are to be initiated.

## Animal Health

Since the Second Five-Year Plan, efforts have been made to control diseases, namely Rinderpest, Foot and Mouth disease, Hemorrhagic Septicemia, Black Quarter and Anthrax. Although Rinderpest has been eradicated from the country, the prevalence of the other diseases continues to be one of the major problems in the animal production programme. Some of the emerging diseases like PPR, Blue Tongue, Sheep Pox and Goat Pox, Classical Swine Fever, Contagious Bovine Pleuropneumonia, Newcastle disease and Gumboro are causing substantial economic losses. The programme for creation of disease-free zone was sanctioned in the Ninth Plan but was not implemented. The Department of Animal Husbandry and Dairying is also not well equipped with the necessary infrastructure and qualified technical manpower to execute the programmes and perform its mandatory duties and responsibilities like disease diagnosis and accreditation as per the international standards, development of an effective surveillance and monitoring system for disease, mass immunisation against the most prevalent diseases, etc.

Dovetailing the animal research institutes of the ICAR with the department would not only improve its efficiency but also provide it with an effective delivery machinery to cary out its regulatory and certification authority functions, including the conservation of endangered breeds of livestock. The suggestion for establishment of an Indian Council for Veterinary and Fisheries Research (ICVFR) by carving out the animal science and fishery institutes from ICAR has not yet materialised.

## Fodder Development Programmes

It is an obvious fact that the health and productivity of livestock and forage production are directly and closely related. The grazing lands are shrinking because of competing demands for food and forage under the increasing population pressure. In our country the available grazing lands are over grazed, denuded and deteriorated. There is a little forage conservation to sustain the livestock in periods and years of lean supplies. For the most part of the year, farm animals are forced to subsist on crop residues and byproducts such as straw, dry stalks, stubbles and sparse vegetation from wastelands. Consequently livestock productivity is low. The shortfall of green fodder is estimated as 75% and that of dry fodder about 49%. To overcome the shortfall an integrated approach in fodder development work was envisaged and various schemes are being implemented.

The various animal husbandry programmes in independent India have brought about tremendous change in animal husbandry leading to manifold increase in meat, milk, egg and fish production, directly benefiting the rural masses particularly the down-trodden. Improvement in production due to livestock development programmes has led to better education, health, housing and clothing. Coupled with this, the working of the democratic system has led to the physical emancipation of vast numbers of rural masses. But the impact is not up to the mark. Any number of development programmes would be of no worth unless people (clientele system) are motivated to adopt scientific animal husbandry practices. Here comes the role of extension education, which has to educate the farmer so as to bring about desirable behavioural changes in them. Thus, extension is considered as an important tool and prerequisite for successful implementation of a scheme. Further, by removing the existing constraints in implementing animal husbandry programmes and rooting out pilferage at the middle level and better financial allocation is bound, in course of time, to lead to near revolution in production, lifestyle and social emancipation of the rural masses.

## CONSERVATION AND IMPROVEMENT OF NATIVE ANIMAL GENETIC RESOURCES (2002)

Initiatives were taken to maintain diversity of breeds and preserve those showing decline in numbers or facing extinction. The improvement programme of indigenous breeds possessing desirable characteristics like disease resistance, heat tolerance, efficient utilisation of low quality feed, etc. were taken up. This is essential even for a sustainable crossbreeding programme. Steps were taken to coordinate all the activities related to the efficient utilisation of draught animal power and animal by-products. Similarly, efforts will be made to conserve indigenous birds. States where a breed exists should take necessary steps with the active involvement of institutions, Gaushalas, Non-governmental Organisations (NGOs) and Breed Societies. The efforts should, however, be effectively coordinated centrally.

### National Agriculture Development Programme

National Agriculture Development Programme (NADP) is also called Rashtriya Krishi Vikas Yojana (RKVY) is a special Additional Central Assistance Scheme which was launched in August 2007 to orient agricultural development strategies, to reaffirm its commitment to achieve 4% annual growth in the agricultural sector during the 11th plan. The scheme was launched to incentivize the states to provide additional resources in their State Plans over and above their baseline expenditure to bridge critical gaps.

NADP is a State Plan Scheme. How much assistance would be provided to a state from centre would depend upon the amount provided in State Plan Budgets for Agriculture and allied sectors, above a baseline expenditure on these sectors. The NADP funds are provided to the states as 100% grant by the Central Government.

The states are mandatorily required to prepare the District and State Agriculture Plans that comprehensively cover resources and indicate definite action plans. The more the states encourage the agriculture and allied fields, the more incentive they get from central government. However, high level of flexibility has been provided to the states including at the level of the State Government.

The nodal department for the scheme in the states is the State Agriculture Department. The department is required to take appropriate steps for identification of the projects that are important for agriculture, animal husbandry and allied sector development. If the government of the state is in hurry, it can also constitute an agency by notification for implementation of the NADP. This agency or the state department of agriculture will ensure the preparation of the DAPs (District Action Plans) and preparing the SAP (State Action Plan). A DAP for each district should be formulated as per the Planning Commission guidelines. The DAP should include clear roadmap of the sectors. Then, the comprehensive SAP should evolve out of the DAPs. Finalized SAP should be placed by the State Planning Department before the Department of Agriculture/Planning Commission, as a part of the State Plan Exercise. The determination of eligibility is done by Planning Commission. How much money should be allocated is also determined by the Planning Commission. Once the state becomes eligible, the Distribution of Funds is done by the Department of Agriculture (DAC), under the Ministry of Agriculture. The money is released to the state governments. For further flow of the money, the State Government is required to create a State Level Sanctioning Committee (SLSC) constituted under the Chairmanship of the Chief Secretary of the concerned State Government/UT. This SLSC approve the projects under NADP to the agency. Here we should note that the money that is released is in two streams. Up to 75% of the money is released under stream 1 only by the SLSC whereby the money is used for project based funding with definite timelines. For expenditure of this money, states will have to prepare DPRs for undertaking projects that are consistent with the SAPs and DAPs. Rest maximum 25% of the funds can be spend for strengthening the existing schemes. However, there are options that all money is used as per stream 1.

SLSC is chaired by the Chief Secretary of the state and its vice chairman is Principal Secretary of agriculture in state departments. It has representations from the DAC, DAHD, and Planning Commission. The quorum for its meeting is incomplete without at least one GoI representative. It must meet in a quarter for at least once.

The total outlay of this scheme was kept ₹ 25,000 crore for the 11th plan period in the form of Additional Central Assistance (ACA). Thus, it became the biggest scheme in the agriculture sector. Despite the fact that India has not been able to achieve the targeted growth in farm sector, the scheme has been continued with increased outlays and increase number of sub schemes every year. Areas of focus of these schemes have been seeds, fertilizers, IPM testing laboratories, horticulture, farm mechanization, extension, crops, marketing and cooperatives, animal husbandry, etc.

## NATIONAL LIVESTOCK MISSION (NLM)

This scheme was implemented since 2014–15. With the aim to ensure quantitative and qualitative improvement in livestock production system and capacity building of stakeholders. The multiplicity of small schemes in these livestock sectors has been a major constraint since this limits the capability of states to effectively access funding under various schemes. In order to provide greater flexibility to states in formulating and implementing various projects, it is proposed to merge these schemes with the main objective of achieving sustainable development and growth of the livestock sector. The NLM will have an important mini-mission of feed and fodder and development of small ruminants, but also covering poultry, piggery and other minor livestock species. Other issues that NLM will address include livestock insurance and extension and any innovative initiative proposed by states for development of the livestock sector, for example, to deal with unhygienic slaughtering and processing and also to provide minor veterinary services and supplement the livestock-extension activity in the states.

## NITI AAYOG

The National Institution for Transforming India, also called NITI Aayog, was formed via a resolution of the Union Cabinet on January 1, 2015. NITI Aayog is the premier policy 'Think Tank' of the Government of India, providing both directional and policy inputs. While designing strategic and long-term policies and programmes for the Government of India, NITI Aayog also provides relevant technical advice to the centre and states.

The Government of India, in keeping with its reform agenda, constituted the NITI Aayog to replace the Planning Commission instituted in 1950. This was done in order to better serve the needs and aspirations of the people of India. An important evolutionary change from the past, NITI Aayog acts as the quintessential platform of the Government of India to bring states to act together in national interest, and thereby fosters Cooperative Federalism.

At the core of NITI Aayog's creation is two hubs: **Team India Hub** and the **Knowledge and Innovation Hub**. The Team India Hub leads the engagement of states with the Central Government, while the Knowledge and Innovation Hub builds NITI's think-tank capabilities. These hubs reflect the two key tasks of the Aayog.

## ANIMAL HUSBANDRY PROGRAMMES LED BY NGOs IN INDIA

Rural development is a multi-disciplinary concept which needs coordination between government institutions, departments, research stations, univer-sities, extension officers and Non-governmental Organisations. Non-governmental Organisations popularly called NGOs, play a significant role in rural development. This lesson focuses on NGOs which are pioneered in Animal Husbandry Programmes.

### Bharatiya Agro Industries Foundation (BAIF)

BAIF development research foundation (formerly registered as the Bharatiya Agro Industries Foundation) is a reputed voluntary organisation, established in 1967 by Dr Manibhai Desai, a disciple of Mahatama Gandhi at Urulikanchan, near Pune to promote sustainable livelihood in rural India. BAIF Dairy Development programme has been providing doorstep breeding services over 5 million families spread over nearly 80,000 villages in 12 states. BAIF central cattle breeding farm maintain animal of exotic females, bulls and bull calves of various breeds of cattle and buffalo.

As a part of dairy development, BAIF maintains molecular genetics and reproduction biotechnology, Krishna valley breed *ex situ* conversation project, animal nutrition laboratory and production unit, All India coordinated research project on improvement of feed resources and utilization, Forage Crop Seed Production Programme (http://www.baif.org.in).

### JK Trust Gram Vikas Yojana (JKTGVY)

Raymond was the first organisation in India to introduce embryo transfer in sheep (1977). A well equipped Raymond Embryo Research Centre (RERC) for cattle was set up during 1983 at Gopal Nagar near Bilaspur. JKTGVY was launched in 1997 to facilitate the transfer of technical expertise gained over 3 decades to the farmers more effectively.

The mission of JKTGVY is to significantly improve the quality of life in India's rural areas through Cattle Breed Improvement Programme (CBIP). The Cattle Breed Improvement Programme is structured under the concept of "Integrated Livestock Development (ILD) Centre".

The programme operator "Gopal" who monitors each centre, is an unemployed youth extensively trained for 6 months to carry out AI in cattle and buffaloes by qualified veterinarians at Raymond Embryo Research Centre in Gopal Nagar. The Gopal is provided with a motorcycle to perform AI and provide other veterinary services at the doorstep of the farmers. Duties of these programme operators are supervised and monitored by veterinarians. One veterinarian monitors the work of 10 ILD centres (http://www.jktrust.org).

### MYRADA

Mysore resettlement and development agency (MYRADA) was founded in 1968 to assist the government in resettling Tibetan refugees. From 1987 the mission of MYRADA focused on the poor and marginalized in rural areas. Animal health promoter training was imparted by MYRADA along with its KVK since 2002. Under this training, animal health services which include livestock upgradation, forecasting and prevention of seasonal disease, first aid, vaccination, pregnancy test, etc. were imparted to unemployed youth. The six months training is a collaborative effort of KVK, Erode District Co-operative Milk Producers Union Ltd., government veterinary hospital, milk producers co-operative societies, self-employment training institutes located in this area (http://myrada.org/myrada).

### Scan Foundation

It is a non-profit organisation dedicated to freeing the homeless animals, and bringing our 'best friend' into the home and family. Protecting animals through advocacy and education, from neglect, abuse and exploitation is the primary objective of this trust.

The goals of voice for animals is comprise the following six principles: Advocate and become a voice for animals living homeless; educate society to evolve a higher ethical and moral standard for the treatment of animlas living under these conditions; to improve the quality of life for these animals; provide low-cost or no-cost house training for dogs and cats whose caretakers wish to bring them into the home, temporarily foster and find new homes for dogs and cats whose caretakers wish them to have a better life but are unwilling or unable to provide that for them ( http://www.voiceforanimals.info).

### ANIMAL WELFARE BOARD OF INDIA[1]

For the promotion of animal welfare generally and for the purpose of protecting animals from being subjected to unnecessary pain or suffering, in particular, Animal Welfare Board of India was established by the central government.

1 http://awbi.org/awbi-pdf/draftawact2011.pdf

The Board, shall be a body corporate having perpetual succession and a common seal with power, subject to the provisions of Animal Welfare Act, 2011 to acquire, hold and dispose of property and may by its name sue and be sued.

### Constitution of the Board

1. The Board shall consist of the following persons, namely:
   a. The Inspector General of Forests, Government of India, ex-officio.
   b. The Animal Husbandry Commissioner to the Government of India, ex-officio.
   • Two persons to represent respectively the Ministries of the Central Government dealing with Home Affairs and Education, to be appointed by the Central Government.
   • One person to represent the Indian Board for Wild Life, to be appointed by the Central Government.
   • Three persons who, in the opinion of the Central Government, are or have been actively engaged in animal welfare work and are well-known humanitarians, to be nominated by the Central Government.
   c. One person to represent such association of veterinary practitioners as in the opinion of the Central Government ought to be represented on the Board, to be elected by that association in the prescribed manner.
   d. Two persons to represent practitioners of modern and indigenous systems of medicine, to be nominated by the Central Government.
   e. One person to represent each of such two municipal corporations as in the opinion of the Central Government ought to be represented on the Board, to be elected by each of the said corporations in the prescribed manner.
   f. One person to represent each of such three organisations actively interested in animal welfare as in the opinion of the Central Government ought to be represented on the Board, to be chosen by each of the said organisations in the prescribed manner.
   g. One person to represent each of such three societies dealing with prevention of cruelty to animal as in the opinion of the Central Government ought to be represented on the Board, to be chosen, in the prescribed manner.
   h. Three persons to be nominated by the Central Government.

i. Six Members of Parliament, four to be elected and two by the Council of States (Rajya Sabha).

2. The Central Government shall nominate one of the members of the Board to be its Chairman and another member of the Board to be its Vice-Chairman.

## Functions of the Board

The functions of the Board shall be:

a. To keep the law in force in India for the prevention of cruelty to animals under constant study and advise the government on the amendments to be undertaken in any such law from time to time.

b. To advise the Central Government on the making of rules under this Act with a view to preventing unnecessary pain or suffering to animals generally, and more particularly when they are being transported from one place to another or when they are used as performing animals or when they are kept in captivity or confinement.

c. To advise the government or any local authority or other person on improvements in the design of vehicles so as to lessen the burden on draught animals.

d. To take all such steps as the Board may think fit for 11(amelioration of animals) by encouraging or providing for, the construction of sheds, water-troughs and the like and by providing for veterinary assistance to animals.

e. To advise the government or any local authority or other person in the design of slaughterhouses or the maintenance of slaughterhouses or in connection with slaughter of animals so that unnecessary pain or suffering, whether physical or mental, is eliminated in the pre-slaughter stages as far as possible, and animals are killed; wherever necessary, in as humane a manner as possible.

f. To take all such steps as the Board may think fit to ensure that unwanted animals are destroyed by local authorities, whenever it is necessary to do so, either instantaneously or after being rendered insensible to pain or suffering.

g. To encourage by the grant of financial assistance or otherwise, 12 (the formation or establishment of pinjrapoles, rescue homes, animal shelters, sanctuaries and the like) where animals and birds may find a shelter when they have become old and useless or when they need protection.

h. To co-operate with, and co-ordinate the work of, associations or bodies established for the purpose of preventing unnecessary pain or suffering to animals or for the protection of animals and birds.

i. To give financial and other assistance to animal welfare organisations functioning in any local area or to encourage the formation of animal welfare organisations in any local area which shall work under the general supervision and guidance of the Board.

j. To advise the government on matters relating to the medical care and attention which may be provided in animal hospital, and to give financial and other assistance to animal hospitals whenever the Board thinks it necessary to do so.

k. To impart education in relation to the humane treatment of animals and to encourage the formation of public opinion against the infliction of unnecessary pain or suffering to animals and for the promotion of animal welfare by means of lectures, books, posters, cinematographic exhibitions and the like.

l. To advise the government on any matter connected with animal welfare or the prevention of infliction of unnecessary pain or suffering on animals.

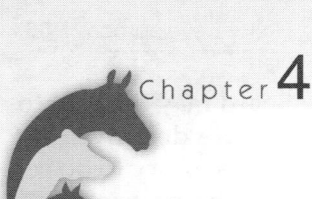

# Chapter 4

# Extension Education Systems

Effective animal husbandry/agricultural extension service supported by research relevant to farmers' needs is essential for sustained livestock production and income. For this, several extension systems were developed and implemented. Training and Visit, Broad-based Extension, Farming System Research and Extension, and Participatory Rural Approach and Extension are a few extension systems widely followed.

## TRAINING AND VISIT SYSTEM

Daniel Benor, a World Bank expert, developed the Training and Visit (T&V) system for extension services for a wide range of agricultural/animal husbandry and administrative environments in developing countries. The purpose of Training and Visit system of extension is to build a professional extension service that will be capable of assisting farmers to raise production and increase their incomes and of providing appropriate support for agricultural/animal husbandry development. A key means to this end is the creation of a dynamic link between farmers, professional extension workers and researchers.

## Important Features of Training and Visit
### Professionalism

Appropriate advice through an extension service by professionals at all levels would help farmers to increase their income. Extension staff must keep in close touch with relevant scientific developments and research in order to formulate specific recommendations. This can be achieved only if each extension worker is fully and continuously trained. The T and V system fulfils this requirement.

### Single Line of Command

The extension service must have single line of technical and administrative command, i.e. under the Department of Agriculture. Though, support is required from teaching and research institutions, input supply, other allied organisations and local government bodies but all the administrative and technical responsibilities vest in one department.

### Concentration of Effort

Only by concentrating on the tasks at hand the impact of extension becomes visible and progress can be sustained. Non-extension education activities like supply of inputs, data collection, etc. dilute the concentration of effort. The supporting activities should be the responsibility of other trained staff in these fields.

### Time-bound Work

Technical information and skills must be imparted to farmers in a regular, timely fashion, so that farmers make best use of the resources at their command. Subjects are for learned for two fortnights by the subject matter specialist (SMS) at monthly zonal workshops. These recommendations are then presented to Village Extension Workers (VEWs) at the two fortnightly training sessions.

### Field and Farmer Orientation

VEWs visit the farmers regularly on a fixed day once in a fortnight and transfer the techniques. This contact must be regular and on a schedule known to farmers. All other extension workers, including SMS, are to spend a large part of their time in farmers' field.

### Regular and Continuous Training

Regular and continuous training of extension staff is required both to teach the techniques and discuss it with them. The training sessions (fortnightly training and monthly workshops) are the key means of bringing actual farmers' problems to the attention of researchers.

### Linkages with Research

Effective extension depends on close linkages with research. Linkage is a two-way process. Problems faced by farmers that cannot be solved by extension workers are passed on to researchers for an immediate solution on investigation. The joint effort of research and extension staff helps to formulate production recommendation.

### Working Pattern

In India, the Training and Visit system was first introduced in 1974 in Rajasthan and Madhya Pradesh followed by 13 states. All the states extended this system in 1985.

## Organisational Pattern of Training and Visit

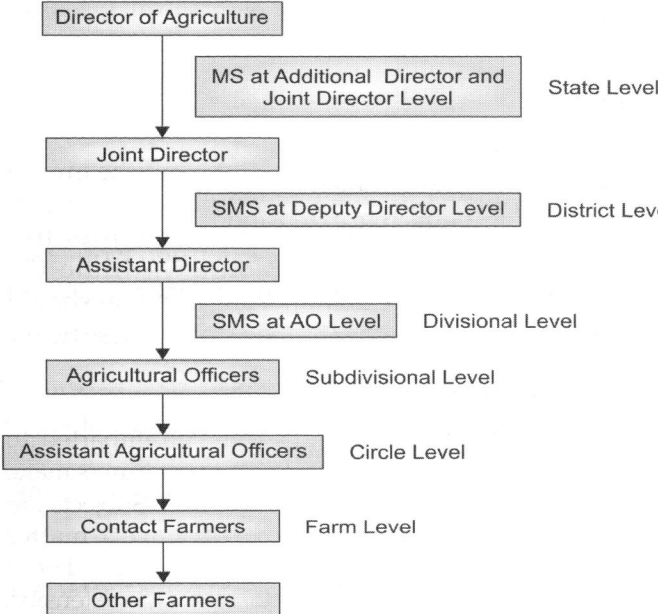

### Training Pattern

The monthly zonal workshop is the main venue of in-service training for SMS and of regular contact between extension and research workers. The chief means of continuously upgrading and updating the professional skills of VEWs and AOs is the fortnightly training session.

### Preseasonal Training

Before the commencement of Kharif and Rabi seasons, preseason training is conducted every year at the research stations and the latest techniques related to the season are passed onto the extension functionaries.

### Monthly Zonal Workshop (MZW)

The monthly zonal workshop is held at a convenient location for two days to build up the technical skills of SMS regularly in the field of their specialisation.

### Objectives of Workshop

1. To review the rate of adoption.
2. To note the difficulties faced by SMS.
3. To formulate and discuss recommended practices.
4. To review the climate, input and marketing situations.

5. To train SMS to carry out recommended practices themselves.
6. To discuss the progress and results of farm trials.

The Assistant Directors and SMS at the district and division level are the participants. The Joint Directors will be the co-ordinator and responsible for overall effective planning of the workshop. Scientists from SAUs and research stations will be the trainers.

### Fortnightly Training

All Village Extension Workers (VEWs) and Agricultural Officers participate in this one-day training every fortnight. This is the chief means of continuously upgrading the professional skills of extension workers and of infusing them with confidence to meet farmers.

### Objectives

1. To present specific recommended practices.
2. To act as a link between field level extension staff and research SMS.
3. Also to regulate the input supply.

## Visit Schedules

### Contact Farmers

Frequent contact between VEW and all farmers in his area is not possible. Therefore visit of VEW focuses on a small, selected number of farmers called 'contact farmers'. The contact farmers normally constitute about 10% of the farming community. The farmers selected are based on the following criteria:

1. They must be the representative sample of their farming community.
2. They should be practising farmers and willing to adopt the recommendations and allow other farmers to observe the practices.
3. They must come from different families and their farms should be dispersed.

### Purpose of Visit

1. To advise/teach and motivate the farmers to adopt improved technologies.
2. To enable extension staff and researchers to be closely and continuously acquainted with farm conditions and problems, so that research is need based.

### Formation of Circle

The first step to organise the visit schedule of VEW is to define the circle of his operation. It should be compact, continuous and manageable by VEW. The number of farm families per VEW may range from 300 to 1500. In hilly tracts 400 is desirable.

### Scheduling Visits

Once VEW circles are established and contact farmers identified the visit can be scheduled easily. His circle is divided into eight groups. The VEW visits each group once in a fortnight. All the farmers in the circle must be fully aware of the day, time, place and purpose of the VEW's visit. Alternative Fridays or fixed days are used by the VEW for depot review and to report to SMS or AO.

### Conduct of Visits

The VEW should visit the farmers when they are in fields during forenoon and in the afternoon make himself available in a common place in the village so that farmers who wish to discuss anything with him may do so.

### Limitations of Training and Visit System

1. The approach is too intensive and may lack sufficient staff.
2. The emphasis is only on the development of agriculture, thus neglecting other aspects of family and rural development.
3. The approach is mainly confined to farmers, the youth and farm women are almost neglected.
4. There is a problem of co-ordination with the research institution and supply agencies.

## BROAD-BASED EXTENSION SYSTEM

In order to further strengthen the technology transfer efforts of the state Agricultural Departments with the active involvement of other departments, the country proposed the Broad-based Extension System (BBES) in the place of T and V system in the year 1991. The concept of broad-based extension education lies in formulating and delivering composite messages to the farmers to meet the needs of their full agricultural environment. This system is an improved one over Training and Visit system. The role of subject matter specialists is amplified in this system as they are instructed to generate/formulate messages suitable to their area of the specialisation and season based activities. The village extension workers have full time job by transferring the technologies.

### Principles

1. Adoption of an integrated farming system approach.

2. Broadening the range of subjects from agriculture to all allied subjects.
3. Improved communication for effective transfer of information to farming community.
4. Introduction of resource based grassroot level planning.
5. Encouraging participation of NGOs in all extension activities.

### Objectives

1. To increase the farm income.
2. To solve farmers' problems.
3. To make cost effective extension.
4. To upgrade the quality of the extension workers.
5. To popularize integrated farming system approach.

### Scope

The activities of all land-based departments are unified in the long run. Duplication of efforts and unhealthy competition is avoided. Officials extend their full support to the activities of all the allied departments.

### Methodology

Broad-based Extension System (BBES) helps the farmers in getting multiple messages needed to improve their overall economy besides helping to grow agricultural crops. Thus, the farmers are encouraged in animal husbandry, fodder development, fish farming, sericulture, etc. These activities enable the farming community to get extra income.

### Need

This system was formed to encourage the activities of the farmers. Different departments compete with one another and they have proposed to increase the staff component to contact as many farmers as possible. The World Bank and Government of India thought to utilise the well-established extension agencies and bring all extension and land-based activities together.

### Role of SMS

Subject matter specialists have to expand their horizon. For instance, SMS of agronomy has to expand his activities to areas like fodder cultivation, sericulture, horticulture, etc. In areas where SMS is not available, trainers from that particular department will act as SMS in that particular subject.

### Organisational Set-up

The extension system created under Training and Visit system is maintained with VEW, AO, Taluk level SMS,

District level SMS operating in it. There are only marginal changes in the strength of field functionaries. The ratio of one VEW to farm families brought down and thus there is marginal increase of VEW.

## Operational Guidelines

The monthly zonal workshop, fortnightly training and fixed programme of field visits is continued without any change. In the monthly zonal workshop the SMS helps in fourmulating messages which are location specific.

## Implementation

In India, Tamil Nadu is the pioneer state which implemented this system from 1993. An agreement has been signed with World Bank for executing a seven-year contract. The Government of India and the State Government have organised regional level workshops to discuss and finalize training programme. Ultimately the VEW were trained fully in all aspects Broad-based Extension System.

## Training Programme

Comprehensive training programme is envisaged in this system. All land-based departments will identify five state level and district level trainers who are SMS. They are responsible for conducting classes fully or partly. The district level trainers attend the monthly zonal workshop. They help to solve the field problems faced by the extension agents. Trainers from animal husbandry and other sister departments may be made to participate in this programme.

## Role of Nodal Department

Broad-based extension involves the co-ordination of allied department with the Agricultural department. Agriculture department serves as a nodal department and initiates activities.

The Broad-based Extension System will help the farmer to obtain composite messages suitable to his agriculture as well as to his allied activities. The extension system will work in close co-ordination with sister and allied departments. The farmer is expected to derive maximum benefit from this system. However, due to lack of adequate linkage, co-ordination is not achieved at all levels.

## ▌FARMER PARTICIPATORY SYSTEM

The generation and transfer of technology in animal husbandry/agriculture was mainly based on the premise that the technology has been developed exclusively by the scientists. It is to be transferred by the extension agency and the farmers would be the recipients of the technology. Thus, the three sub-systems, viz. Research, Extension and Clientele were considered as separate sub-systems. However, the experience of last several years has shown that this cannot be the strategy in future and all these three sub-systems have to be conceived as integrated holistic sub-systems, each having a role to play at every stage.

The inter-dependents and intra-dependents and harmonious synchronization of efforts at different salient stages of technology generation, technology transfer and technology use have to be the main planks of animal husbandry/agricultural development exercise. Technology generation through research the world over, has been the monopolistic domain of agriculture/animal husbandry research stations/universities. The technology so generated is passed on to the users for adoption. However, there has been a growing realization that in this process farmers for whom the technology is generated, remain passive and are, by and large, at the receiving end. They have hardly any say in the type of technology that is needed to be generated and the improvement that is to be brought about in the entire technology domain for their better acceptability by the low economic group farmers in order to cross the barriers to higher productivity.

This way, farmers hardly feel involved in the technology generation process and no wonder that the final outcome in the shape of technology which is passed on to farmers quite often has no relevance to the specific location/area. Blanket recommendations of technology even for different zones have sometimes proved to be irrelevant to the problems the farmers of that area are faced with. This is why a strong need is being felt that instead of concentrating and confining all the research activities at the Research Stations, some of the researches of purely applied nature and of direct utilitarian value should be conducted at the farmers' fields with the active involvement of farmers and for their benefit. This type of research and extension is called Farmer Participatory System. There are three types of participatory system.

1. Farming System Approach.
2. Participatory Rural Appraisal.
3. Decentralised and Participatory Extension System.

## Farming System Approach (FSR)

Farmers throughout history have been engaged in what we regard as FSR. It describes the process farm families and farming communities go through to meet multiple objectives, despite being constrained by limited resources in an uncertain environment, through the application of inputs and technologies (Norman, despite being (FSR) 1982). Until very recently, agricultural innovations, technology generation, and adaptation and adoption of new practices were carried out almost entirely by farmers themselves. The phenomenon of organised agricultural research is a fairly recent historical event.

The gradual development of scientific animal husbandry/agriculture, first in universities and then by scientifically trained farmers and later by research stations, gradually shifted the process of generation of technology away from farms and onto research stations, universities and laboratories.

### Evolution of FSR

Several converging forces in the 1960s and 1970s led to a resurgence of interest in research client linkages and the fact that green revolution technologies were not emerging for other crops and in less-favoured areas. Many innovations being proposed were not being adopted by farmers (Simmonds, 1986) and the main reason for non-adoption was that innovations proposed were generally not suitable for the socioeconomic situation of the farmers it was felt that research should be determined by explicitly identified farmers' needs springing from an understanding of farming systems rather than by the pre-conceptions of researchers.

### Farmers' participation in research

The FSR/E terminology revolves around the principle of 'farmers' participation' in which farmer comes first and not towards the end. The Farmer Participatory Approach as the name suggests, ensures that the farmers are actively associated at different stages like selection of the field for research, selection of the need-based problems, prioritisation of the problems by the farmers themselves, taking stock of the past and the present and the future needs, developing alternate plan and choosing the enterprises related to animal husbandry/agriculture and allied sectors and then farmers continuing to remain active partner in the entire process of technology generation and its final release.

All the experimental/research activities are performed by the farmers in presence of scientists working with them. Thus FSR/E is by the farmers, for the farmers and of the farmers and in farmers' situation—farmers everywhere from beginning to the end and the process goes on.

Since the farmers are involved, there is a check on the research not becoming futile and a waste, and an assurance of the relevance of technology from the very beginning. Thus, the farmers feel morally obliged to adopt such technology in their farming system more so because they had a say in the development of the technology. Such technologies are also location-specific, need-based, problem solving and have a little chance of failure and rejection. The farmers who have once adopted such technology do not revert to their earlier practices.

This turned the traditional 'top-down' or 'research push' approach upside down to a 'bottom up', 'down stream' or 'farmer-pull' approach with an having farmers' needs and knowledge as inputs for setting the research agenda. This led to formulation of the FSR approach to agricultural research, extension and development. Much of the early work in developing the philosophy, terminology, procedures and methodologies was carried out by the International Centres of Agricultural Research under the Consultative Group for International Agricultural Research (CGIAR).

During the 1990s a good beginning was made, in a few states of India by adopting the Ford Foundation-supported farming system research/extension methodology for technology generation and technology transfer.

### Types of FSR

There are six types of FSR approaches, distinguished mainly by the objectives underlying the research. There are as follows:

i. **FSR *sensu strico*:** It is the in-depth study of existing farming system as they exist.

ii. **On-farm research with farming system perspective (OFR/FSP):** It is a form of research done in fields with heads and flocks of farmers and their families acting as partners in research and extension (Collinson, 1987). It seeks to test socioeconomic suitability of research ideas a farm before recommending the technology for extension.

iii. **New farming systems' development (NFSD):** It is based on the assumption that many existing farming systems are unsustainable and radical changes may be necessary to correct the underlying problems. The objective is to evolve, test and introduce new farming systems and introduction of new animal species or new crops in the area. It may require government intervention.

iv. **Farming system research and extension (FSR/E):** It is a multi-disciplinary methodology for technology development, evaluation and delivery which merges researchs and extension efforts. It is often called by other names such as On-Farm Adaptive Research (OFAR) with a farming systems perspective.

v. **Farming system approach to infrastructure support and policy (FSIP):** It is more macro than FSR/E. Since it deals with policy, the variables treated by it are mainly outside the farm gate and involve more socioeconomic scientists than agro-biological scientists.

vi. **Farming systems research and development (FSR/D):** There are two basic and complementary components of FSR/D as recognised by Norman (1982) under different terminology, viz. FSIP and FSR/E. These two components together comprise the farming systems approach to research and development.

### FSR/E Approaches

1. **Farmer base approach:** Where practitioners pay close attention to farmers' conditions, and where they integrate farmers' ideas into the research and development process.

2. **Problem solving approach:** It seeks opportunities to develop and guide research and identify ways to make local services and national policies more attuned to the needs of small farmers.

3. **Comprehensive research and development approach:** Where all farm activities are included in the search for improvements in the farm families' output and welfare.

4. **Multidisciplinary approach:** Where researchers and extension staff work with farm families' which come from a different backgrounds.

5. **Interactive approach:** Where research results are used to better understand the system and to design improved research and implementation approaches for the future.

6. **Dynamic approach:** Where modest changes are first introduced to the farm families' routine and if these are successful and acceptable to the families, more significant changes are encouraged.

7. **Society-based approach:** Where the long-term interests of the general public are kept in mind in addition to the concerns of affected farmers.

### Stages of FSR/E

Researchers agree on four broad stages of FSR/E, viz. (i) Diagnostic stage, (ii) design stage, (iii) testing stage and (iv) dissemination stage. However, one more stage is also observed between third and fourth stages in some projects such as the Operational Research Project (ORP), that is 'Pilot Development Programme' which is found useful for livestock research and development.

1. **Objectives of FSR/E:** In order to remove various misconceptions about the concept and approach various inter-related objectives of FSR/E were delineated by Dillon et al (1978). There were slightly modified by Singh et al (1995) for the following objectives:

   - To understand the physical, biological and socioeconomic environment of the farming system within which agricultural production and household decisions are taken by farmers.

   - To gain an understanding about the farmers' skills, problems, constraints, goals and preferences.

   - To analyze the inter-relations among problems and causes and to identify and evaluate possible solutions for interventions in the existing farming systems for improving the focus of agricultural research.

   - To evaluate the existing farming systems along with practices and enterprises.

   - To provide direction to the agricultural research and extension organization to conduct and evaluate relevant on-station and on-farm research focusing on priority areas.

   - To assess technical feasibility and economic viability of new technologies and modifications to existing farming systems.

   - To monitor farmers' perceptions of new technology and their translation through rates of adoption.

   - To provide feedback to researchers, extensionists, planners, and policy makers to better focus research and development efforts.

### Farmers' Participation in Extension

As for technology transfer, farmers, who are active participants in the research process, assume the role of change agent and disseminate the technology in the neighbourhood at a faster speed such transfer of technology has a greater acceptance value because it comes from within the very social system. The followers do have a conviction that the technology that is being passed on to them by their fellow neighbours has a much greater relevance to their situations than the technologies coming from change agents. It is true that a local legitimization is very important for a technology to be accepted and acted upon.

## Advantages

Even if we accept the premise that the quality of research would suffer if research is conducted in farmers' fields, the benefit and the result that we get by conducting research in farmers' field is so much that the minus side becomes insignificant. After all, the ultimate objective of any research, more so in an applied science like animal husbandry, is the ultimate uplift of the socioeconomic status of farmers. This cannot be possible and realistic if something is thrust upon them from outside the social system on a long-term basis.

## Inter-disciplinary Group

FSR/E could be a good model of research and extension in the coming times. Inter-disciplinary groups of scientists identified as Nodal Scientists from different sister disciplines like animal breeding, livestock production, management, animal nutrition, parasitology, pathology and social sciences like extension education (poultry science, fisheries science, home science and other scientists can be included according to the location) forming a core group could work jointly together in an orchestrated synchrony with the farmers, mixing freely with them while identifying their problems, defining their objectives based on needs, planning the experiments and need-based research and so on and so forth.

## Participatory Rural Appraisal

Participatory Rural Appraisal is the talk of the day for development. Usual method of understanding the village and villagers by survey techniques is gradually being replaced by an alternative technique called Participatory Rural Appraisal (PRA). It makes one aware of the situation, usually a village, within a short time. One can learn everything about a village within a week's time, provided one has aptitude, knowledge and skill of using PRA techniques and utilises every minute of stay in the village for learning the purpose of crop or livestock production.

**Definition:** There are umpteen number of definitions. A comprehensive definition is what Dr V.E. Sabaratnam has given in his book entitled R/R/PRA (PLA) for Agriculture: Rapid, Relaxed and Participatory Rural Appraisal (Participatory Learning and Action) for Research and Extension in Agriculture (for Crops and Livestock) (2002) is worth remembering:

PRA is a flexible, low-cost and time saving set or family of approaches and methods used to enable the rural people to collect and analyse information in terms of the past, present and future situations to understand about the rural people and the conditions existing in rural areas which would provide a thorough and comprehensive idea regarding problems, potentials, resources and solutions to formulate realistic development programmes by the villagers themselves, but facilitated by PRA practitioner, feasible to achieve within a specific period of time by the villagers of a rural locality or the use of information and analysis by researchers to formulate need-based research programmes to solve problems of rural people. PRA (PLA) is useful provided one understands its principles and the PRA techniques. The validity and reliability of PRA has been proved beyond doubt empirically. PRA (PLA) has to be used by using a logical sequence of the various activities of PRA.

**Activities of PRA:** According to Dr Sabaratnam formulation of a cohesive team, preparation of the checklist for each technique, selection of the village/area, identification of key informants and rapport building are the activities which could be considered as forerunners for conducting PRA. The techniques of basic information, time line, seasonal analysis, climatic diagram, boundary transect, general transect, agro-ecological map, social map, resource map, time trend, daily routine diagram, mobility map, Venn diagram, technology maps (for crops and livestock) direct matrix ranking for technology decision behaviour of farmers, decision tree, consequence diagrams (for crops of animals), farm household map, bio-resource flow diagram, wealth ranking, livelihood analysis, livestock progeny history diagram (LPHD), ethnoveterinary flow diagram, browse ranking, success ranking, problem identification, problem tree ingenious technical knowledge map, technology assessment, measuring agricultural sustainability action plan preparation are to be carried out sincerely by devoted PRA practitioners and the key informants for effective implementation of the action plan. Evaluation of the PRA (PLA) is essential for betterment of PRA.

All the techniques of PRA are to be carried out if rural appraisal is to be realistic. Omission of any of the PRA techniques, a casual approach to PRA, lack of practicality of PRA, leaving out of any item on content of any PRA technique will reflect in the action plan preparation, which will jeopardise the whole process of PRA and its impact.

## Decentralised and Participatory Extension System (DPES)

Multi-disciplinary team of existing scientists working at Regional Research Stations/Sub-stations and Krishi

Vigyan Kendras could be utilised for FSR/E. They could be motivated to adopt FSR/E system and to give emphasis on "On-Farm Research' while forming the inter-disciplinary group, those who have aptitude for working with farmers alone should be included.

The decentralised and participatory extension apporoach is adopted in order to exploit the opinion leaders in the rural areas and form para extension services for effective extension work on agro-climatic zone basis. Maintaining functional and organisational linkages with sister departments will be very useful in transfer of technology (TOT) relating to whole farm approach if our efforts are concentrated on agro climatic zones. Zones are being earmarked under NARP for research purpose. The same zones can be considered for implementing this extension system. Districts having similar crops, livestock, nearness to the neighbouring zones are grouped into one for better TOT. This will facilitate perfect matching of research and extension components in dissemination of technologies (Chandrakandan and Palaniswamy, 1999).

### Salient Features of the DPES

1. Agro-climatic regional planning, monitoring and evaluation with effective supervision and span of control.

2. Farmer-led participatory method using model farms and model villages as powerful tools for transfer of technology.

3. Bottom-up approach and shift from higher productivity to profitability.

4. Better co-ordination of line departments by positioning subject matter specialists at regional/ district levels.

5. Better research—extension-client interface through periodical meetings and deliberations such as need-based seasonal zonal workshops and trainings and annual regional/district level seminars-cum-workshops.

6. Pre-season campaigns in village clusters well in advance of each season and group approach—weekly schedule of visits and purposeful follow-up visits by extension officers.

7. The Veterinary Assistant Surgeon and Extension Officer of animal husbandry to be available on afternoons of some fixed days in their respective office for farmers' office calls.

8. Joint diagnostic field visits by researchers, extension team as and when needed. Mid monthly meeting of research team with the joint directors and subject matter specialist's team at district levels.

9. Thrust on broad-based and profit-oriented farming with focus on actual farm operators who are involved in decision making including farm women and youths.

10. Better use of mass media in a co-ordinated manner.

11. Better co-ordination among production, processing, storage and marketing systems.

12. Advisory and financing through co-operative/ financing institutions by proper linkage and self-help group method.

13. Farm plan based micro level planning and livestock species/farming system based recommendations with flexibility for the local extension workers.

14. Motivating farmer groups to take up to modern farming/market linked approach.

15. Documenting resources and potentials of different sub zones through SWOT and yield gap analysis.

16. Scientific management of state Animal Husbandry/ Agriculture by adopting management principles with accountability at all levels in the hierarchy.

17. Promotion of agro and livestock industries through entrepreneurial development.

18. Promotion of concepts of opinion leaders who act as para extension staff in the villages.

19. All viable voluntary and Non-Governmental Organizations can be involved in this task in an effective way.

### Merits of this System

1. The decentralised and participatory extension system will pave the way for decentralised agro-climatic region-based planning besides ensuring the clients' participation and accountability of extension functionaries at all levels.

2. Further to compliment the efforts of extension officers under Broad-based Extension System, the concept of promotion of opinion leaders who act as para extension workers in the villages will be promoted so as to concentrate its issue on positioning of subject matter specialists on agro-climatic region basis besides formation of group of opinion leaders/conveners in the villages for effective technology transfer.

## TRANSFER OF TECHNOLOGY PROJECTS OF ICAR

ICAR's TOT projects are also referred to as front line extension projects, initiated to improve and act as a catalytic agent for the existing extension system. The major aim of the project is to demonstrate the highest production potential of improved technological advances by the scientists to actual users and to enable extension methodologies and suitable approaches. These include National Demonstration Scheme (NDS), Operational Research Projects (ORP), Lab to Land Programme (LLP), Krishi Vigyan Kendra (KVK), Pilot Project on Technology Assistance and refinement through Institution—Village Linkage Programme (VLP) and National Agricultural Technology Project (NATP).

The latter has been initiated with the aim of working out appropriateness of technology, keeping in view the management of micro-environment and production system, farmer's perspectives for utilisation of technology and developing methodology and capacity building for more effective extension approaches for natural resource management in micro-environments. The technological interventions and family modules are developed in participatory mode to provide food economic security to the household and to increase sustainability of technologies with farmers.

a. **National Demonstration Scheme (NDS):** This scheme was launched during the year 1965 with the objectives of introducing demonstration of the genetic production potential of the major food crops in the field conditions, and to develop the farmers into local leaders to serve as agents of change in their area. The NDS essentially provides an opportunity to the scientists to demonstrate the validity and relevance of their experimental findings at the farmers' fields. This scheme was taken up initially in 100 districts of the country mainly through the sate agricultural universities. In each project location, there are four scientists of different disciplines for conducting demonstrations, and offering specialised support from the scientists of the implementing institutions.

This project has provided the farmer an opportunity to assess for himself the suitability of a new agricultural technology to the growing conditions in his farm. The results have shown that blanket recommendations for the entire block or even village are not appropriate and also indicated the potential of for increasing yields of various crops by 2–3 times over the national average yields. The results also indicated that the gap between potential and actual yields could be reduced through scientific management of land, water and crops. The field based data on production performance available from this project, are being used by

both government and non-governmental agencies for developing crop production strategies.

b. **Operational Research Project (ORP):** Based on the result obtained in NDS, the ICAR decided to introduce the concept of an area on watershed basis (whole village or cluster of villages) to tackle some of the common agricultural problems on the community basis using inter-disciplinary approach. The project, started in 1975, envisages testing of technologies in the field conditions and to identifying agro-ecological, socioeconomic and institutional constraints in addition to technological constraints which act as barriers to adoption.

*Objectives:* The objectives of the ORP are:
  i. To introduce technologies on area basis and evoke appropriate cropping patterns
  ii To educate and train the farmers on the adoption of technologies
  iii. To identify constraints and farming problems and evoke community participation.

*Types of ORPs:* There are three types of ORPs, namely (a) watershed resources, development in dryland areas, (b) problem-oriented ORPs (disease management), and (c) audience-oriented ORPs (SCs, STs, etc.)

*Implementation:* There are 46 such projects in operation in 146 centres in different parts of the country. It includes 46 operational research centres for total resource development in watershed areas. In addition, specific and specialized areas like mixed farming, crop improvement, integrated pest management, reclamation of acidic, saline and alkaline soils, plantation crops, post-harvest technology, water management, dry land agriculture, watershed resource development, stock, fisheries, etc. are also included.

*Farmer interaction:* There is purposeful interaction between the scientists, extension personnel and farmers under this project which enables the scientists to gain insight into the socioeconomic constraints that affect the adoption of research results.

c. **Krishi Vigyan Kendra (KVK):** The Education Commission (1964–66) recommended the establishment of specialised institution called "Agricultural Polytechnics" to provide vocational education in agriculture and allied fields at the pre- and post-matriculate levels for boys and girls from rural areas. As a follow-up of this recommendation the ICAR established KVK (farm science centres) as an innovative institution for vocational training of farmers, farm women, youth, fishermen as well as field extension functionaries. The first KVK was established in 1974 at Pondicherry.

*Functions*

1. Farm advisory services.
2. Organizing Front Line Demonstration (FLD).
3. Vocational training of farmers, farm women and school drop-outs.
4. In-service training of the field level extension functionaries of the state governments.
5. On-farm trials and farming system research.

*Organizational structure:* Extension education specialist in the cadre of associate professor holds the position of Training Organizer (Head, KVK). An inter-disciplinary team in the cadre of assistant professor is employed as training associates. The discipline may be Agronomy, Animal Husbandry, Extension, Horticulture, Agricultural Engineering or Home Science.

*Transfer of technology:* Vocational training for practicing farmers, farm womens and youth is a critical input for accelerating agricultural production as long-term strategy. The basic aim of KVKs is to improve the farmer's technology, literacy and they are designed to impart skill-oriented training through work experience and learning by doing. Residential and non-residential courses of varying duration, which are tailor-made and need-based, are organised in the areas like Animal Husbandry, Crop Husbandry, Horticulture, Fisheries, Forestry, Home Science, post-harvest technology, etc.

d. **Trainer's Training Centres (TTCs):** To train the KVK trainers eight TTCs were established. The TTCs offer in-service training courses for the trainers/instructors of the Extension Training Centres, Farmers' Training Centres, Agricultural Schools, KVKs and vocational courses, teachers from schools. Two TTCs have been established for exclusively for women trainers and teachers, one at Indore and another at Nagaland. The training courses of the TTCs are mostly ad hoc in nature and are tailored to the needs of the specific interest groups, in service trainees. Major part of the training is centres on imparting work experience and the rest by discussions and lectures.

e. **Lab-to-Land Programme:** To commemorate its 'Golden Jubilee', an innovative extension programme called LLP was launched by the ICAR in 1979 to extend and promote new technologies among the small and marginal farmers and agricultural labourers and also to test the relevance of technologies in their socioeconomic conditions. There are 142 LLP centres with 1500 scientists working in them on part-time basis. The farm families adopted under this scheme receive support for a period of two years with follow-up guidance at least for one more year.

The scientists are permitted to spend ₹ 2,000 per family in two years on critical inputs. This amount, though too small, has been a good motivational force for the farmers to listen and learn about the low cost technologies which would improve their production and income. This programme also brings the scientists in close interaction with the farmers and gives them first hand feedback to reorient their research priorities to suit farmers' needs.

Of the adopted families in 2,103 villages in 303 districts, 13.2% belonged to landless agricultural labourers, 51.2% to marginal farmers and 36.6% to small farmers. During the Seventh Plan period (1989-90) resource constraints reduced the families adopted under this programme and two sub-projects, Land-to-Land and the Roving Extension Advisors have been initiated as part of the LLP to strengthen the feed back mechanisms.

f. **National Agricultural Technology Project (NATP):** National Agricultural Technology Project was launched during the Ninth Plan (1997–2002). The broad objective of the project is to sustain and strengthen the research and extension capabilities in the country.

**Specific objectives of NATP**

a. To improve the efficiency of organisation and management system of the Indian Council of Agricultural Research.

b. To enhance the performance and effectiveness of research scientists in responding to location-specific needs of farmers.

c. To pilot test innovations to improve the management of technology dissemination activities with greater accountability and participation by the farming community.

**Components of this project**

1. Development and Management System of the ICAR.
2. Support for Agro-Ecosystem Research.
3. Innovations in Technology Dissemination (ITD).

### Objectives of ITD components

1. Increase the effectiveness of technological support service by making them more demand drivers and responsive to location-specific problems of farmers.
2. Develop and strengthen institutional linkages.
3. Empower farmers through farmers' organization/ associations to play greater role in the management of the system.
4. Increase the financial sustainability of the public technology discrimination system.
5. Develop new partnerships with the private institutions including NGOs.

### Broad features of ITD

- Strengthening the district level technology discrimination capacity.
- Strengthening research-extension-farmer linkages.
- Adopting an integrated extension delivery system at the district level by establishing Agricultural Technology Management Agency (ATMA) as a registered society by involving all the state holders responsible for generation assessment and transfer of technology.
- Improving financial sustainability of extension services.

Major investments under the project are likely to be built around strengthening district level technology dissemination capacity. Based on the agro-ecological considerations, the project initiatives are proposed to be piloted in Andhra Pradesh, Bihar, Himachal Pradesh, Maharashtra, Orissa and Punjab.

g. **Front line transfer of technology projects:** ICAR started four TOT projects, namely National Demonstration Project (1964), Operational Research Project (1975), Krishi Vigyan Kendra (1974) and Lab-to-Land project (1979) but all of them have been merged into KVK. The KVK performs farm advisory services, vocational training and on-farm research/operational research.

h. **Institutional Village Linkage Programme (IVLP):** IVLP was launched by ICAR in 1995, for greater linkage between scientists and farmers in a 'bottom-up approach'. In IVLP villagers' problems are identified, solved and solutions are implemented through participatory approach.

Apart from the various ICAR institutes, State Agricultural and Veterinary Universities and IRMA, Anand are also engaged in the animal husbandry development in India.

**National Agricultural Education Project (NAEP):** National Agricultural Education Project was launched by ICAR in 2012 with an aim shaping higher agricultural education towards sustainable development. The goal of the National Agricultural Education Project would be "To improve and sustain quality of higher agricultural education for addressing emerging challenges for livelihood security and sustainable development".

In pursuance of this goal, the objectives would be to bring improvements, achieve excellence, enhanced relevance and high efficiency in the agricultural higher education system, and the agricultural universities to offer enhanced services to benefit farmers, rural women and other stakeholders. The project objectives would be achieved through two components with distinct modes.

**Systemic Reforms**—funded in a non-competitive investment mode—would include (a) reforms in governance and increasing system's internal efficiency; (b) ensuring compliance with ICAR's quality assurance policies, criteria and procedures, and strengthening accreditation and quality monitoring capacity; (c) human resource need assessment and strategic planning, and (d) attracting young talent to agricultural education.

**Institutional Development**—institutions would be funded through a selection mechanism. Selection criteria will be developed during project preparation—these will reflect institutions' willingness to reform, and their potential and vision for development. This component would support (a) restructuring and modernization of undergraduate and postgraduate programmes in various specializations; (b) promotion of academic excellence in critical/emerging areas at postgraduate and doctoral levels; (c) increasing scope and effectiveness of networking with educational institutions and research organizations within India and abroad; and (d) enhancing reach and effectiveness of agricultural education to agri-business, farmers and rural women. Efforts would also be made to increase public–private partnership in agricultural education through the increased role of the private sector in curriculum design, faculty and students development, research and development, institution's governance, and providing a window for direct project support for other specific initiatives.

**Farmer FIRST:** 'Farmer FIRST' is an ICAR initiative launched in year 2015 to move beyond the production and productivity and to privilege the complex, diverse and risk prone realities of majority of the farmers through enhancing farmers scientists contact with multi-stakeholders—participation. Many aspects are multiple or multi; multiple stakeholders, multiple perspectives, multiple realities, multi-functional agriculture, multi-method approaches. There are concepts and domains that are new or new in emphasis like food systems, trade, market chains, value chains, innovation pathways and most of all innovation systems.'Farmer FIRST' aims at enriching farmers-scientists interface for technology development and application. It will be achieved with focus on innovations; feedback; multiple stakeholders participation, multiple realities, multi-method approaches, vulnerability and livelihood interventions.

The project is conceptualized to deal with focus on:

i. *Enriching Farmers—scientist interface:* Enabling involvement of researchers for continuous interaction with farm conditions, problem orientation, exchange of knowledge between farmers and other stakeholders, prioritization of problems and setting up of research agenda.

ii. *Technology Assemblage:* Application and feedback integrating components of technology for application in different agro-ecosystems with focus on innovations and feedback.

iii. *Partnership and Institutional Building:* Building partnerships involving different stakeholders; development of rural based institutions; agro-ecosystem and stakeholders analysis and impact studies.

iv. *Content Mobilization:* Using the platform of the project having commodity institutions as partners to develop commodity specific contents for e-enabled knowledge sharing.

**Attracting and Retaining Youth in Agriculture (ARYA):** Realizing the importance of rural youth in agricultural development of the country, ICAR has initiated a programme on "Attracting and Retaining Youth in Agriculture" in year 2015.

The objectives of ARYA project are:

i. To attract and empower the Youth in Rural Areas to take up various Agriculture, allied and service sector enterprises for sustainable income and gainful employment in selected districts.

ii. To enable the Farm Youth to establish network groups to take up resource and capital intensive activities like processing, value addition and marketing.

iii. To demonstrate functional linkage with different institutions and stakeholders for convergence of opportunities available under various schemes/program for sustainable development of youth.

ARYA project will be implemented in 25 states through KVKs, one district from each state. In one district, 200–300 rural youths will be identified for their skill development in entrepreneurial activities and establishment of related micro-enterprise units. KVKs will involve the Agricultural Universities and ICAR Institutes as Technology Partners. At KVKs also one or two enterprise units will be established so that they serve as entrepreneurial training units for farmers. The purpose is to establish economic models for youth in the villages so that youths get attracted in agriculture and overall rural situation is improved.

Skill development of rural youths will help in improving their confidence levels and encourage them to pursue farming as profession, generate additional employment opportunities to absorb under employed and unemployed rural youth in secondary agriculture and service-related activities in rural areas. The concurrent monitoring, evaluation and mid-term correction will be an integral part of project implementation.

**My Village My Pride (Mera Gaon Mera Gaurav):** The "My Village My Pride" has been conceptualized (2015) in which scientists of ICAR and Agricultural Universities will identify villages in the vicinity of the institutions for providing advisories and consultations to farmers for increasing farm productivity and production. The objective of this scheme is to provide farmers with required information, knowledge and advisories on regular basis by adopting villages. Under this scheme group of scientists will select villages and will remain in touch with that village and provide information to farmers on technical and other related aspects in a time frame through personal visits or through telecommunication. In this way, 20,000 scientists of national agricultural research and education system (NARES) can work directly in villages.

Chapter 5

# Animal Husbandry Co-operatives

When human beings began to associate with each other co-operation come into existence.

Co-operation, otherwise known as co-operative movement, in general refers to the conscious association of the weak, the powerless and the poor to achieve the advantages which are available to the rich and the powerful. It is an institution of economic democracy for the promotion of common economic interests of the members. It has greater significance in the developing countries like ours.

A co-operative society is a voluntary organisation and all are welcome to join in it. Every member of the society has equal rights and responsibilities. The association is for the mutual benefit and help and not for getting individual profit. The animal husbandry co-operatives that are in vogue are dairy co-operatives, sheep co-operatives, poultry co-operatives, etc. and they play an important role in the socioeconomic transformation and development of livestock farming community.

## Meaning

Co-operation means working together. Co-operation is looked at from different angles. It is viewed as a form of economic organisation, a method of working, an instrument of change, a way of life, a business coupled with ideology and social purpose, practical philosophy and a means of social control and ownership.

## Definition

It is difficult to define co-operation precisely because the movement is born out of adversity and the nature of adversities in different countries. There are many definitions of cooperation given by different authors. According to Co-operative Planning Committee 1946, co-operation has been defined as a form of organization in which persons voluntarily associate together on the basis of equality for the promotion of their economic interests. Those who come together have common economic aim which they cannot achieve by only concerted action because of the weakness of the economic position of large majority of them. This element of individual weakness is overcome by the pooling of their resources, by making self-help effective through mutual help, and by strengthening the bonds of moral solidarity between them.

Co-operative society may be defined as a voluntary democratic association of persons for conducting united trade for the benefit of all its members. It is done by eliminating middle men in the purchase of all the inputs and consumable articles at a bargained price from the primary producers and the sale of produce from the members at a fair price directly to the consumption centres or wholesale buyers (Mathialagan, 1996).

Some of the other quoted definitions are as follows:

Co-operation has been defined by H. Calvert as a form of an organisation in which persons voluntarily associate together as human beings on the basis of equality for the promotion of their economic interests.

Hough defined co-operation as a voluntary association in a joint undertaking for mutual benefit, admittedly a lower ideal than a joint effort directed at the common good, but a long step in advance of seeking more.

According to Tyagi, a co-operative organisation is an association which furnishes an economic service with entrepreneur's profit and which is owned and controlled on a substantially equal basis by those for whom the service is being rendered.

Lambert states that a co-operative society is an enterprise formed and directed by an association of users, applying within itself the rules of democracy and directly intended to serve both its own members and the community as a whole.

Herrick defined co-operation as the act of persons voluntarily united for utilizing reciprocally their own forces, resources, or both under their mutual arrangement to their common profit or loss.

Fay defined co-operative society as an association for the purpose of joint trading, originating among the weak and conducted always in an unselfish spirit such that all those who are prepared to assume the duties of membership may share its rewards in proportion to the degree in which they make use of the association.

## OBJECTIVES OF CO-OPERATIVES

1. **Economic objectives:** As an institution a co-operative caters to the members' need and that of the society on the basis of self-help. It needs the mutual co-operation of its members and workers for their own benefits and for the benefit of the community as a whole. The overall economic objective of co-operatives is the welfare of the members of the society through supply of cheap credit; spread of banking habits; securing better prices for farm produce; eliminating exploitation by middlemen and creation of storage facilities for the produce until it is sold at an opportune time.

2. **Social objectives:** To develop democratic leadership and to motivate people to opt for voluntary participation and group action. All the members are treated as equals. Individuals are not discriminated on the basis of wealth or poverty. Everyone has equal rights and opportunities. They bring about harmony among the village people. It also aims at industry, self-reliance and mutual help. It fosters a sense of responsibility and integrity. It brings a sense of security among the members.

3. **Educational objectives:** To bring about knowledge of co-operatives to its participants and to develop responsibility and honesty among the members.

## PRINCIPLES OF CO-OPERATION

The co-operation movement made its first appearance in England. It was started to give relief to persons exploited by middlemen during the Industrial Revolution. When 28 poor weavers of Rochdale came together with a capital of 1 pound each to open a small retail shop in 1844, they adopted a set of rules which were later known as the Rochdale principles. The principles, which are laid down by Rochdale pioneers, have generally been accepted all over the world.

### Rochdale Principles

1. Democratic control.
2. Open membership.
3. Limited interest on capital.
4. Patronage divided.
5. Cash trading.
6. Political and religious neutrality
7. Promotion of education.

### Reformulated Principles of Co-operation

With the eventual growth in science and technology and diversification in co-operative business, it was felt that these principles needed some modifications, clarifications and adjustments. Consequently, the International Co-operative Alliance (ICA) appointed a sub-committee in 1934 for this purpose. The committee, in its 1937 report, classified these principles into two broad groups:

1. Essential principles
   a. Open membership
   b. Democratic management
   c. Limited interest on capital
   d. Payment of dividend in proportion to transactions.

2. Non-essential principles
   a. Religious and political neutrality
   b. Cash trading
   c. Education of members.

These principles did not leave enough scope for interpretation and understanding. Accordingly, the ICA again appointed a commission in 1964 and this commission submitted its report in 1966. The report has two characteristic features. Firstly, it did not classify the principles as essential and non-essential and, secondly, the principles were explained as accurately as possible. The reformulated principles were accepted as below.

1. **Voluntary association and open membership:** Membership of a co-operative society shall be voluntary and available without artificial restriction or any social, political, racial or religious discrimination to all persons who are keen to make use of its services and are willing to accept the responsibilities of membership. There is no compulsion on any one to join a co-operative society and one may withdraw from membership as and when he wishes. The principle of voluntarism is considered to be cordial and vital to the co-operative character of the society.

2. **Democratic control:** Co-operative societies are democratic organisations. Their affairs are to be administered by persons elected from among members in a manner agreed to by the members and accountable to them. Members of primary societies should enjoy equal rights of voting (one member, one vote) and right to participate in taking decisions affecting their societies. In those other than primary societies the administration should be conducted on a democratic basis in a suitable form.

3. **Limited interest on capital:** Share capital shall receive a strictly limited rate of interest, if any. The main purpose of limited interest is, of course, to

safeguard the non-profit character of the co-operatives. But it has another meaning, that within the co-operative economy capital has to serve, not to dominate.

4. **Equitable division of surplus:** The economic results arising out of the operations of the society belong to the members of that society and shall be distributed in such a manner that it would avoid any member gaining at the expense of others. This may be decided by the members as follows by providing for:

   a. development of the business of the co-operative,

   b. common services, and

   c. distribution of surplus among the members in proportion to their transactions with the society.

5. **Co-operative education:** It has been widely acknowledged that the strength and success of co-operative movement depend on the existence of enlightened membership. Hence, all co-operative societies shall make provision for the education of their members, officers, and employees and of the general public, and teach them the principles and techniques of co-operation, both economic and democratic.

6. **Co-operation among co-operatives:** All co-operative organisations, in order to serve the interest of their members and communities, shall actively co-operate in every practical way with each other at local, national and international levels. In the competitive conditions the whole trend of modern economy is towards closer economic integration and larger units. To realise the benefits of science and technology the principle of unity is vital not only among individuals but also for co-operative institutions.

7. **Concern for the society:** Co-operatives are not only concerned about the individual members of the institution but also the society.

## SERVICE CO-OPERATIVES

The National Development Council in1954 recommended a radical reform in the pattern of organisation of co-operative societies at the village level. As per the recommendation of this committee, the policy of organizing large sized societies like Service Co-operatives were introduced. The priniciple of co-operation was brought into practice through co-operative societies. The co-operative society is an association of unlimited number of persons formed on the basis of quality for the promotion of members' interests and managed by members themselves.

The service co-operatives were to serve as a store, a bank, a distribution agent, a supply and marketing unit for the members. After successful introduction of Amul pattern, co-operative societies that aimed at rural dairy farmers, sheep and poultry farmers were established. Presently all the livestock development programmes are routed through these co-operative societies.

Service co-operative societies brought the villages under a single institution, which in turn helped them to develop leadership, the democractic processes and self-employment and their socioeconomic status.

### Activities of Livestock Farmers' Co-operatives

The main function of co-operative societies is to accept livestock products, milk, egg, meat, etc. from their members and to market them independently or through their product-supply unions. The societies may also undertake activities concerned with the development of livestock breeds, their improved feeding, management and disease control. They are also a medium through which financial assistance is made available to their members for various productive purposes such as purchase of livestock, construction of sheds, etc.

### Dairy Co-operatives

The sheer dominance of the traditional milk traders and the limitations in the procurement and processing capacity of the organised dairy industry has kept our country's potential milk production below the desired level. The milk producers were compelled to sell their milk at throw away prices to the private traders. The traders involved indulged freely in malpractices like under weighing of milk, delayed payment and giving less than fair price for the milk.

After the introduction of the Indian Co-operative Act, 1912, the co-operative dairying, i.e. milk production's collection and sale by co-operatives, was first attempted by Katra Co-operative Dairy Society in Allahabad as early as 1913, for the purpose of eliminating middlemen in all spheres. In Tamil Nadu, the first dairy co-operative, Ayanavaram Dairy Co-operative, was established in the year 1927. First Milk Union— Lucknow Milk Producers Union established in the year 1937.

### Anand Pattern of Dairy Co-operatives

The dairy co-operative did not make much headway until the farmers of Kaira district of Gujarat agitated and forced their government to set up a state supported dairy co-operative in 1946, namely District Co-operative Milk Producer's Union, Latercome to known as AMUL.

Tribhuvandas Patel was elected by the farmers as the first leader of this co-operative. The AMUL collecting milk from villages and selling in cities like Bombay (now Mumbai), it fetching the dairy farmers proper price for their milk. Unlike the traditional milk co-operatives. Co-operative dairies on the Anand pattern are fully integrated vis-à-vis all the activities connected with milk such as production, processing, marketing and exporting.

The system of collective ownership, operation and control of milk trade by farmers came to be known as "Anand pattern". This system included milk production, procurement, processing and marketing through farmers' co-operatives. Dr Verghes Kurien set up the Anand model of co-operative dairy development.

The three-tier system in the co-operative dairies on the Anand pattern are: (1) Primary milk producer's co-operative society (village level), (2) district dairy co-operative union (district level), (3) milk producers' co-operative federation (state level).

### Primary Milk Producer's Co-operative Society

The first and basic unit of the Anand pattern is the village primary milk producers' co-operative, which is under the District Co-operative Milk Producers' Union. The functions of a milk producers' co-operative society can be broadly classified into managerial, operational and input services.

i. **Managerial:** All the members form the general body, which has supreme power. The society has a managing committee of 11 members elected among themselves. The managing committee in turn elects a president. The committee decides the policies and forms guidelines and also employs paid staff such as secretary and assistants for efficient running of the society as per Tamil Nadu Co-operative Society Act and Rules and bylaws of the society. The committee holds its meetings every month.

ii. **Operational**

   a. *Reception of milk*: Every society has a milk collection centre, and the milk producers (farmers) bring milk to the society every morning and evening. A sample of milk is taken for quality testing and the quantity of milk supplied is measured properly.

   b. *Testing of milk*: Once sufficient number of samples are collected, they are tested for fat percentage. After the test results are recorded by serial number, the left over samples' milk is disposed of. The entire milk is collected, mixed together, and a sample is drawn from the pooled milk for testing the fat and solid non-fat.

   c. *Despatch of milk*: Each and every morning the truck of the union comes to the society for milk collection. The milk cans, secured tightly, are loaded on the truck after making necessary entries in the truck sheet. The truck also does the job of unloading the empty cans for societies' use for the next collection.

   d. *Payment for the milk*: The payment is made on the basis of both quality and quantity. The price of milk fixed by District Milk Producers' Co-operative Union and the producers is paid weekly in cash by the society. The entries of payments are made both in producer's pass book and society's records.

   e. *Accounting*: The job of accounting starts right from the time a producer enters the society with milk. There is a set of standard registers, most of which are to be posted twice daily. There are separate records for different transactions. The accounts reflect the financial standing of the society at any time. A society prepares its balance sheet on a yearly basis.

   f. *Cleaning*: Daily cleaning of all the pieces of equipment in the society is done to avoid contamination and spoilage of milk.

   g. *Distribution of profits*: Apart from the regular payment of milk price, the society, at the end of the each year, also pays bonus to members, if it is running in profit, and dividends for the shares. Besides the above mentioned operations, the societies also perform activities such as disposal of sample milk, local sale of milk, standardisation of equipment, chemicals, etc.

   h. *Input services*: The next important work of a society after milk trading is the input services provided to the producers (farmers). These services include artificial insemination, veterinary first aid, selling cattle feed, providing quality fodder seeds at cost prices, organising meetings, arranging educational tours, cattle insurance, etc.

### Organisation and Registration of a Milk Producers' Co-operative Society

The first and foremost step is the survey of a village and data analysis. The villages are graded on the basis of milk potential. Then the Gram Sabha is organised.

**Gram Sabha:** The steps involved in organising a Gram Sabha are:

1. A milk procurement officer/supervisor from the union visits the selected village and arranges a meeting.

2. A socially respectable person from the village is requested to preside over the meeting.

3. The supervisor/officer explains the purpose and advantage of organising a milk society.

4. Once the villagers have decided to form a milk society, a chief promoter is selected from amongst them.

### Organisation of society neeting

A general body meeting of the members is called to elect the president of the milk society and to pass resolutions regarding the area of operation and to constitute an ad hoc managing committee comprising 11 directors for a proposal.

### Procedure for registration

The proposed milk co-operative society is allowed to function as such for three months. Then the union supervisor puts forth the proposal for registration. The proposal is recommended by the milk procurement section's head and forwarded to the competent authority in the Dairy Development Department. Before registering the society.

1. The application form is filled as per the Act and Rules. Specimen of the form is given in the Act.

2. All members of the society sign the application form as promoters.

3. The application is submitted along with:
   a. Seven copies of the bye-laws signed by the chief promoter.
   b. A list of members with number of shares held by each of them.
   c. One copy of all the resolutions passed at the society's meeting.
   d. A copy of accounts for the period it has worked as a proposed society.
   e. A certificate regarding jurisdiction of the respective village Panchayat.

The Registrar, after satisfying that the proposed society is in conformity with rules and regulations in force and the principles and philosophy of co-operation, and that the proposed will have reasonable chance of success in future the appointed society chief promoter who is authorised to collect the share of ₹ 10 along with ₹ 1 as entrance fees from all members. Promoter deposits the amount in the suspense account the after receiving the challan and member list.

The society is considered to be a registered only when a registration certificate with a registration number and also the management of society (the interview board) is issued by the registering authority. After registration, the secretary of the society in consultation with the president of the society calls a general body meeting to consider certain agendas such as acceptance of the registered bye-laws, election of a managing committee, regularisation of membership, affiliation of the society with the Milk Producers' Co-operative Union, District Co-operative Bank, etc. and appointment of local auditors for auditing the accounts.

### District Dairy Co-operative Union

The second-tier in the milk producers organisation having Anand pattern is the District Dairy Co-operative Union. Each and every village milk co-operative society becomes a member of District Dairy Co-operative Union with a share capital and an entrance fee.

### Organisation and Registration of Milk Union

The district level milk producers' union comprises minimum 25 organised and registered village societies, which form the basic units of union. The organisational function is regulated by the approved bye-laws of the District Registrar of Co-operative Societies at the district level. In some cases, the implementing agency (Government/Corporation/Federation) may nominate the union's directors to organise the societies. The application for registration is made on the prescribed form available with the District Registrar along with seven copies of bye-laws duly signed by promoter members, a copy of minutes of organisation's meeting, bank balance certificate, etc.

### General Body Meeting

After the registration, the chief promoter must issue an indicating the date, time, place, and purpose of the meeting for holding the first general body meeting of the union. The meeting's agenda should be the selection of president of the meeting, acceptance of registered bye-laws, election of regular board, approval of accounts, fixing the borrowing limit for union and other works. The office-bearers are elected according to norms prescribed in the bye-laws/Rules and Acts of the state.

### Management

The Dairy Co-operative Union is controlled by a board of directors having 17 members out of which twelve are elected representatives of the village societies. The remaining five members comprise the managing director, an official of the union as a member secretary, one or two representatives of financial institutions, a representative of the Registrar of Co-operative Societies and a representative of the state federation but these five members are not eligible for contesting the post of chairman. The general policy of the union is framed by the board. The board employs the Managing Director. While the board determines the number, type and scales of the post, it is the Managing Director who appoints the junior staff.

## Functions

The union carries out five important functions:

i. Procurement of milk.

ii. Processing and marketing of the milk.

iii. Providing technical inputs, such as animal health, artificial insemination, feeds and fodder development.

iv. Strengthening of milk co-operators' movement.

v. Organisation of extension activities and rural development services.

The District Dairy Co-operative Union owns and operates a dairy plant for processing milk and other by-products, a cattle feed plant for mixing feed and selling it to the farmers at cost price, bull mother farms, semen collection banks, and a headquarter centre for animal husbandry activities.

### Milk Producer's Co-operative Federation

The third tier of the Anand Pattern of milk producers organisation is the Co-operative Milk producer's Federation operating at the state level. The District Dairy Unions become members of the federation by subscribing at least the minimum prescribed share capital. The federation is responsible for the implementation of the policies of co-operative marketing, product-price, provision of joint services (A.I. health cover, etc.) and co-operative marketing of technical inputs to members.

## Management

The board of the federation consists of the elected chairmen of all the co-operative unions and the federation's Managing Director. Other members are the representative of the Registrar of Co-operative Societies, a representative of financing agency, nominee of NDDB (National Dairy Development Board) and one nominee of the State Government. These members elect a chairman of the board and the board evolves the federation's policies on all its functions. The federation's Managing Director is the committee's chairman the

General Manager, and its Secretary. The committee meets once every month and implements policies and plans.

The federation controls the centralised technical input programme (milk production enhancement programme) which covers essential activities such as animal health, artificial insemination, feed and fodder development and extension activities. The facilities available with the federation for performing these activities are a central diagnostic laboratory, frozen semen banks (production and supply), liquid nitrogen production and delivery system and a centralised publication unit for publishing news of various dairy activities.

### Extension Programmes of Dairy Co-operatives

Technical knowledge and skill are the most essential inputs which the dairy co-operatives provide through their extension education programmes to the milk producers. Unless the milk producers are properly educated about the advantages of adopting modern scientific practices, they will be reluctant to adopt newer techniques. Hence, the extension work is considered to be an important tool and pre-requisite for successful implementation of a scheme.

The dairy extension programmes aim at inducting and orienting the milk producers towards dairy development on co-operative lines and seeking their participation in building up a strong co-operative base.

## Role of federations

The Co-operative Dairy Federation is actively involved in the centralised publication of news bulletins, posters, leaflets, folders, handbills, etc. These printed materials are prepared in the simple local languages. The publications do represent the farmers' problems, reactions of farmers on various issues, latest information on scientific developments, adoption of various methods, package of practices of various Animal Husbandry activities, etc.

## Role of unions

The District Dairy Co-operative Union engages a wide range of extension activities such as arranging field tours, farmers' visits to union's infrastructure, successful village societies, etc. The unions also undertake screening of motion films through projectors in villages, organise calf rallies and livestock shows. It also helps the farmers in establishing demonstration units such as dairy farms and fodder farms, which serve as a live-lab as well as model farm for a wide number of farmers.

By visiting these model demonstration farms, the farmers' interest is stimulated, leading to adoption of newer technologies at a faster rate. The staff employed in the union popularise new technologies through campaigns such as infertility camps, vaccination camps, rallies, etc. The other extension services are provided in the form of incentives for artificial insemination of cattle and sale of cattle feed at cost price.

### Role of societies

The most pivotal role in the area of extension service is played by the village Milk Co-operative Societies. They act as the vital link through which the union communicates its programmes to the milk producers. Societies have an impeccable effect of creating a better impact on farmers and encouraging their active participation in societies. They also engage in the organisation of talis of local farmers, animal health camps, livestock shows, competitions, etc.

Thus, all the three-tiers of the dairy co-operatives play an important role in the dissemination of scientific knowledge to the grassroot farmers. Though illiteracy is a big obstacle, extension serves as a vital tool in creating conditions for better growth and development of farmers.

### Problems in dairy co-operatives

The dairy co-operatives are confronted with numerous difficulties in the day to day affairs of milk production and distribution. They are as follows:

1. The societies are not absolutely loyal to the unions in the supply of milk and in the absence of binding contract to deliver a specified supply, the unions are faced with acute shortage in the reception of milk during the lean (dry) season and surplus during flush season.
2. Shortage of supply of milk to the plants leads to underutilized capacity of plants.
3. Malpractices such as adulteration of milk by the milk producer.
4. Delay in payments to societies by the dairy plants leading to dissatisfaction among the producers.
5. Inappropriate testing of fat by the fat testers/secretary.
6. Intervention by middle men/milk vendors.
7. Curdling of milk due to delay in transportation.
8. Failure to increase the milk yield per animal by the co-operatives.
9. The demand for milk is steady and continuous, but the supply is often subjected to fluctuations.

10. The co-operatives are at a disadvantage when compared to private vendors in the qualitative aspect of collection, testing, transport and storage.

### Suggestions

1. The supply of minimum quantity of milk by the society to the union should be insisted.
2. Arrangements should be made for pasteurisation of milk in the nearest production centre so as to prevent spoilage.
3. Attention should be given to the crossbreeding of dairy cattle, cultivation of fodder, purchase and distribution of concentrates at wholesale rates by the unions and societies.

The Co-operative Planning Committee (1946) made the following suggestions for the development of milk co-operatives:

1. Societies should be formed within a radius of 30 miles from towns with a population of 30,000 or more.
2. A minimum daily quantity of 3,000 litres of milk should be supplied.
3. The societies should inform the union at the beginning of each month the quantity of milk its members can supply daily so that disbursement of payment is in time.
4. Milking of cattle should be carried out in the presence of secretary or members of a society in a common shed for which the funds should be provided by the state.
5. The financial needs of the members should be met by giving loans through the primary credit society or milk supply society.
6. The milk unions should suggest appropriate milk collection centres in the village from where the milk may be collected and transported easily to the milk union.

## Sheep Breeders' Co-operative Societies

In India, sheep rearing is an important small-scale activity predominating the domain of villagers such as marginal farmers and poor landless labourers. It does play a major role in economy of rural poor by supplying various products such as meat, skin, wool and manure. It also provides subsidiary occupation for the small and big farmers and primary occupation for the unemployed and agricultural labourers. Nearly 55.5 million sheep (1987) are distributed throughout India, which has a significant impact on the nation's economy.

After launching a series of rural development programmes the Government also realised the importance of starting the Sheep Breeders' Co-operative Societies (SBCS). Hence, the Government agencies have come forward to motivate sheep rearing farmers to start co-operative societies.

## Administrative Control

In Tamil Nadu, the Animal Husbandry Co-operatives, such as the Sheep Breeding Co-operative Societies, Poultry Breeders' Co-operative Societies and Cattle Breeders' Co-operative Societies, etc. were initially under the administrative control of the Registrar of Co-operative Societies (Department of Co-operation), Chennai. The officers of the Co-operative Department had a close link with the officers of Animal Husbandry Department for proper organisation and working of Sheep Breeders' Co-operative Societies and sought help in the areas related to breeding, feeding, management, disease control and asset creation.

The Tamil Nadu Government felt that the Animal Husbandry Department should play a vital role in organising and administering the affairs of Sheep Breeders' Co-operative Societies and hence, the administrative control was transferred to them from the Co-operative Department with effect from January 1964.

The State Director of Animal Husbandry is vested with the powers of the Registrar of Co-operative Societies, Chennai, and the Regional Deputy Directors and Assistant Directors of Animal Husbandry are vested with the powers of Joint Registrars and Deputy Registrars of Co-operative Societies respectively.

## Objectives

The multi-faceted objectives of the Sheep Breeders' Co-operative Societies are as follows:

1. To adopt improved scientific methods of sheep breeding, and weaving wool into finished products.
2. To arrange for the procurement and sale of sheep for the members of the society.
3. To arrange for grazing of sheep for the benefit of the members.
4. To provide facilities for the purchase of raw materials required for wool weaving.
5. To arrange for the manufacture of blanket and other finished products out of the wool of sheep.
6. To receive or purchase finished goods from members for sale.
7. To act as an agent for the purchase of domestic and other requirements to the members.
8. To purchase and arrange or hire the improved appliances connected with the wool industry.
9. To impart business and technical training to the members.
10. To provide loans for essential purposes to the members of the society.

## Organisation and Registration

1. Initial survey for assessing the potentiality of the area.
2. Enrolment of members and collection of share amount.
3. Meeting of the enrolled members.
4. Adoption of bye-laws.
5. Constitution of an ad hoc management committee and election of a chairman.
6. Appointment of society staff and securing surety from them.
7. Opening of bank account in the name of society and authorisation to secretary and chairman to operate the account jointly.
8. Selection of a suitable building for the society to function.
9. Registration of the society.
10. Signing of an application form by all enrolled members and submission of the following to the Assistant Director of Animal Husbandry through the Veterinary Assistant Surgeon.
    a. Four copies of bye-laws signed by the chief promoter.
    b. Four copies of the list of members.
    c. One copy of the resolutions passed at the society's organisational meeting.
    d. A copy of accounts.
    e. Certificate regarding jurisdiction of village Panchayat under which the village falls.
11. Once the society is registered, the first general body meeting needs to be organised by the secretary with the consent of the chairman and the following agenda items such as selection of chairperson, acceptance of the bye-laws, election of a managing committee, approval of the accounts, etc. are to be considered.

The Veterinary Assistant Surgeon of that area will be the ex-officio director of the society. The remaining procedure for functioning are similar to that of Milk Producers' Co-operative Societies. The members will market sheep and wool instead of milk through the society. They do receive farm inputs, financial assistance and also avail credit facilities and technical service.

### Impact

1. A sense of awareness and perceived knowledge is evident among the sheep farmers.
2. Adoption of scientific farming practices is increased.
3. The number of people availing scheme loans and subsidies through these societies has gone up.
4. Development of leadership qualities.
5. Increased employment opportunities.
6. Socio-economic status improved.
7. Standard of living improved.

### Limitations

1. A number of Sheep Breeders' Co-operative Societies are dormant and the failure of these societies is attributed to the poor involvement of the members of the society compared to Milk Producers' Co-operative Society. The Sheep Breeders' Co-operative Societies were started by members only to avail loans under IRDP, DPAP, etc. and poor repayment has been reported.
2. Unlike the Milk Producers' Co-operative Societies, the members of the Sheep Breeders' Co-operative Societies market their produce on their own because of the sellers' market.
3. Due to untrained leadership, improper functioning of Sheep Breeders' Co-operative Societies has been noticed. Out of 1,693 Sheep Breeders' Co-operative Societies in Tamil Nadu, only 1,419 are functioning and they too are not healthy and well developed.
4. The insurance claims were not properly made due to lack of contact between the society and members leading to heavy losses to the farmers.

## Poultry Co-operatives

The success of Anand pattern of dairy co-operatives led to multifarious suggestions to replicate their experience to promote poultry enterprise. Hence, Poultry Egg Production and Poultry Meat Production Co-operatives emerged in a few states.

In the livestock sector, poultry has emerged as a rapid growing industry in India, and recently India was listed as one among the leading nations of the world in poultry production. Poultry farming in India progressed further after the initiation of poultry Co-operatives. After spread of poultry egg and meat production on the European model, due to expertise of extension agencies and early co-operatives, the trade has been taken over by large farmers and traders. The co-operative societies, catering to small farmers, had an asphyxial death due to inefficiency and corruption on the part of leadership. Where the small farmers form themselves into unregistered private co-operatives without the state control there is prosperity.

### Objectives

1. To launch activities for production of eggs and poultry meat.
2. To provide facilities for more profitable marketing of farm produce.
3. To undertake various extension and poultry husbandry activities.
4. To develop manpower for poultry industry.

### Formation of Co-operative Society

The steps followed for formation of dairy co-operatives is applicable to the starting of a poultry co-operative also. All the poultry farmers are eligible to become members of the society. The society is be run by a duly elects managing committee. The chairman elected by the society appoints a secretary, who in turn acts as a manager. He should have a thorough knowledge of poultry husbandry activities. The members of the society decide regarding the source of supply of chicks, feed, and also disposal of birds, whereas the union takes care of loans, repayment, insurance, loss due to unforeseen causes, etc.

At the district level, nearly 150–200 societies form one union. The union should have hatchery, feed manufacturing plant, egg cold storage facilities, packing, service and training centre. The union should be run by a duly elected chairman, vice-chairman and board members. A number of Poultry Producers' Unions come together to form the State Poultry Producers' Co-operative Federation, which may be linked with the national organisation.

Unlike the dairy co-operatives which emerged due to the initiative from the dairy farmers for marketing their milk, the poultry co-operatives have emerged mainly due to the government's initiative. The poultry co-operatives were started with an intention to provide employment to the weaker sections of the community. The degree of people's participation and involvement in poultry co-operatives is poor when compared to that in Milk Producers' Co-operative Societies. The farmers took interest in the poultry co-operatives mainly to obtain loans and avail subsidy. The poultry market is not always steady and the price of the produce keeps fluctuating.

The expectations from poultry co-operatives are manifold, namely:

1. They are often considered to be institutions for transfer of technology.
2. Provision of cheap quality feed.
3. Bargaining for good price for the output.
4. Considered as institution to promote socio-economic change of weaker sections.

## Status of poultry co-operatives

At present there are about 2,595 poultry co-operative societies in India. Out of the nine states with well developed poultry industry, the co-operatives are performing well only in two states. The two states are Gujarat and Maharashtra. The number of societies doubled during the period 1972–92 but the percentage of dormant and loss-making societies constitute about 80%. Even after three decades of intensive poultry development , the poultry co-operatives have not been able to establish themselves on a strong footing. The current status of some of the successful poultry co-operatives are:

i. **Gujarat Poultry Co-operative:** In the state of Gujarat, some voluntary agencies introduced the industrial estate concept for poultry industry. A flock of 100 to 150 birds were put in a compartment and assigned to the beneficiary, who had to perform activities like visiting the hen house three times a day for cleaning, feeding and watering the birds. The society also provided feed and made arrangements to market the eggs and subsidy was also offered for the construction of sheds under tribal development programme.

Though co-operatives are performing satisfactorily in Gujarat, the poultry development is still in the primitive stage. But in this context, it is important to mention that Gujarat is the only state where a strong co-operative federation exists.

ii. **Maharashtra Poultry Co-operatives:** The co-operative societies in Maharashtra have set up a centralised poultry shed, where chicks are reared up to 20 weeks and when the birds are ready for laying, they are given to the members in flocks of 100–200 birds to rear near their homes with subsidies for constructing pen house. They also supply feed and arrange for marketing. Though the society pays uniform price for the eggs throughout the year, the farmers are reluctant to supply these when the market prices are higher.

Though the number of poultry co-operatives in the state is increasing, they still have a long way to go to flourish as an industry. But the emphasis in Gujarat and Maharashtra is for developing a viable industry for the socially backward class.

iii. **Poultry co-operatives in other states:** The poultry co-operatives in Tamil Nadu, Kerala, Andhra Pradesh, Karnataka, Uttar Pradesh, West Bengal, Rajasthan, Madhya Pradesh, etc. are still poorly developed. The concept of developing poultry schemes for the economically weaker sections led to the development of poultry units at scattered and far off places, and to some extent succeeded in persuading the farmers to purchase their feed at reasonable prices, to seek medical cover, and to sell their eggs on their own.

The beneficiaries were new entrants to these schemes and they had poor knowledge to check mortality and to prevent various emerging diseases in the birds. In many states, the poultry co-operatives assumed a mercantile role of merely buying and selling eggs and feed.

## Institutions supporting the poultry co-operatives

Several institutions lend a helping hand in the development of poultry co-operatives in India. They are:

1. **National Co-operative Development Corporation (NCDC):** To hasten poultry development, NCDC sought expert guidance to formulate viable schemes. In this the primary poultry co-operatives were promoted to rear and supply layer birds and feed, and collect the eggs for marketing. NCDC promoted this integrated poultry scheme and the supply of ready to lay birds to the members under a lease programme. During the Eighth Five-Year Plan, NCDC modified the scheme particularly with respect to farm level production. It also proposes to sanction 90 more projects with a contribution of Rs. 100 crores.

2. **National Scheduled Caste and Scheduled Tribe Finance and Development Corporation (NSFDC):** This organisation was set up on 8th February, 1989, under the Companies Act, 1956, to promote economic development of the members of Scheduled Castes and Scheduled Tribes whose family incomes are below twice the poverty line limit. NSFDC provides seed capital and term loans to members of Scheduled Castes and Scheduled Tribes through state Governments.

3. **National Agricultural Co-operative Marketing Federation (NAFED):** This organisation has been entrusted with the responsibility of operating a Market Intervention Scheme to enable the farmers

to get reasonable price for eggs. NAFED is expected to buy two crore eggs in a year which is less than one-third of a day's egg production in the country.

### Poultry egg and meat production co-operatives

In the case of poultry industry, the egg and broiler production are two distinct sub-sectors and the role performed by co-operatives in these sectors are also entirely different. Hence, there are two separate co-operatives, namely Egg Producers' Co-operatives and Poultry Meat Producers' Co-operatives.

i. **Egg production co-operatives:** At present in the egg producing industry, poultry farmers get all the inputs, namely chicks, feed, etc. from the co-operatives. At the marketing end, the National Egg Co-ordination Committee (NECC) fixes the price and hence all the producers get the same price. The eggs produced directly reach the consumers without any sort of processing unlike in the case of milk. The co-operatives can also oversee the marketing aspect, but the main problem is that they have to handle a large volume of eggs. The cost of feed accounts for nearly 70% of egg production and hence the co-operatives have to concentrate on this operation with high managing capability. Hence, the failure of some of the co-operatives is primarily due to small size of operation and poor management.

ii. **Poultry meat production co-operatives:** In the case of developed countries, the three main forces that have propelled the poultry meat industry are:

   a. Market ownership and margin control
   b. Bio-security and quality
   c. Economics of scale and optimization of capital resources.

In India, most of the broiler units sell live birds and they are transported to far off places especially to major consuming centres. The broiler co-operatives in India do have very little scope for conferring huge benefits to the farmers, who usually sell the birds to middlemen. In the private sector a few poultry processing units have been set up and they too are handicapped for want of supporting infrastructures like refrigerated transit facilities and absence of retail outlets for processed chicken. The poultry co-operatives can play a significant role in meat processing but this would call for huge capital investment and strong marketing capability.

### Future Strategy for Poultry Co-operatives

The future strategy for growth of poultry co-operatives is that they should have market orientation. The role of co-operatives is generally assumed to be cost reduction and appropriation of value addition. For achieving the prosperity of their members, the co-operatives should take special care of risks, namely sudden fall in productivity, violent price fluctuations etc.

A sound management information system (MIS) is needed to overcome those risks and to promote profitability of the members. An organised development of poultry co-operatives is needed. There is also a proposal to set up a National Poultry Development Board. The poultry co-operatives should concentrate both at the grassroot level production and at specialised marketing.

## IMPACT OF ANIMAL HUSBANDRY CO-OPERATIVES

The advent of various Animal Husbandry Co-operatives, such as dairy, poultry and sheeps co-operatives, has been a boon to the traditionally poor farmers. These have provided a sustainable income to their members throughout the year from their produce, namely milk, meat and eggs. The main source of income for small farmers is from the animal husbandry sector. The co-operatives have played a substantial role in the transformation of social and economic status of the poor livestock farmers.

1. A sense of togetherness was developed among the livestock farmers.

2. Social evils such as untouchability, etc. have been considerably reduced.

3. Age-old superstitions prevalent among the farmers in the management of livestock were markedly reduced.

4. Increased productivity was evident because of the adoption of improved scientific practices advocated by the co-operatives.

5. The members of the co-operatives obtained a profitable price for their produce through co-operative marketing which resulted in a steady flow of income making the farmers more self-reliant.

6. Employment opportunities for rural youth and farm women were considerably increased.

7. Leadership qualities of the members were developed.

8. A considerable portion of the profit obtained from the co-operatives was utilised for the development of schools, hospitals, etc.

9. An overall improvement in the status of living such as increased material possession, providing better education to children, etc. was evident.

The Animal Husbandry Co-operatives were initiated with the object of improving the living standard of the rural population by providing them with additional employment and increased income. These co-operatives, in addition to performing routine duties and functions like procurement, processing, manufacturing finished products, marketing and providing inputs, were also engaged of in transferring the technical knowledge and skill for improving the productivity. Though there is considerable socioeconomic impact of these co-operatives on the farming members, the present status of some of the Animal Husbandry Co-operatives is not appreciable as they are dormant. The failure of these co-operatives is attributed to the poor involvement and association of the members of the society. Hence, various measures such as formulating suitable strategies for procurement, marketing, reduction of cost of input, avoiding price fluctuations, providing sound information system, are on the anvil to overcome these shortcomings and help in improving the non-functional co-operatives for serving the farming clientele in a better way.

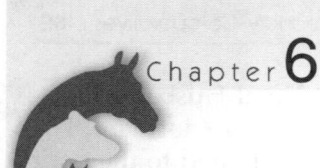

# Chapter 6

# Extension Teaching Methods

The basic function of an extension worker is to create environment or situation in which farmers learn. Learning is an active process on the part of the learner. He/she should be interested in knowing things and involve himself/herself otherwise nothing is accomplished. It is the duty of the extension worker to "provide people with an opportunity to learn, and stimulate mental and physical activity that produces the desired learning." Effective teaching methods fulfil these criteria.

Desired learning results by effective teaching. Effective teaching depends upon the aptitude of the teacher, method of teaching adapted and handled by the teacher. Proper 'selection' and 'combination' of teaching method and 'skillful handling' will bring out expected behavioural change. This expected behaviour change is called education. Education enables the people to understand their problems and solve those problems by themselves. To help people to help themselves is the core idea of the extension education. Extension education is not service. Service makes people more dependent on others but education makes them more self-reliant. By providing free eggs, you can feed a person for a day or two. But by providing knowledge and skill on poultry rearing you can feed him and his family throughout life.

## Definition

"Teaching methods are the devices used to create situations in which communication can take place between the instructor and the learner.[1]

"Extension teaching methods are the plans used by the extension workers to communicate their ideas to the clients".[2]

## Functions of Extension Teaching Methods

1. To provide communication so that learner may see, hear and do the things to be learnt.

2. To provide stimulation that causes the desired mental and/or physical action on the part of the learner.

3. In brief, to take the learner through one or more steps of the teaching-learning process, viz. attention, interest, desire, conviction, action and satisfaction.

In this part is set forth some basic guidelines for extension teaching. Extension education is of such scope and complexity that one has to study and have experience beyond the material presented here. But some lines are laid down that point towards useful direction.

## Classification of Methods

Many bases can be used to classify the methods according to use, form and function.

### I. Classification according to use

| Individual contact | Group contact | Mass contact |
|---|---|---|
| • Farm and home visit | • Method demonstration | • Printed meterials |
| • Telephone calls | • Group discussion | • Radio programmes |
| • Personal letters | • All types of meetings | • TV programmes |
| • Result demonstration | • Training courses | • Exhibition |
| • Office call | • Tours | • Film shows |
| • Farm Clinic | • Minikit trail | • Campaigns |
| | • Field day/ Farmer's day | • Circular letter |
| | • Farmer field school | • e-mail |
| | • Result demonstration meetings | • Internet |
| | • Drama and puppetry | • Video text |
| | • Tom-tom | |
| | • Video lesson | |
| | • Computer multimedia | |

### II. Classification according to form

| Written | Spoken | Visuals |
|---|---|---|
| • Printed materials | • All types of meetings | • Result demonstration |
| • Personal letters | • Farm and home visits | • Method |

*Contd...*

1. J.P. Leagans." Extension Education in Community Development". op. cit.
2. P. Mathialagan. "Extension Teaching Methods and Aids-Manual", op. cit.

| Written | Spoken | Visuals |
|---------|--------|---------|
| • Circular letters | • Office calls and Telephone calls • Radio talk (broadcast) • Tom-tom | • Demonstration • Exhibition • TV telecast • Meetings with AV aids • Film shows • Drama and puppetry • Video text • Internet |

## III. Classification according to function

| Telling | Showing | Doing |
|---------|---------|-------|
| • Lecture • Meetings • Audio lessons • Farm & home visit • Radio talk • Extension talk • Tom-tom | • Motion picture • Exhibition • Tours demonstrations • Internet • Video text | • Practicals • Workshop • Method • Result demonstration • Do it yourself |

## INDIVIDUAL TEACHING METHOD

Individual contact is defined as the direct contact by the extension worker with an individual (farm, farm woman, youth, etc.) or the members of his family for a specific purpose. The individual contact may be established through the farm and home visits, office calls, informal contacts, telephone calls, personal letters, etc.

### Farm and Home Visit

It is a face to face type of individual contact by the extension worker with the farmer and/or the members of his family at the latter's farm or home for one or more specific purposes connected with extension.

### Objectives

a. To develop good relationship with farmers and to gain their confidence.

b. To obtain and give first-hand information on matters relating to the development of farm and home.

c. To discuss individual farm and home problems.

d. To identify the local leaders and demonstrators.

e. To teach skill.

f. To discuss and find out the unfelt needs and take suitable action.

g. To contact those farmers who could not be reached by other methods.

h. To promote good public relations with the extension agency.

Points to be considered while adopting this method:

1. The visit should be made with a definite purpose.
2. Be punctual.
3. Save time—by proper planning.
4. Remote farms and homes should be given first preference.
5. This method should be used to reinforce other methods when other methods alone cannot be adopted.

### Demonstration

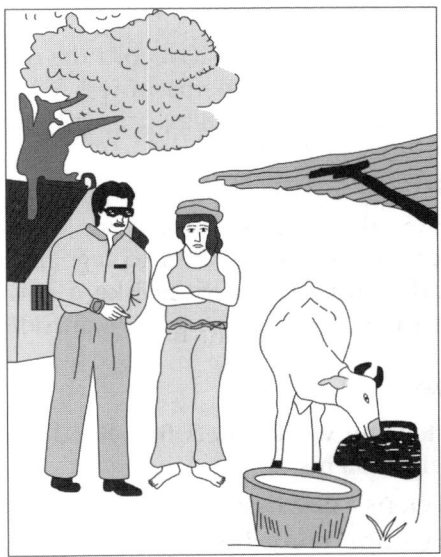

**Fig. 6.1:** Demonstration of farm and home visit

*Suggestions to make an effective farm and home visit*

1. Greet the person properly and use common social courtesies. Try to develop sound and favourable relations.
2. Identify the topic of interest of the farmer.
3. In order to start discussion, begin the conversation with a question put in such a way that it cannot be answered by merely saying 'yes' or 'no'.
4. It is not necessary to tell the person immediately and directly the purpose of the visit. Even though that is the main objective, the purpose of the visit should be explained in such a way that appears as beneficial for the farmer.
5. The extension worker should know everything about the subject about which efforts are made. He should be accurate and correct in his statements.

6. Allow the farmer to do more of talking, do not interrupt him in the middle.

7. The extension worker should speak when the farmer is willing to hear and talk according to the interest of the farmer. Use the simple language of the farmers' family and common terms with cheerful nature. Avoid argument. Try to learn from the farmer.

8. Find something to praise. Never talk down the farmers.

9. Take some printed matter to be handed over to the individual.

10. Avoid writing the conversation in the farmer's presence.

11. Leave the farm or home with genuine friendliness and appreciation.

12. Immediately after the visit, record the date of visit, purpose of visit, problems noted for follow-up action. Keep the promises by proper follow-up.

### Application

By employing this method the existing farm practices can be improved, e.g. deep litter to cage, floor cage to raised platform, new practices like disinfection of poultry house with flame gun can be introduced.

### Advantages

1. The extension worker gets first-hand information on rural problems.

2. He develops a goodwill with the farmer.

3. He develops confidence when his ideas are accepted by the farmers.

4. Help in locating local leaders and co-operation.

5. The interest of the people in extension services is created.

6. Those farmers who could not be contacted by other methods can be contacted by this method.

7. Percentage of adoption is high.

8. Visits are a source of material for news stories.

### Limitations

1. It consumes much of extension worker's time and energy.

2. Limited contacts of farmers.

3. Neighbours and friends to the farmers will blame the extension worker of favouritism, if they are not visited.

4. Sometimes visit may not be opportunistic to the farmer.

5. Tendency to visit the same farm again and again may be created.

6. It is a costly method.

### Office Call (Fig. 6.2)

It is a call made by a farmer or a group to the extension worker at his office for obtaining information and for inputs or other farm helps needed or for making acquaintance with him. The volume of office calls is related to the degree of public interest in the programme of the extension service, the relationship existing between the local extension worker and the villagers, and the accessibility of his office to rural people.

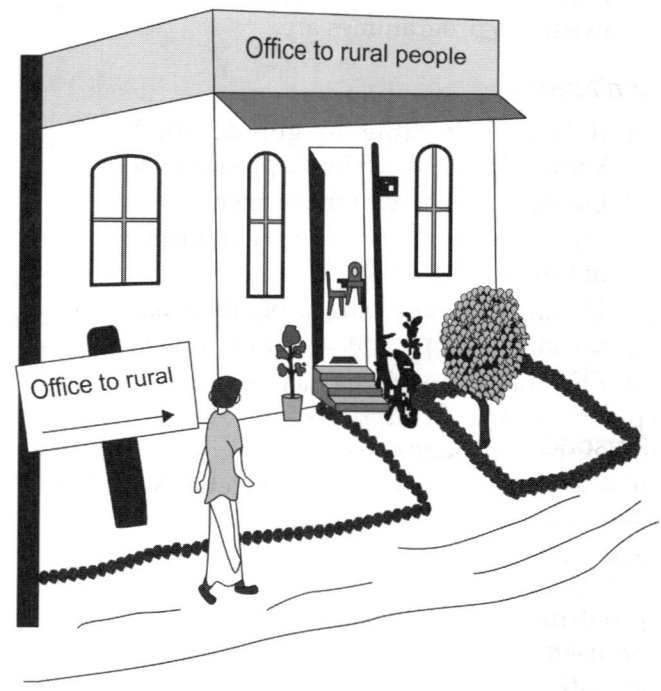

**Fig. 6.2:** Office call

### Suggestions for Making Successful Call

1. The office hours should be fixed.

2. The office should be kept neat and tidy and at a convenient location.

3. A signboard or notice board should be put up.

4. The farmer should be cordially received with a smiling face, treated properly and with satisfactory information.

5. The office should be equipped with extension teaching materials, charts, models, etc.

6. The assistants should be trained properly to receive the farmers and should be provided with adequate information to satisfy the farmers.

## Advantages

1. Economic use of extension workers' time and energy.
2. Farmer is in the receptive stage of mind and ready to follow or put the new idea to the practice.
3. It develops goodwill and confidence.
4. It reinforces other methods.
5. It is the sign of confidence that the farmer has in the extension worker and respect for his ability.
6. A careful record of office calls provides a basis for follow-up activity and may serve as one measure of public participation in extension activities, i.e. it is a parameter to show how much influential the extension worker is and how important the extension programmes are.

## Limitations

1. It is not possible to get detailed first-hand knowledge of the farmer's problems and activities.
2. Limited contact with the farmer.
3. Waiting for visitors who are not turning up is waste of time.
4. Unbusiness-like handling of office call will result in unconcerned person using the office as lounging place.

## Personal Letter (Fig. 6.3)

It is a personal and individual letter written by the extension worker to a farmer in connection with extension work. In practice personal letters are used to answer enquiries from farmers regarding specific farm problems, supplies, services, etc. This method can also be used to seek farmer's co-operation in extension activities.

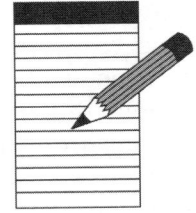

**Fig. 6.3:** Personal letter

Points to be considered in using this method:

1. When sought for, information should be answered promptly because the person writing the letter has more interest in the matter and will like to receive information immediately. Remember the saying that "Information delayed is information denied".

2. One should have the empathy and write the letters in a useful way to the farmer.
3. The letters should be complete, concise, clear, and correct in courteous language.
4. The writing should be neat, free of overwriting, striking, spelling and grammatical mistakes.
5. It should be easy readable.

## Advantages

1. Individual problems can easily be solved.
2. Cheap method.
3. To seek farmer co-operation for extension work it is a good method.
4. Useful to educate farmers.
5. The best method to reach farmers who could not be reached by farm and home visit and office call methods.
6. To develop good relations and confidence this is one of the best method.
7. Percentage of adoption is very high.
8. Extension worker gets first-hand information about rural problems.

## Limitations

1. It is a time-consuming method.
2. Since majority of the farmers are 'illiterates' this method has limited usage.
3. It is difficult for the extension worker to answer 'each and every' individual problem.
4. Only few persons can be contacted.

## Phone Call (Fig. 6.4)

It is a contact between the extension worker and farmer over the telephone for one or specific purposes connected with extension.

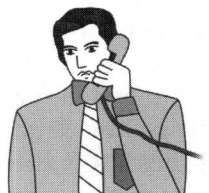

**Fig. 6.4:** Phone call

## Advantages

1. Although face to face contact is missing they have the advantage that it may be initiated by either the farmer or the extension worker.
2. They are useful in society for giving specific information such as:

a. First aid treatment of some disease condition can be done by the farmer before the arrival of the veterinarian, e.g. uterine prolapse

b. Control of lice infestation

c. So stress medication in poultry farms it is much useful in energy contact.

3. They provide a means of follow-up and evaluation of the effectiveness of radio broadcasts or television telecasts. People will call the extension office to request for a certain news bulletin or circular mentioned in the radio announcement.

4. Extension office in highly developed services sometimes finds it necessary to employ special telephone number and taped recordings to answer the flood of inquries after especially interesting programmes or announcements.

5. Economical, it creates goodwill and proper human relation.

### Limitations

1. Use of phone call is very limited in our country.
2. The extension worker cannot see the farmer's face and his farm.

### Result Demonstration

"When you teach by method demonstration, you show someone how to do a new job, or you show him how to do an old job better."[1] The strength of the demonstration lies in its obviousness—its appeal to logic and reason. It is there before your eyes. It works better than the old method. Its use would bring improvement. Extension uses two types of demonstrations method and result. Method demonstration is a group method, whereas result demonstration is an individual method. But result demonstration meeting is the group method.

Result demonstration is a demonstration conducted by a farmer, home maker or other persons under direct supervision of an extension worker to prove the worthiness of a recommended practice or combination of practices. The new practice is compared with the old one on the farmers' field. It is convincing because the farmers learn by seeing and doing.

### Objectives

a. To show the advantages, applicability and profitability of a new practice.

---

1. Using Visuals in Agricultural Extension Programs—ESC-561 International Cooperation Administration and Federal Extension Service, US Dept. of Agriculture.

b. To establish the confidence (farmer and extension worker).

Types of result demonstration:

a. Short duration: Deworming.

b. Long duration: Crossbreeding.

c. Single practice: Debeaking.

d. More practices: Complete package of practices.

### Organising and Conducting

1. **Analysis the situation:** Study the local problem. Select the practice. Analyse whether the farmers feel the need for the demonstration. Plan the demonstration. While planning, define the objective. Discuss the plan with the selected farmer and make a detailed written plan.

2. **Selection of the farmer:** Consult the local leaders and select the farmer. He should have the ability to conduct demonstration successfully and is respected by his neighbours. A responsible co-operative and average farmer with a field where most of the villager can go should be selected. Make sure that the water and other conditions are typical of the area.

3. **Prepare the action plan:** After selecting the farmer, prepare a plan of action with him. A copy must be given to the demonstrator. Help the farmer in procuring the necessary inputs.

4. **Conducting the demonstration:** Before starting make sure that all the necessities are procured. Extension worker should help the farmer to carry out the activities. It must be ensured that all the work is being done as planned. Help the farmers in keeping the records.

5. **Supervision of the demonstration:** Extension worker should pay regular visit to the demonstration farm. Give specific suggestions, furnish new information when needed, check progress and see the succeeding steps are performed as planned. Give farmer recognition and provide him opportunities to meet the scientists and other extension specialists.

6. **Recording the results:** The results must be carefully observed, measured and recorded especially in the presence of leading farmers. Invite other farmers to see the effect of new method.

7. **Follow-up:** Extension worker should publicise the result through all mass media. The impact of result demonstration is measured by number of people who are persuaded to try the practice.

## Suggestions for Effective Control

1. Proper selection of the practice, farmers and the place.
2. It is better to conduct one good demonstration than many unsuccessful ones.
3. Conduct the 'meetings' at the site of demonstration.
4. Avoid selecting the same farmer for several times.
5. Give wide publicity to the results.
6. Help the farmer to keep the proper records.
7. Fix signboards to attract visitors.
8. Encourage other farmers.
9. Better to conduct more than one demonstration in the same village on the same subject.
10. The place selected should be at the roadside.

## Advantages

1. It is seen by the eye and effectively reaches the 'show-me' individuals.
2. It gives extra assurance.
3. Increases the confidence and also more number of people will understand.
4. Useful for introducing new technologies.
5. Contributes to discovery of the local leader.
6. Provides teaching materials for further use, in the future meetings, news items, pictures, radio talk, etc.
7. Helps in developing local leadership.
8. Furnishes cost data and other basic information.

## Limitations

1. Requires a lot of time.
2. A costly teaching method.
3. Difficult to find good demonstrator who will help perfect records.
4. Unfavourable weather and other factors may destroy the value.
5. Unsuccessful demonstration may create strong unfavourable condition.

## Farm Clinic

Farm clinic is a facility developed and extended to the farmers for diagnosis and treatment of farm problems and to provide some specialised advice to individual farmers. The extension agency may set up farm clinic in the village and/or in the organization's headquarters and subcenters, where the relevant subject matter specialists in collaboration with the extension agents, discuss, diagnose and issue prescription treatment to farmers' problems, meeting those persons individually on fixed place, day and time.

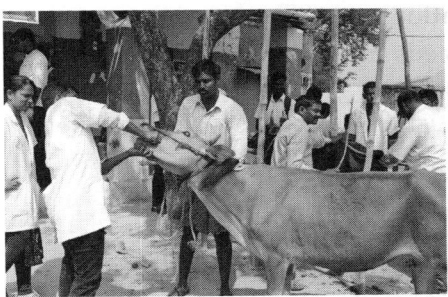

**Fig. 6.5:** Farm clinic

## GROUP TEACHING METHOD

Many of the important problems of villagers can be solved through group action, according to Leagans/ Legans (1961), 'a group is a body of individuals drawn together around a common interest'. Such a group (about twenty in number) discussion, is utilised to promote an objective group reaching collective decisions, through co-operative methods are (Fig. 6.6):

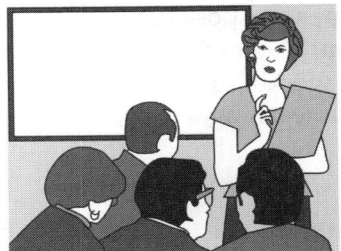

**Fig. 6.6:** Group teaching

| | |
|---|---|
| A. Minikit trial | B. Method demonstration |
| C. Field trip | D. Meetings |
| E. Field days/ Farmer's days | F. Farmer field school |

### Adaptive or Minikit Trial

- It is a method of determining the suitability or otherwise of a new practice in farmers situation. The objective of this method is to test innovative practices under the resources, constraints and abilities of the farmer.
- This is the first stage an innovation passes through, before it is taken up for result demonstration and method demonstration for large scale adoption. His trail involves selection of promising innovation, selection of innovative farmers, explanation of objectives to the farmers, implementation of trail in the farmer's field, follow-up, discussion with researchers and farmers, if required extending time,

exploring the suitability of the innovation to the farmers field and decision making on adoption.

- Limitations
  - Needs more time and energy of the extension worker
  - Satisfactory results may not be obtained if the practice or the farmers are not carefully chosen.

## Method Demonstration

This is the oldest form of teaching. Long before the language was developed, men taught their children how to hunt, how to milk the animal, etc. by demonstrating it. "It is relatively a short time demonstration given before a group to show how to carry out an entirely new practice or old practice in a better way."[1]

It is not providing the worth of the practice, but it tells how to do it. It is not an experiment, but it is a teaching effort. Here the extension worker shows the step by step procedure of the practice. The farmers watch the process and listen to the oral explanation to clear up points. To increase the farmers' confidence in their ability, in the presence of the extension worker, as many farmers as possible are asked to repeat the demonstration. The method demonstration is given by the extension worker himself or by a trained leader for the purpose of teaching a skill to a group.

### Objectives

1. To enable the people to acquire new skills.
2. To enable the people to improve upon their old skills.
3. To give confidence about the practicability.
4. To bring the research findings to the farmers.
5. To uphold the principle of seeing is believing, and learning by doing.
6. To make the learners do things more efficiently.

### Conducting the Demonstration

1. **Analyse the situation and determine the need:** Decide exactly what you want to accomplish with the demonstration. Check these objectives against such factors as whether or not the practice really is important and whether people can afford to practise it, whether supplies and services and equipment are available in sufficient quantity to permit its widespread use. Decide the number of demonstrations to be conducted.

2. **Consult the local leaders:** Talk over the problems with a few local leaders. Explain the purpose of demonstration to the farmers. Secure their approval to conduct demonstration.

3. **Plan the demonstration:** Decide the day to conduct the demonstration, select the site and the farmers. Invite the village leaders and leading farmers to witness the demonstration.

4. **Preparation for demonstration:** Plan your presentation step by step. Include inventory and summary portions. Gather all information. Familiarise yourself with the subject matter, check the research findings. Identify the key points for emphasis. List out the required materials and equipment.

5. **Rehearse the demonstration:** Practise the demonstration until you are thorough with all the steps. Memorise exactly what you should say or do at each step. Make sure that the points are clear from the audience point of view.

6. **Execute the demonstration:** When farmers have assembled to watch the demonstration explain how it is applicable to local problems. Show the step by step operation.

Invite persons in the audience to help you with different tasks. Use simple words. Make sure that all the audience can clearly see and hear. Emphasise the key points. Solicit questions. Repeat difficult steps. Then give opportunity to the learners to learn. Check the effectiveness of your instructions by having participants do one or more of the steps. Summarise the importance of the practice. Distribute supplemental teaching materials such as leaflets, bulletins, etc. Get the names of the participants who propose to adopt. This would help for the follow-up.

### Follow-up

Prepare a write-up about the demonstration for office record. Disseminate the demonstration details through press and AIR. Make a sample check to assess the extent of adoption. Visit the participant farmers' farm frequently to give necessary assistances. Often the method demonstration paves way for the result demonstration.

### Suggestion for Effective Conduct

1. Find out the audience's level of knowledge and literacy to plan the demonstration.
2. Find out the resources available.

---

1. J.P. Leagans, "Extension Education in Community Development". op. cit.

3. A poor demonstration is worse than none at all.
4. Do not try to show too much.
5. Location should be suitable for both the farmers and the extension workers.
6. Keep the records, photos, slides, news write-up, etc.

### Advantages

1. It is very effective in teaching new skill.
2. It stimulates action.
3. Builds confidence.
4. Serves publicity purpose.
5. It introduces a change of practice at low cost.

### Limitations

1. Suited only to the 'skill involving technologies'.
2. Transporting the materials and equipments to the demonstration plot is difficult.
3. It causes a setback if whole programme is improperly co-ordinated.

### Difference between Result and Method Demonstrations

| Result demonstration | Method demonstration |
|---|---|
| 1. To prove the value of a recommended practice in the local farm is the main purpose | To teach a new skill or old one in an improved way |
| 2. Here, the farmer is the demonstrator. He conducts the result demonstration under the guidance of extension worker | Extension worker himself or trained local leader conducts the demonstration |
| 3. The farmer who conducts the demonstration and other farmers who visit the demonstration farm may be benefited | Participants of demonstration may be benefited |
| 4. Maintenance of record essential | Not essential |
| 5. It requires long time to complete the demonstration | Relatively short time is required |
| 6. It involves much cost | Relatively cheap |
| 7. Environmental factors may have significant effect on the results | May not be affected |

## Field Trips and Tours

Tours and field trips are methods of extension teaching which appeal to man's desire to go places and see things.[1] A group of interested farmers, accompanied and guided by extension worker, goes on tour to see

and gain first-hand knowledge of improved practices in their natural setting. This visit may be to the research farms, demonstration plots, farms of progressive farmers, institutions, etc.

### Purpose of Tour

a. To stimulate interest, conviction and action in respect of a specific purpose.
b. To impress the group about the feasibility and utility of a series of related practices.
c. To induce a spirit of healthy competition.
d. To help people to recognise problems, to develop interest, to generate discussions and to promote action.
e. To see the results of new practice. Operation of new tools and implements and to see the accomplishments of other villages, college farms etc.

### Procedure

1. Planning
2. Conducting
3. Follow-up

#### Planning

Plan the trip on the basis of dimension of places, things to be seen and learnt, necessary permissions, date, time, transport, size of the group, food, accommodation, refreshments, instructions to be given to the participants, advance visit if possible, etc.

#### Conducting tour

a. Prepare and give tour programme to the participants.
b. The extension worker should keep the interest of the group always in mind.
c. Once they reach the places of visit the extension worker should allow every one of the group to see, hear and discuss at the place of visit.
d. Allow sufficient time to put questions and get answers from the concerned authority.
e. Encourage the farmers to take notes of achievements seen.
f. The programme should not be overcrowded because the farmer may lose interest.
g. Provide recreation and keep the group cheerful.
h. Contact the farmers both individually and in group and discuss.

---

1. Using Visuals in Agricultural Extension Programs—ESO-561 International Cooperation Administration and Federal Extension Service. op. cit.

i. Recognise the bright and successful among the group taken on tour.

j. Adhere to the schedule.

### Follow-up

Record the trip with regard to the participant's name and other details in order to facilitate follow-up. In the follow-up action, make post-trip contact with the participants, arrangements for necessary supply and services, aim for desired action, recognition to successful members, publicity materials building, etc.

### Suggestion for Successful Tour

1. Planning for all arrangements should be made in advance.
2. Participants should be homogenous.
3. Number of participants should be limited to 30.
4. Distribute responsibility to the leading members of the group.

### Advantages

a. Participants gain first-hand knowledge of improved practices and are stimulated to action.

b. Best suited to the 'show me' type of people.

c. Adoption percentage is high.

d. Widens the vision of farmers.

e. Caters to group psychology and leadership.

f. It has the entertainment and site seeing values.

g. It develops better personal relationship between the participants and extension worker.

### Limitations

1. It is the most expensive method.
2. It involves time, transport and other number of preparations.
3. It is difficult to fix up season and time suitable for all.
4. Frustration may result if the tour is badly conducted.
5. There is risk of accident.
6. The recreational aspect may mask the educational aspect.

## Meetings

Meetings are one of the oldest and the most important group methods of extension teaching. If properly arranged and conducted, they rank high in ratio of practices adopted in relation to cost as compared with other methods. The term meeting includes all kinds of meetings held by extension worker. In size the meeting varies from small committee meeting to large special occasion meetings with meals or festivals and attended by thousands.

### Types of Meetings

Kelsey and Hearne[1] (1963) identify five general types of meetings involved in extension work:

1. Organization meetings (board of directors' meet, youth clubs)
2. Planning meetings (village planning meeting)
3. Training meetings (rural leaders' training)
4. Special interest meetings (special meeting about dairying)
5. Community meetings (community meet for general problems).

### Other Classifications of Meetings

1. General meetings, 2. Lecture, 3. Group discussion, 4. Debate, 5. Symposium, 6. Panel, 7. Forum, 8. Buzz sessions 9. Workshop, 10. Seminar; 11. Conference, 12. Institute, 13. Syndicate studies,14. Brain trust or Brain storming.

### Planning the Meeting

Plan the meeting with the representatives of the people for whom it is held.

1. Select the topics, 2. Timing, 3. Place, 4. Speaker and chairman 5. Publicity and material arrangements.

Consider these factors in planning meetings:

1. Size of the audience.
2. Character of the audience.
3. Comfortable physical facilities.
4. Be time conscious, do not overcrowd the programme.
5. Do not allow unrelated announcements and unscheduled speakers to prolong the programme and distract the audience.

Subsequently the extension worker has to conduct the meeting following the procedures specified for each type of meeting. The last step is follow-up. It includes summary preparation, and sending press reports, displays and evaluation.

### General Meeting

General meeting is broadly a meeting of heterogenous participants wherein certain information is passed on

1. L.D. Kelsey and C.C. Hearne, "Co-operative Extension Work", op.cit.

for consideration and future action. This is employed effectively to reach and serve large numbers to prepare the people for other methods of extension work; to find the reaction of the people to certain activities.[1] Plan the meeting in advance as mentioned before.

## Conducting the meeting

While conducting the general meeting the following points are to be borne in mind:

1. Hold the meeting preferably in a central place having all physical facilities.
2. Preferably the meeting should be held in a days notice during summer/off seasons for light farm work.
3. Be prompt in starting and closing the meeting.
4. Though giving allowance for liberal discussion, focus attention on the purpose of the meeting.
5. Avoid sharp conflicts.
6. Use visual materials if available.
7. Take advantage of group psychology and employ appeals to arose interest and stimulate action.
8. Give recognition to all sections and groups participating.
9. Associate local leaders for welcoming the gathering or thanking the participants if not for presiding.
10. Acknowledge services briefly and then indicate the follow-up work, if any.
11. Prepare news reports of the meeting and publicise.
12. If possible arrange exhibition and film shows.
13. Distribute relevant folders or pamphlets at the time of break.

## Application

This meeting could be employed:

1. To introduce the community development programme or any welfare programme.
2. To present the annual programme of extension activities.
3. To enlist people's participation in community work.

## Advantages

1. Large number of people can be reached.
2. Serves as a preparatory stage for other methods.
3. Group psychology can be used in promoting the programme.

4. Reactions of the people to a programme can be assessed.
5. Adoption of practices can be accomplished at low cost.

## Limitations

1. Meeting place and facilities are not always adequate.
2. Scope for discussion is limited except possibly for a few questions and answers.
3. Handling the topic becomes difficult because of mixed composition of audience.
4. Circumstances beyond control like fractions and weather might reduce the attendance.

## Lecture (Fig. 6.7)

Lecture is the most commonly used method. Lecture is the best method for presenting information to large number of persons in short period of time. Its weakness is that it is a one way communication method. The range of subjects that can be covered by this method is unlimited. It has the advantage of large group communication; when it is necessary to cover a large quantity of information in a given time, at the time of initiating new programmes to arose interest; for giving factual information; when providing a common background of information as a basis for further study; to supplement other methods, etc. Lecture is not effective for skill teaching; when group members participation is needed; when problems are to be solved; etc.

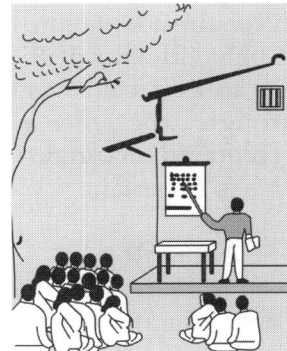

**Fig. 6.7:** Lecture

## Extension Talk (Fig. 6.8)

Most of us spend about seven out of every ten working hours communicating with others. Three-fourths of our communication is done by speech. Research reveals that an average person speaks some 34,020 words per day. That is equal to several books a week, more than

1. J.P. Leagans, "Extension Education in Community Development", op. cit.

120 lakh words a year. Speech is 'essential' to some seven out of ten jobs in our country.

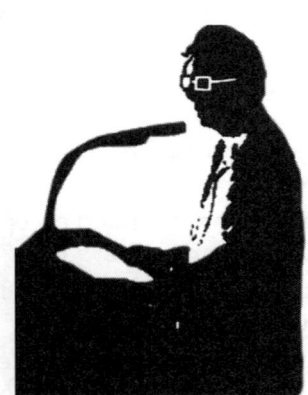

**Fig. 6.8:** Extension talk

There are countless situations in which we interact with other human beings and strive to get their valued co-operation and support. Interaction requires interpersonal communication in a variety of ways. Extension talk (public speaking) is one of the most powerful ways through which we can communicate with others.

Public speaking is an art. If one wants to be successful in any walk of life, he should learn the art of public speaking. One of the essentials for it is to have a burning desire is to become a great public speaker. Public speaking is the shortcut to distinction. If you are so inclined you can certainly acquire the skills, and master techniques required to make a speech that is effective, informative, eloquent and entertaining.

Becoming an effective communicator in inter-personal relationship involves a wide range of skills. Most of the skills require adaptation, i.e. moulding our communication behaviour to fit the circumstances. Almost all of them are perfected over the time, through experience. Through experience we learn what is required and not required for certain situations, people and message—this is important.

### a. Need for public speaking

Often the extension workers have to address the public in their project area. The need to speak in a manner that is both impressive and expressive, is felt today by people in all walks of life but not only the extension personnel also the professionals.

Businessmen, dignitaries, politicians, students, teachers and members of social organisation have felt all the growing need to improve their art of speaking. The need to deliver a speech can arise in almost any line of work at one time or another, especially if one wishes to move upwards in one's profession. The

inability to speak before groups cannot only be embarrassing, it can cost you a promotion or spoil a chance to demonstrate your expertise at your job. Therefore, if you want to be successful in any walk of life you should learn the art of public speaking.

If you are a leader of the state or nation and you deliver a speech, people will listen to you though you may not a good speaker, but that is because you are the leader. Otherwise you have to make an impressive speech if you want people to pay attention to you with interest. The most effective way of projecting one's personality is through speaking.

### b. Qualities of a good speaker

Those who want to become a good speaker should have the following qualities:

1. He should be a voracious reader and have deep and wide knowledge of various subjects.
2. He should be a good listener. Whenever chances occur, he must attend good speaker's meeting.
3. He must be a creative thinker and also have presence of mind.
4. He should have attractive voice and know the art of voice modulation.
5. Since words are the tools to express ideas, good speaker must be fluent in the language in which he wants to become a public speaker.
6. He should have good memory.
7. He should know the group psychology.
8. He should have conviction, courage, confidence and convincing power.
9. He should have pleasing appearance.

When we communicate with others, besides the force of our utterance, our gestures, our personality, our voice, our philosophy of life, our past experiences, our capacity to draw others' attention to us, our general reading, etc, also help us considerably.

**Reading:** To acquire knowledge one has to read lot of books, and journals. Not only for information but also to acquire more words. People used to say about the popular speaker and the then Chief Minister of Tamil Nadu. Anna Durai, that the entire Chennai Kannimara Library was in his brain. The sound knowledge he acquired due to his voracious he bit reading habit helped to win the hearts of the people.

**Thinking:** As a speaker speaks he simultaneously keeps on thinking. So, speaking and thinking are inter-connected.

**Listening:** When others are talking the speaker's has to listen to them attentively in order to determine how he is going to respond or find out how they are reacting to his words. So, a third dimension is added to speaking and thinking.

**Talking:** So, now the speaker's circle of inner activities is made up of reading, thinking, listening and talking. To make these activities more effective he has constantly to draw upon practice or experiences. Now the efforts are in five directions, viz. reading, thinking, listening, talking and practising. These activities do not take place one after the other. They are closely related and are carried on simultaneously.

**Conviction:** As a speaker, one will be required to deliver his ideas on a subject. He must have conviction in what he says. He must sincerely believe in his own words. If he is dishonest, how so ever strongly he might preach the advantages of honesty, no one is going to be convinced. Abraham Lincoln strongly believed that slavery was a blot on the face of humanity. So, when he spoke against slavery, people were moved with pity for the unfortunate slaves and supported Lincoln in his mission of abolishing slavery. Gandhiji believed that non-violence could be a powerful tool to win freedom. Both Lincoln and Gandhiji derived their strength from their conviction.

**Courage:** However, conviction alone will not help to become a good public speaker. He might have conviction in a certain point of view, but to be convincing, he should also have the courage to start it. Conviction and courage sustain each other. Conviction without courage is lame or cripple. Courage without conviction is rudderless. Just as one needs well defined goals in life, speaker has well defined goals. He must be clear about what he wants to say. He must have conviction in it and the courage to say it. Swami Vivekananda once addressed his fellow Indians in the following words: "You are not sheep. You are not a goat. You are a lion. So, be bold. Be fearless."

**Confidence:** The next essential requirement is confidence. As a human being the speaker has unlimited potential. He is an inexhaustive reservoir of energy, and talent, but he does not know himself. He must realise himself, his potential and buildup of self-confidence. Our dormant self, is a mighty storehouse. If he has confidence in himself, he can carry mammoth crowds with him. If he lacks confidence, he will simply make a fool of himself, for he will become nervous when he goes to the stage and people will only laugh at him.

**Convincing:** If one has conviction, courage and confidence then convincing others is relatively easy. It will inevitably follow, as spring follows winter.

**Memory:** Good memory is very important for a public speaker. Human memory is just fantastic. It you start developing it, only sky is the limit. A good memory is a great asset. When an experienced speaker stands up to speak; he is relaxed. He stands in an easy way. He had made his speech flexible. He has great trust in his inner potential, his past experiences, his creative thoughts which come from his gray matter and help him to deliver his speech impressively. Many ideas, thoughts, examples come to his mind and contribute significantly to make his speech remarkable. This is because of his memory.

Speaker with poor memory often forgets his points. Some time he confuses the facts. He scratches his head, fumbles and falters and on the whole makes a fool of himself. He finds himself in a situation that is not only embarrassing but also humiliating. Our mind is just like a horse. A trainer trains the horse to do great things. In the same way we can train our minds to increase our memory.

"When we concentrate on something, it goes very deep into our minds and gets registered in our memory bank. Power of suggestion also helps us to improve our memory (self-hypnosis). Repetition is also an important aid to memory. When we associate new things with old ones by mental filing system, it becomes easy for us to remember them. Numerical mental exercise also improves memory. It is better to commit things to memory when we are fresh, for example in the morning after a sound sleep. These periods of freshness may be called green periods. Loud reading also helps us to memories things.[1]

You can yourself be the best judge of what devices to use to develop your memory. A sharp memory is a very powerful aid. It is possible for you to sharpen your memory provided you are keen to do it.

**Group psychology:** Knowledge of group psychology is also essential for the public speaker to measure the audience response as to change his style, mode and other techniques of presentation and to have control over the audience.

**Time Consciousness:** Time consciousness is an important attribute required to let an effective public speaker. The speaker should know how to cut short or prolong his speech depending upon the availability of time.

---

1. P. Mathialagan. "How to Develop Your Memory", Athiyaman Pathippagam, Namakkal, India, 1995.

**Cheerfulness:** Having a cheerful face is an essential quality for the successful speaker.

### c. Various dimensions of public speaking

1. **Selection of topic:** Success of public speaking begins with the selection of the topic. Making an early selection should be a very big advantage. It will give you sufficient time for preparation. It will eliminate strain and tension and keep you relaxed.

   Choose a theme on a specific topic. Before selection of subject find out the characteristics of the audience you are to speak to and what they want to know. What is their intellectual level, what kind of allusions will be intelligible to them, what kind of style they would be able to appreciate. Hence, the topic selected should be relevant to the audience and to their interest. If the topic is a subject of tropical interest or reflects current information, it will be easier for the speaker to catch the attention of the audience.

   As an extension worker of animal husbandry you can select the topic related to current problems in livestock or poultry farming in that area. Sometimes you may be asked to deliver speech at some special functions in schools, other clubs, etc. because extension worker is an important person in the rural area. On such occasions the subject you choose should carry your individual stamp. You may even talk about your successes, your desires, your failures, in fact, any of your experiences which you think could interest and benefit others. With such a subject, you will not be delivering a dry discourse mechanically.

2. **Collection of facts:** Once you have selected your topic, begin planning your speech. Give it a deep thought, that way ideas will come gradually over a period of time. Ponder over it. Sleep with it, and dream with it. Transact through all available related books and journals. If you want to become a good speaker collect cuttings of any interesting or useful pieces of writing you come across. File these cuttings systematically. Make an index of the file to facilitate easy access to the desired information when needed. Discuss it with idea that comes to your mind, do not ignore it, however little it might be. Remember that it is only little drops of water that make mighty oceans. Therefore collect all facts.

   Keep on asking all kinds of questions like how, why, when, where, who and what related to your topic. Answers to these questions will help you to get new ideas. Collect a more material than you intend to use in your speech. It is unwise to attempt to formulate your speech just the night before you are due to deliver it. The more time you give yourself the clearer your thoughts will be.

3. **Planning and organising a talk:** Organisation has something to do with the sequence of ideas. How is the talk to be started, put forward and concluded.

   *Methodology:* The methodology of organisation of talk varies with the speaker, audience and subject. Speech on the same topic will have to be organised differently when delivered to two different groups, e.g. college students and rural farmers.

   *Discarding:* After collecting the facts, if suppose you are having hundred ideas, discard ninety of them. Develop additional ideas and thoughts to keep in reserve. It will give you great confidence.

   *Message:* Whatever be the subject, you should be absolutely clean about one point; your talk must have a real message in it. A message from your heart, a message that reflects you, a message that is yours.

   *Inject humour:* Include in your speech a few stories and personal anecdotes that will help to make the speech more entertaining. Inject humour where you can, but only if really relevant and really funny.

   *Short speech:* Know the time allotted to you and prepare. Keep the speech short. No speech will ever be criticized for being too short; the same cannot be said if it is too long! Before your speech find out exactly how long you will be required to speak, and then make every effort to keep it within the time frame.

   *Accuracy:* Be accurate and authentic. If you are not sure about facts, verify them from same reliable source.

   *Visuals:* Prepare some suitable visuals related to your speech. The visuals enhance the value of your speech. It will make the speech more informative, more lively, more intimate. It will also give you relief during your talk.

   *Key cards:* After organising the speech, well go through the script for few times to remember the main points. Those who are not confident enough of their memory can prepare 'key cards'. For example, if you are going to make a speech before a group of people about 'personality development' and you wish to cover ten good points in 20 minutes allotted to you take 10 cards—on the basis of the one card one-point for the ten points you intend to cover. Think hard on the points and reduce them to one-word phrase each (keyword). Suppose one of the points you want to discuss is the role of interpersonal communication skill in personality development. Take one of the 10 cards and write 'communication'. Do the same thing with the other points as well.

*Rehearsal:* Rehearse or go over the talk yourself. Try it out on your family. The more you practise the more confident you will feel, the more confident you feel the more relaxed your eventual performance will be. It is only when you are in complete command of yourself and your material that your speech will be spontaneous. Speaking effortlessly is hard work. Many world great speakers had this habit of practising before delivering the speech, e.g. Winston Churchill.

If it is a technical meeting, better rehearse under conditions similar to those under which you will actually speak. Consider the physical facilities like capacity of the auditorium, the seating, lighting arrangements, the voice amplification system, the use of podium, whether you will be standing or sitting, etc. Rehearse with your visual aids so that you are able to handle them easily, efficiently and naturally. If possible, request same of your friends to listen to your rehearsal and get feedback from them.

*Voice:* The voice should be sweet and entertaining. To have good voice and voice modulation tongue twister may be practised. Which is as follows: "Betty botter bought a bit of butter, the butter was bitter so betty botter put some better butter to make the bitter butter better". Voice modulation is important to maintain the interest of the audience, avoid monotone, and emphasise the points. This art can be acquired by practice. But it is a difficult thing to do. A better rule to simply follow is to vary your speed. When you are making an important point make it slowly and intentionally.

*Speed:* To correct the speed of speech delivery, time and to check and change the pronunciation an audiotape recorder can be utilised so that you can make adjustments, if necessary.

*Travel:* If you have to travel for a long time to reach the meeting spot plan and make advance arrangements to reach the place well in advance.

4. **Effective presentation techniques:** In a speech, there are three factors involved—who says it? What he says in it? How he says it? And these three, the third factor is the most important. For effective presentation or communication the following techniques can be followed:

1. Walk in confidently, do not to exhibit the fear, stand up right and keep the feet apart, clear the voice, check the mike by giving it a mild tap.

2. Before giving your speech make a survey of the audience, size, age group, composition, tolerance time, etc. and make sure that everyone can see and hear you. If some persons are standing in the rear and there are seats ask the organisers to make them be seated.

3. The opening sentence of the talk should arouse curiosity in the audience to know more from you. So, start with an interesting story, quotation, jokes, anecdotes, etc. Be careful with these as it is the rare person who can deliver a story successfully. Nothing is less humorous than a supposedly funny story poorly told. When delivering your speech, be warm, be humane and be natural and never be discouraged. Treat your audience as a group of intimate friends and speak to them not to dictate but to share.

Speak in a loud and clear voice. Come direct to the point. Choose your vocabulary carefully, make direct statements. Use simple language. Use transactional phrases between ideas as a clue to the listeners of what is to come, e.g. "Now, lets see the causes of the emerging diseases", as an introduction to the new topic. Cultivate an informal style especially while addressing the rural people. These days, only speakers with a conversational ring are considered to be effective.

4. First, the audience must feel that there a message is being delivered from the heart of the speaker and it is going directly deep into their hearts.

5. Have a series of specific points to follow. Tell the audience in advance what you are going to do. This lets them realize where you are in your talk, and where the end is to come. Repeat the point wherever possible.

6. Illustrate your talk with more personal examples and, if possible, use suitable visuals.

Maintain eye contact with each of the listeners present in the hall. Keep your eyes moving over your listeners. It may be difficult to develop eye contact with all the audience. Move from left to right, then forward to backward, section to section. At least pick out few friendly faces, who seem to indicate that they are following you, and focus on them".[1]

7. After you have made an important point in your speech, you should pause for a few seconds. When you tell a story or some events before, telling the climax keep silent for a few seconds. This will stimulate the interest and everybody will be attentive. This sudden silence will have the same effect as a sudden noise. Remember that there are moments when silence is more articulate than words. Pause is a very powerful tool which a speaker should never forget to use effectively. A meaningful pause after well made point will help you to drive home the point successfully. As an extension speaker you can use this pause when you ask a question, real or rhetorical. Let the group think about their answers for a few seconds.

8. Use natural gestures. Movement of head, a wave of the arm, raising the eyebrows, turning the head, etc. are gestures. These should be spontaneous. They should give life to talk by suitable articulation and emotional expressions.

9. By watching the audience's body language and faces you can know their interest, approval, disapproval, lack of interest and drowsiness. Closed signals like crossed arms, turning away, fidgeting usually indicate there has been some annoying change in the room's environment. Audience's facial expressions are the best guide for the speaker to gauge success or failure of his talk. If your audience begin to yawn, respect their fatigue. Then windup as quickly as possible and if the audience is not reacting to a humour, then drop it. Keep a specially careful eye on the people at the back. If they are shifting around while every one else is still, then reason is most possible that they can not hear you properly. Speak up. Keep the speech as brief as possible without actually leaving out valuable points. Better to stop, while the audience's interest is high than to keep on until they become restless and bored.

10. Express, argue and appeal: Write it and order the selected ideas. Buildup your speech around a central theme. Good talk can be organised in the following ways:

    **a. Express your facts**

    **b. Argue for your facts**

**c. Appeal for the action at three stages—introduction, body and conclusion.**

11. Inform the audience beforehand whether they can ask questions in the middle or at the end of the speech. Try to be courteous when someone asks a question you have just finished answering. In big gathering or where time may not permit questions, you may suggest that people come afterwards and you would be happy to speak with them.

12. Be careful with the conclusion at the end of your talk. Try to spell only the major points discussed, not a complete review. Your conclusion should consist of one or two important sentences. Some commonly used techniques for wrapping up a presentation are: Summarizing the main points briefly. Re-emphasizing the reasons why the subject is important to the listeners. Suggesting something the listeners can do to put the ideas that have been presented into action.

13. Your ending is more important than beginning. End your speech with a laugh or a thought-provoking remark. Your success as a public speaker largely depends not on how you start but how you finish your talk which the audience will take home with them. Before you conclude your talk which the audience will take home with them, acknowledge the organizers and audience in your speech.

*Other points*

1. Speaker's dress should suit the occasion. It should be neat and acceptable to audience. Old time speakers used to put on a coat even in the hot summer afternoon. Nowadays, it is just not done. People come to platform wearing all kinds of informal dresses. It is a healthy practice, since it removes the barriers between the speaker and the audience.

2. In village condition you may not be able to provide chair to all the rural audience. At least ensure that sufficient floor space is provided for comfortable seating.

3. In rural condition all meetings will be first attended by the small children. Usually they are the first row audience. The actual target group of our talk may be seated at back. The children must be tactfully managed otherwise they will spoil the entire atmosphere of the meeting.

4. Microphone should be in good working condition. Many times improper selection of public address

1. R.K. Samanta. "Semantics in Scientific Communication". Training Coursc Reading Material, NAARM, Hyderabad.

system distracts the audience's attention and spoils the charm of the meeting.

5. The distance between stage and the audience must be close otherwise the speaker will not be able to see the faces of the audience.

6. Persons on the stage must sit calmly. They should not talk with others while the speaker is delivering the speech. That will distract the audience's attention from the speaker.

### Don'ts in public speaking

1. Do not cover too many points—be brief—especially learners should not speak for more than two or three minutes. Don't underestimate two or three minutes' duration. Don't speak beyond your allotted time.

2. Do not say anything that does not carry the mark of your conviction. Don't start with an irrelevant joke or story. To many presenters turn out to be entertaining but the audience is left wondering what was the message? While presenting jokes the speaker himself should not laugh. Allow the people to enjoy. But you can smile. While people enjoy your speech, say by laughing or clapping, do not speak continuously, please wait for a few second to let and then is finish what you are saying.

3. Avoid distracting mannerism like scratching your nose, putting your hand near your face, playing with shirt buttons, rotating the hand watch, etc.

4. Do not exhibit your nervousness. Don't worry about being nervous.

5. Do not apologie for your shortcomings and limitations except as good manners require, for example, for being late. If this is necessary, be convincingly brief.

6. Do not use a lot of unnatural gesture. They will probably look foolish and pointless to the audience.

7. Do not memories or read a speech script. Use your key cards for reference.

8. Do not repeat the same words or phrases each time you give the presentation, the ideal are the same and your choice of words will be free and natural.

9. Do not come to the stage with dirty dress, i.e. do not come dressed for the field.

10. Do not speak too loudly. Do not stand very close to microphone. Do not hold or touch or tap the mike. If you like to check it, do by making a simple blow of air.

11. Do not talk down to the audience, people are smarter than we give them credit for.

12. Do not belittle the introduction you were given by the local man who introduced you.

13. Do not play down a member of the audience. You do yourself more damage by this than the one you are trying to hurt. This is especially important to remember when questions are being asked. Try not to get angry or provoked, and if you do, try not to express it. Avoid being pedantic.

14. Do not be late. Reach the meeting place well in advance so that you can avoid tension, you need not lose your balance.

15. Avoid distributing handouts or supplying tea and biscuits or any drinks when someone is delivering his speech. This may distract the audience's attention from the speaker.

### Discussion Type of Meetings

**Group discussion** (Fig. 6.9): Group discussion is a method by which two or more persons meet, express or convey their ideas, clarity and bring about a solution to the commonly felt problems by their own efforts.

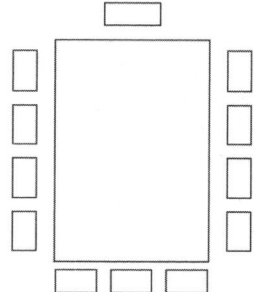

**Fig. 6.9:** Group discussion

### Objectives

1. Democracy in action involves group functioning.

2. Systematic discussion among representative persons promotes the analysis of commonly felt needs.

3. We can solve many important problems or meet the needs only through group action.

4. Group discussion provides opportunity to the members of the group to exchange their experience or their points of view.

5. It promotes the habit of group thinking, group planning, group action and expression.

6. Most of the problems in many villages could be solved by group action which means that there should be organised group in the village with a group leader.

7. Organised group may not always be available in a village. Lack of organised group by itself is a

challenge for the extension worker. The village group must be identified first than the public interest should be focussed on a problem to mobilise the villagers to action.

8. Group discussion is a miniature democracy giving equal rights, privileges and opportunities to every members to discuss an issue.

**How to conduct a group discussion?**

1. The extension worker or village leader should locate and identify the individuals interested in a particular problem through individual contact and invite them informally to meet for informal group discussion.

2. The time, date, place and the topic should be informed to the people concerned well in advance.

3. The seating arrangements should be in a circular or semi-circular fashion, so that the speaker face the audience.

4. The extension worker should receive the member with a welcoming smile and see that they are comfortably seated.

5. He should find out whether any one member of the group is capable of leading the discussion and request him to start the discussion. If nobody prefers to lead the discussion, the extension worker himself take the lead.

6. The atmosphere of the meeting should be kept friendly and informal.

7. The group leader should be elected democratically.

8. At the beginning of discussion, ideas should be invited from members of the group and the problems should be defined. If the person goes on talking the extension worker should politely ask him to end his speech. The easiest way to avoid this is for the extension worker to tell him, "You have given a nice idea and spoken nicely. Shall we hear others' opinion also?

9. Extension worker should not dominate the discussion.

10. Extension worker should encourage all the persons of the group to express their suggestions, because the objective of group discussion is to get maximum participation by the members present.

11. The discussion should promote recognition of problem by the group and also create the desire for a solution. All the available information about the problem should be presented before the group, preferably with some visual aids.

12. The extension worker should not give the impression that his solution is the best and should not condemn the existing and suggested practices. Even a shyperson of the groups should be persuaded by the extension worker to give his suggestion. It is quiet possible that his suggestion may be the best of all suggestions.

13. At the end of group, discussion made the summary of the problem; solution arrived at by the members through discussion and the actions that are to be taken should be given.

14. Appreciate the members for their valuable contribution.

15. Undertake a systematic follow-up.

**Application**

- Intensive deworming for sheep.
- Disease prevention measures.
- Formation and working of co-operation.

**Advantages**

1. Every participant shares the pride of having helped in solving the problem.
2. Helps in deciding the debatable issues.
3. Leaders, group interests and problems are discovered.
4. Group planning and group action results.
5. Fairly large numbers can be reached.

**Limitations**

1. Group factions in the village might hinder the effective working of the method.
2. 'Traditional leaders', who are not functional, come in the way of group activities.
3. Possibility of creating rivalries.
4. Difficult to avoid unconnected persons' attendance.

2. **Debate:** The common pattern is to have two teams, one representing positive or affirmative and the other the negative side of the topic. Thus, there is a team of speakers for the each side. Each speaker is allowed a definite period of time. The great danger in this method is that the debate may become highly antagonistic and in the interest of winning talkers may distort the information. The big advantage in a debate is that more than one side of a question is presented.

3. **Symposium** (Fig. 6.10): This is a short series of lectures, usually by 2 to 5 speakers, on the various aspects of a single subject or a problem, each with a different view point. Subject is not necessarily

controversial. A moderator controls subject matter and time. The speakers are experts of the subjects on which they speak. The speakers may be followed by a forum to facilitate mastery of information. The main advantage of this method is two or more experts present the same topic favourably.

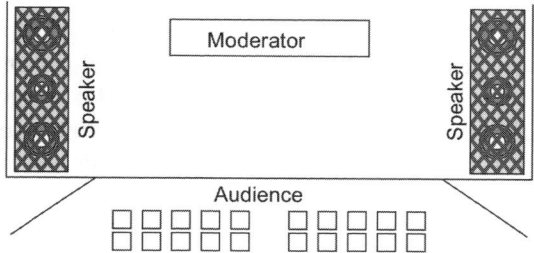

**Fig. 6.10:** Symposium

4. **Panel discussion** (Fig. 6.11): This is an informal conversation before audience by a selected group of persons (3 to 6) under a moderator. It is excellent for presenting controversial subjects and varying points of view. The panel members are usually seated in a semi-circle so that they can see each other and also face the audience. The leader introduces the topic and puts some questions. There are three types of panels:

   i. **Question-answer:** Panel discussion in which the presentation is actually a series of questions by the leader and the answers by members.

   ii. **Set-speech panel:** In which members deliver speech.

   iii. **Conversational panel:** In which members hold conversation among themselves on the topic, with questions and comments going from one member to another.

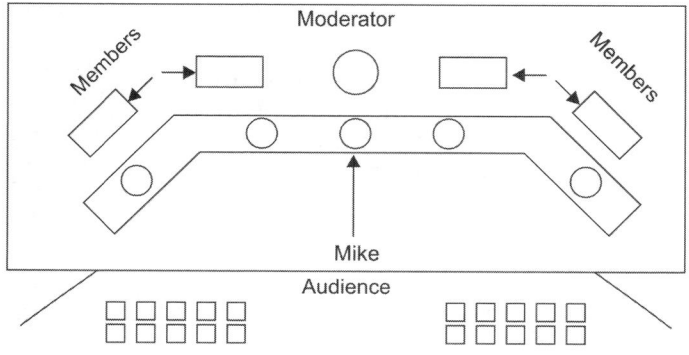

**Fig. 6.11:** Panel

The third type is more near to the definition of panel discussion than the other two. Any topic is suitable for panel discussion. The special advantage

is the spontaneous conversation on some subject may have more interest than the lecture.

5. **'Huddle' method (Discussion 66 or Philips 66):** This is a device for breaking down a large group into small units to facilitate discussion—six persons discussing a subject for six minutes.

6. **Forum** (Fig. 6.12): It is a discussion period that may follow panel discussion, symposium, lecture, etc. e.g. lecture forum, discussion forum and film forum.

   Audience ask questions and get their doubts clarified and also get additional information. This helps in understanding information correctly. Forum is rarely used as an isolated technique.

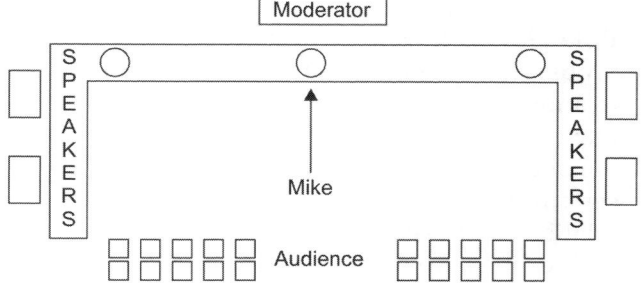

**Fig. 6.12:** Forum

7. **Buzz group** (Fig. 6.13): This method is followed with large groups when limited time is available for discussion. The audience are divided into smaller units for a short period. The secretary for each group records the discussions and presents a report to entire audience, when they all assemble again.

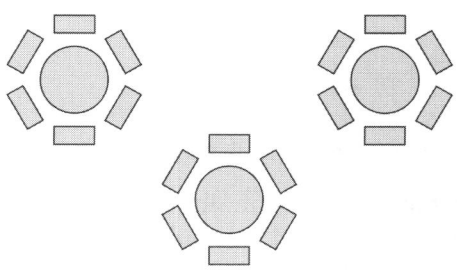

**Fig. 6.13:** Buzz group

8. **Brain storming sessions:** It is a type of small group interaction designed to encourage the free flow of ideas on an unrestricted basis and without any limitations. This newest idea is called a brain trust or brain storming in which questions are posed and the participating 'brains' express their opinions and views. It is a form of creative thinking in which judicious reasoning gives way to creative initiative. Participants are encouraged to list with in a period of time all the ideas that come to their minds

regarding some problem and are asked not to judge the ideas during the brain storming session. Judgement will come at a later period in which all the contributions will be sorted out, evaluated and perhaps later adopted.

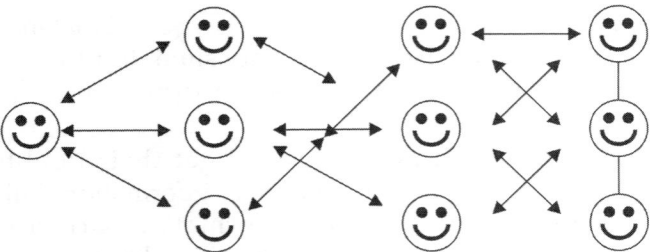

**Fig. 6.14:** Brain storming session

9. **Role playing** (Fig. 6.15): It is the dramatisation of a problem or a situation in the general area of human relations. The technique of role playing is based on our natural inclination to imagine ourselves in a particular situation. This method can bring out certain insights relating to human behaviour and relations and bring to the surface mental reactions and feelings. Roles are usually assigned to various members of the group who act out the problem situation. In most cases no script is used, but considerable briefing and planning proceeds the role playing scene.

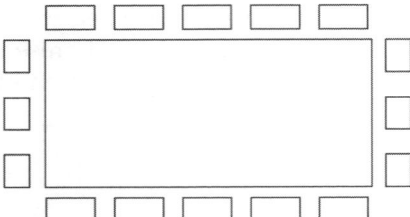

**Fig. 6.15:** Role playing

10. **Workshop:** It is essentially a long meeting of one day to several weeks, involving all participants. There must be a planning session in which the participants are involved in the discussions from the beginning. There must be considerable time for work session. There must be summarising and evaluating session at the closure. The workshop, as the name implies, must produce something at the end a report, a publication, a visual or any other material object.

11. **Seminar:** It is one of the most important forms of group discussion. The discussion leader introduces the topic to be discussed. Members of the audience discuss the subject to which ready answers are not available. This method has the advantage of pooling together the opinions of a large number of persons.

12. **Conference:** A pooling of experiences and opinions among a group of people who have special qualifications in an area.

13. **Institute:** Consists of a series of meetings and lectures. They are a source of new information and new ideas.

14. **Syndicate studies:** This follows the seminar method and focuses on any particular subject or problem. Resource men are utilised for this method. Group discussion, supplemented by the available literature, is the method. The report is brought out at the end. It may take a month's time or more with 10–12 sittings.

## Puppetry

Puppetry is the most suitable for villages. It is not an expensive activity and an easily acquired art. The puppets can hold an audience, provided they are played with a lively sense of drama. Lessons about health, literacy, agriculture, animal husbandry home making, etc. can be taught easily with the help of puppetry. The object of puppetry is teaching and entertainment simultaneously.

### Types of puppets

The puppets are of four types:
1. Glove or hand puppets.
2. String puppets.
3. Rod puppets.
4. Shadow puppets.

### Conducting puppetry

Out of various types, the glove puppet is the simple and easy to be worked with. It is like a three-fingered glove which fits in the hand of the operator. The first finger is inserted inside the head of the puppet and moves it. The middle finger and thumb fit in the hands and move them. The dress covers the hand and forearm. One person can operate two puppets at a time. In a puppet play, the following points should be observed:

1. Never try to teach or preach too much as it makes the audience bore.
2. The lesson should be illustrated by a story.
3. The story should have a dramatic value.
4. There should not be a silent pause when the play is on.

5. Dialogues should be quick and speeches and scenes short.

6. There should be lot of action.

7. Wit and humour should be introduced even in tragedies.

8. Music, songs and poems of short nature, should be repeated at intervals to drive the lesson home and help the audience to remember the lesson.

9. The story, illustrations and situations displayed in the drama of a puppet, should relate to everyday life.

10. In the art of puppetry, voice of different puppets should be different, so that the puppet which is talking can be identified.

## Songs and Drama

### Songs

The villagers have a great fascination for folk songs, dance and dramas. These are very good sources for conveying information in a better way. The monotony of discussion of serious nature, in a meeting, can be broken by light songs.

1. The song should be composed on the subjects which are to be communicated to the people.

2. They should be in the form of a story with a moral. The tune of the song should be popular and local, which villagers are accustomed to hear.

3. It will always be preferred if the song has just message to convey.

4. A few words by way of explanation will be appreciated before the singing is started.

5. The song can be followed with a little explanation of its theme.

6. Seasoned singers are liked by everybody but new voices are also welcome.

7. People should be encouraged to come on the stage to sung. Under no circumstances, should the song writer or singer go unrewarded. It will give further encouragement to the lyricist and singers to compose and sing on their own. Competition for the best songs on a particular subject, which is desired to be communicated to the people, should be singled out for reward. People will come to hear the song and go home with message as well.

8. The chief characters of folk songs and dramas are that they should have local tune, tone and dialogue. They are good sources of attracting the people and as such help extension programme indirectly. They are the parts of cultural programme.

### Drama

Drama is not so common as the song in villages. But when properly announced, the drama is well-attended to by the villagers and by those in neighbouring villages.

**Artiste:** The drama is a source of entertainment and education. The Gram Sevak will find at times that he is unable to get together the artistes required from one single village. It may be possible for him to get the artistes by picking them from different villages. But many literate villagers can be trained in this art, and the villagers seeing the familiar faces on the stage will find additional amusement in what is being put on boards.

**Script:** The first difficulty will be getting somebody to write the script and compose the songs. This again is an art which is not given to all. It may be possible to get copies of popular one-act plays in the local language which suit the local needs.

**School teacher:** You can also get new dramas on some aspect of improved farming or living. In this work you may get help from the village school teacher. He is often good in this art. Generally, it is the schoolmaster who organises dramatic performances on special days. He should be of help in training the actors as well as providing the necessary material for the stage. In case you have no such help, do the work yourself. First select villagers who have a bent for acting. This can be done by having them read or repeat a passage. You will find that a number of villagers have appealing voices.

**Stage:** It is not necessary that you have a well-built stage, any space well located, with a little raised ground or platform, will do. A single piece of cloth will serve as a curtain.

**Night-time:** The drama should be staged at a time when all villagers can come. It is best to stage the dramas on nights when there is moonlight, so the villagers may go back home in the light. If the drama is good, the village worker will find big crowds attending the show. The village song or drama has much drawing power. You can use it to get people together. Then tell them about the village programmes in your mind.

**Remember:** The talks should not be long. The villagers will feel tricked and clamour for the continuation of the show. It is a good idea to say few words before the curtain goes up about the purpose of the drama. At the end of the show speak well of the people who have taken part and others who have helped.

### Tom-tom

Tom-tom is a traditional method employed by the villagers in India, especially in states like Tamil Nadu, to communicate information to the members of the village. There will be a nominated person (messenger) to do this job. He has a small audio instrument (tom-tom) made up of cattle skin covered over a mud pot having wide mouth. If there is any local festival, disease outbreak, mass vaccination campaigns, Gram Panchayat meeting, etc. the local leader calls the messenger and tells the information to be communicated to the village people. The messenges then goes into the village, street by street, and makes a big sound with the tom-tom for few seconds; or hearing the sound the villagers, come out of their house and are ready to hear the message. He then communicates the message in a loud voice. Within a short period the entire village will receive the message. This is still being practised in spite of advancement in modern communication technology.

### Field Days/Farmer's Days

A method of influencing the people to adopt a new practice by showing what has actually been achieved by applying the practice under field conditions. A field day or farmer's day may be held in a research farm or in a farmer's field or home. Field days help farmers and extension workers to consider the state of the crops and to discuss them together. The group should be small (about 10 people).

### Farmer Field School (FFS)

1. **Genesis:** The term "Farmer Field School" was coined from the Indonesian expression **Sekolah Lapangan** meaning field school. The first Field School was established in 1989 in Central Java during the pilot phase of the FAO assisted National Integrated Pest Management Programme. FFS is a participatory approach where farmers are involved in curriculum designing based on the real field problems observed by the farmers from sowing to harvest.

   The Field School was a school without walls that taught basic agro-ecology and management skills. Graduation certificates were awarded to farmers at the end of the course. On the success of FFS on IPM, many Asian countries implemented FFS for rice which then branched out to vegetables, cotton, livestock and other crops. At present, FFS programmes are being conducted in over 30 countries.

2. **The four major principles within the livestock FFS process**
   - Raising a healthy animal
   - Observing the animal regularly
   - Understanding the relationship between ecosystem and productivity
   - Understanding ecology and become experts in their own field

3. **Characteristics of the farmer field school approach**
   - *Farmers as experts:* Farmers 'learn-by-doing', i.e. they carry out for themselves the various activities related to the particular farming practice they want to study and learn about. This could be related to annual crops, or livestock/fodder production. The key thing is that farmers conduct their own field studies. Their training is based on comparison studies (of different treatments) and field studies that they, not the extension/research staff conduct. In so doing they become experts on the particular practice they are investigating.
   - *The field is the learning place:* All learning is based in the field. The maize field, banana plantation, or grazing area is where farmers learn. Working in small subgroups they collect data in the field, analyse the data, make action decisions based on they analyses of the data, and present their decisions to the other farmers in the field school for discussion, questioning and refinement.
   - *Extension workers as facilitators, not teachers:* The role of the extension worker is very much that of a facilitator rather than a conventional teacher. Once the farmers know what it is they have to do, and what it is that they can observe in the field, the extension worker takes a back seat role, only offering help and guidance when asked to do so. Presentations during group meetings are the work of the farmers, not of the extension worker, with the members of each working group assuming responsibility for presenting their findings in turn to their fellow farmers. The extension worker may take part in the subsequent discussion sessions but as a contributor, rather than leader, in arriving at an agreed consensus on what action needs to be taken at that time.
   - *Scientists/subject matter specialists work with rather than lecture farmers:* The role of scientists and subject matter specialists is to provide backstopping support to the members of the FFS

and in so doing to learn to work in a consultative capacity with farmers. Instead of lecturing farmers, their role is that of colleagues and advisers who can be consulted for advice on solving specific problems, and who can serve as a source of new ideas and/or information on locally unknown technologies.

- *The curriculum is integrated:* The curriculum is integrated. Crop husbandry, animal husbandry, horticulture, land husbandry are considered together with ecology, economics, sociology and education to form a holistic approach. Problems confronted in the field are the integrating principle.

- *Training follows the seasonal cycle:* Training is related to the seasonal cycle of the practice being investigated. For annual crops this would extend from land preparation to harvesting. For fodder production would include the dry season to evaluate the quantity and quality at a time of year when livestock feeds are commonly in short supply. For tree production, and conservation measures such as hedgerows and grass strips, training would need to continue over several years for farmers to see for themselves the full range of costs and benefits.

- *Regular group meetings:* Farmers meet at agreed regular intervals. For annual crops such meetings may be every 1 or 2 weeks during the cropping season. For other farm/forestry management practices, the time between each meeting would depend on what specific activities need to be done, or be related to critical periods of the year when there are key issues to observe and discuss in the field.

- *Learning materials are learner generated:* Farmers generate their own learning materials, from drawings of what they observe, to the field trials themselves. These materials are always consistent with local conditions, are less expensive to develop, are controlled by the learners and can thus be discussed by the learners with others. Learners know the meaning of the materials because they have created the materials. Even illiterate farmers can prepare and create simple diagrams to illustrate the points they want to make.

- *Group dynamics/team building:* Training includes communication skills building, problem solving, leadership and discussion methods. Farmers require these skills. Successful activities

at the community level require that farmers can apply effective leadership skills and have the ability to communicate their findings to others. Farmer Field Schools are conducted for the purpose of creating a learning environment in which farmers can master and apply specific land management skills. The emphasis is on empowering farmers to implement their own decisions in their own fields.

4. **Steps in conducting FFS**

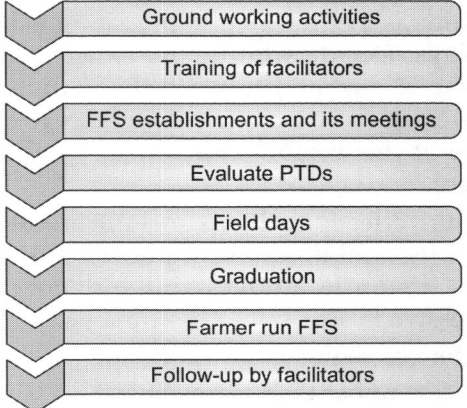

**Fig. 6.16**: Steps in conducting farmer field school

## MASS TEACHING METHODS

Individual, face to face and group methods cannot reach everyone who wants and needs information. So, mass methods such as exhibiting farmers' interest are now in practice. Once stimulated or made aware through mass media, farmers will seek additional information from neighbours, friends, extension workers or progressive farmers in their locality. The above mentioned mass methods may be used singly or in combination, as needed, to meet the proposed objectives.

### Exhibition

An exhibition is planned on systematic display of models, specimens, charts, information, posters, etc. presented to public view for instruction, judging and creating interest or entertainment. An exhibition covers three stages of Extension Education, viz. arousing interest, creating desire to learn and providing a chance to take a decision.

Fairs and festivals are usually taken advantage of, for arranging exhibition. There is difference between exhibits and displays. The exhibits are more of

3-dimensional nature, while displays are mostly 2-dimensional.

### Importance of Exhibition

1. To acquaint the people with better standards.
2. To influence the people to adopt better practices.
3. To create interest in a wide range of people.
4. To promote understanding and create goodwill towards extension.

### Points for Arranging Exhibition

1. Planning is the first step in preparing exhibits and displays. Decide who the audience is, what the message is, what you want the audience to do. Answering these questions will help you plan the scope of the exhibit, the appeal to use and the content.
2. The most effective exhibits are built around a single idea with a minimum of supporting information. Make it simple, understandable, portable and impressive in size.
3. Let there be sequence and continuity.
4. Use a few rather than many objects.
5. Select durable, attractive, and action exhibits. Keep written materials at a minimum. Cluttering is the worst enemy of an exhibit. The fewer elements in your exhibit or display the better. This might be a live object such as a goat in an exhibition.
6. Label the exhibits legibly and briefly.
7. Spacing and decoration should be appearing to the eye and to tell the story without any interpreter.
8. Keep the exhibits at a height not less than 2 feet, and not more than 7 feet from the floor. Place the exhibit of central interest at eye level. This is approximately five feet.
9. Give adequate publicity.
10. Evaluate the effectiveness by the attendance, enquiries and requests.
11. Distribute relevant literature.

### Suggestions in Laying Out Exhibitions

1. Use local materials as far as possible since specimens from locality have greater significance.
2. Take advantage of the local festivals and fairs.
3. Exhibitions can be used for a wide range of topics such as improved home living, model villages, feeding practices, shed construction, product promotion, display of best material in the community etc.

### Advantages

1. Best method to teach illiterates.
2. Most fit for festive occasions.
3. Promotes goodwill towards the extension.
4. It is also for recreational purpose.
5. Can create market for certain products.
6. It has an imaginative appeal.
7. It can fit into festive occasions and serve recreational requirements.
8. It promotes creative abilities to some extent.
9. It can stimulate competitive spirit when used for that purpose.

### Limitations

1. Requires much preparation and investment.
2. It cannot be used frequently or widely.
3. Cannot lend itself to all topics.
4. Normally extension exhibits are arranged in a routine manner, without specific teaching aim.
5. It cannot be used again at the same place without making substantial changes.
7. It cannot represent all phases of work.

### Radio Talk

It is one of the quickest ways of communicating technical information and innovations to the farmers.

### Method of Preparation

There are five important steps involved in preparation of radio talk.

  i. Selection of topic.
 ii. Collection of facts.
iii. Preparing outline.
iv. Buildup script.
 v. Presentation.

  i. **Selection of topic:** The topic selected for radio talk should suit to the area. Know the coverage zone of the AIR station and identify the topic relevant to the farmers of that area. Topic related to season and timely informations are preferred by the AIR programme executives and also by users. Therefore care must be taken in selecting the topic itself.

 ii. **Collection of facts**

    1. Collect all the facts which are related to the selected topic.
    2. Use the real experience and success stories.
    3. Use quotations.
    4. Have the recent research findings.

### iii. **Preparing outline**

1. Know the duration of time allotted by Farm Radio Section. Prepare the speech according to the allotted time. A single page typed in double spacing is sufficient for two minutes' talk. A five-minute talk is ideal.

2. Choose the most appealing mode of presentation like straight talk, interview, question and answer, documentaries, plays, skits, etc.

3. Treat the message according to the level of the target mass.

4. Write down the main idea of the talk.

5. Then add all the important points you wish to emphasize in the talk.

6. Arrange the points in a logical order.

7. Add additional points and illustrate with local examples.

### iv. **Buildup script**

1. The script should be brief, clear and awaken the attention and interest of the audience.

2. Write the script with empathy, keeping the target audience in the mind. Write for the ears not for the eyes. As radio is personal the approach has to be personal, with person to person or a special I and You quality.

3. Write brief introduction about the selected topic and do not cover too many ideas.

4. Use personal words, active verbs and simple familiar language. Scientific words should be translated in the local language.

5. Underline the important words which are to be given emphasis. Round off figures wherever possible to avoid confusion in voice pronunciation.

6. Write complete information and do not end with wanting details.

7. Use widely known abbreviations only like ICAR, YMCA, NABARD and the like.

8. Script should be written in such a way that the audience understands the talk in the first hearing. Prepare the speech well ahead according to the time available and edit it. Write the script in single side of the paper.

### Don'ts

1. Avoid technical jargons, long and confusing numbers, offensive statements and jaw breaking words.

2. Avoid listing names at great length. Often unfamiliar names need not be used at all.

3. Avoid complex sentences.

### v. **Presentation**

*Do's*

1. Rehearse, recheck, pre-record and criticise yourself by listening to tape recording. Correct the pronunciations and adjust the length of the script.

2. The first 30 seconds are the critical period to catch the listeners' attention. Catch it preferably with an interrogative statement.

3. Be friendly, natural and conversational. Speak as if you would to a friend nearby. Talk to the audience. The speed of the speech should be on an average 125 words per minute.

4. Believe in your subject matter and let your interest show it and sound enthusiastic.

5. Be careful in pronouncing pronouns, making certain that 'he' and 'she' actually refers to the person intended.

6. Main and important points should be repeated as many times as possible without boring the listeners.

7. In conclusion, first summarise the main points, tell the audience what you expect them to do.

*Don'ts*

1. Avoid referring back to any statement.

2. Conclusion should not contain any new idea.

3. Do not shout before the microphone.

4. Do not read the script.

5. Do not speak fastly.

### *Television Talk*

Television telecast is a powerful mass teaching method. The visual effect in it has the merit over the radio broadcast. It has great potential as an educational method as it can arouse and sustain interest and also leave lasting impression on the mind of the viewers. It needs less effort than reading the printed matters. Apart from seeing by their own eyes, farmers also respond readily to what is said, especially by other farmers, and if the same point is made and highlighted by extension workers in their inter-personal communications the combination is highly effective.

TV programmes cannot change the entire behaviour of the farmer immediately but the awareness creates curiosity about a new innovation in the minds of farmers and arouses interest to seek further information.

### Factors Involved in TV Programmes

1. The farm programmes should be telecast at a suitable time. It varies according to the target viewer, e.g. farmer, farmwomen.
2. Frequency and length of the farm telecast depends on the farmer's need, season, information, manpower for production, availability of the sorting, editing and other pieces of equipment and budget.
3. Format of the programme depends upon the content and purpose.
4. Content of the programme should be complete, correct and fulfil the timely needs of the farmers.
5. Treatment of the message is related to nature of the target mass, subject matter, time allotted and mode of presentation.
6. Assess the accuracy of the information before production and telecast.
7. Rehearsal is an important aspect to produce the best programme.
8. The specialist who delivers the subject in the programme should wear a dark colour dress.
9. The speakers should avoid distracting mannerisms.
10. The speaker must carry suitable visuals and required quantity of specimens if any.

### Film Show (Cinema)

Film is an influential medium than the print and broadcast media. This method can be very effectively utilized to teach both literate and illiterate masses. Before the advent of TV this was the only medium which was used in the villages for education and entertainment. While playing films in the villages following points should be kept in mind:

1. Selection of the film (subject) based on the teaching objective.
2. Check the cinema projector, film, seating, ventilation, electricity, etc.
3. Just before projection, the participants should be briefed about the subject to be played and points to be observed and noted.
4. The show should end with a discussion with the participants regarding the utility of the subject matter played.

### Campaign

An educational campaign is a well-organized plan for bringing about widespread adoption of a particular practice. It is a continued teaching effort concentrated into a set period of time. The central idea—a better practice is kept before the people constantly during that time. People are shown repeatedly that this is a solution to a problem.[1]

The more the people are exposed to a new idea, the more likely they are to adopt it. Campaign uses this principle. In a campaign, people have their attention focussed on a new practice through many methods.

"Campaign is an intensive teaching activity undertaken at an opportune time for a brief period, focussing attention in a concerted manner towards a particular problem, so as to stimulate the widest possible interest in the community".[2]

Campaigns are launched only after a recommended practice has been found acceptable to the people. It encourages emotional participation of a large number of people and it develops a favourable psychological climate for quick and large-scale adoption of improved practices.

### Steps in Conducting Campaign

1. **Create awareness:** The first step for the campaign is to analyse the situation, identify the local need and create an awareness of the need for the campaign. This awareness is given through the meetings.

2. **Purpose of campaign:** Before planning the campaign, the purpose must be made clear. The campaign should fulfil the need of the people. Be direct towards the solution of a problem the people recognize. Deal with a problem important to a majority of the people. Offer a solution that the people can and will accept. Focus on one idea at a time.

3. **Planning**
   a. Discuss with local leaders and agencies.
   b. Consult the specialists and find solution to the problems.
   c. Ensure technical sources and supplies.
   d. Select a suitable time for launching the campaign.
   e. Schedule events—decide how to involve people.
   f. Give wide publicity about the campaign in advance.
   g. Specify the work to each service person and local leaders.

---

1. Helen A. Strow. Educational Campaign in Extension Work—OIE 24 Federal Extension Service, U.S. Dept. of Agriculture in Cooperation with the Agency for International Development, Washington, D.C.
2. J.P. Leagans. "Extension Education in Community Development" op. cit.

4. **Conducting:** Conduct the campaign with the help of local leaders as per plan. Open your campaign by doing something dramatic that focuses attention on the problem. Hold a meeting under the presidentship of a popular respectable personality and incite everyone interested. After the inauguration, keep the attention of the people focused in the recommended practice continuously. Apply all your creativity and device unusual and interesting approaches.

a. Use meetings of all kinds to carry the message.

b. Make farm and home visit to encourage them and to speed up their progress and to identify their difficulties in adopting the practice.

c. Arrange tours and field trips to show the results.

d. Conduct demonstration to prove to people that the recommended practice will work.

e. Wide publicity can be given by using all mass media. Exhibits are a good way to show the value of the recommended practice. Keep some exhibits in markets.

f. Announce contests to assure interest.

g. Set a definite time to end the campaign. Feature the final day so the people can share the satisfaction of completing the project. Invite an important person. Report results to the people. Recognize community leaders for their work.

h. Evaluate the results—review the objective and if necessary reconsider it. Watch the campaign closely from the beginning to end. Failure should be avoided.

5. **Follow-up**

a. By discussion the reaction of farmers should be found out.

b. The extent of adoption should be assessed.

c. The reasons for failures should be found out.

d. The success stories must be published.

e. The local leaders must be properly recognised for the contributions.

*Points to be considered for effectiveness*

1. The campaign should be organised at the 'right time'.

2. Timely provision of inputs including loan.

3. If the farmers are aware of the need the response would be better.

4. Complete information, including how to use a better practice, should be taught.

5. For any campaign to be successful leading to adoption, there must be constant encouragement up to the adoption.

6. Evaluation of the campaign and correction for the new start would increase the number of beneficiaries.

*Advantages*

1. Specially suited to stimulate mass-scale adoption of an improved practice in the shortest time possible.

2. Campaign exploits the group psychology for introduction of new practices.

3. Successful campaign creates conducive atmosphere for popularising other methods.

4. Builds up community confidence.

5. Best method for the technologies which need the entire community's adoption.

*Limitations*

a. Not suited to individual problems.

b. Campaign would be successful only when all participants co-operate in it.

c. Not suitable to the complicated technologies.

d. Requires adequate preparation, and close association of technical agencies, propaganda technique, etc.

## Printed Media

Printed media is used for communication of techniques that rely principally on combinations of printed words and pictures. This is our oldest formal combination. To apply this method effectively the educational levels and literacy rate of the audience must be considered. Extension programmes can take a broad and creative approach to ways in which to use print medium for conveying news to audience.

Spoken words are forgotten rapidly. To often refresh the farmer's memory there should be some method to remind them from time to time. About 35% of farm information loss was found in between extension worker and farmers. For effective communication, written methods are useful. Thus, the written methods are used in extension teaching to provide facts in such a manner that the subjects' attention is attracted, to make them understand, remember and finally to help them to take favourable decisions. Further the written communication reduces the loss of information during transit and in addition it covers large number of people within a short time.

### Preparing Printing Materials

**Planning:** When preparing printing materials, keep the audience constantly in mind. Write the timely information. Write about things that interest people.

Change the method of presentation as the proposed audience changes (youth, farmers, women). The relevant materials may be collected. They should be arranged in a logical sequence.

**Writing:** The writing should be accurate, brief, clear, couseise and consistent. Avoid exaggeration.

**Illustration:** The importance of illustrations cannot be overemphasized. Even where literacy is not a problem, people interpret words differently because of differences in past experience. Illustrations reduce the risk of misunderstandings and increase the extent of learning. Realistic illustrations are usually the most effective in extension work, although humorous drawings have a definite place, use humour carefully so as not to hurt anyone. Good pictures make any publication easier to understand and more interesting to read, but do not crop up unnecessary details from photographs and keep drawings simple.

**Title:** It should be short, attractive, easily understandable and clearly bring out the subject to create interest among the readers.

**Words and sentences:** They should be very simple and short. Use the familiar words. One sentence should have one idea. Eliminate difficult scientific and technical terms.

**Paragraphs:** Paragraph is a group of related ideas. It should be short. Each para should convey sub-idea of the main ideas. Sub-headings should be given to paragraphs.

**Colour:** Choose colours that are legible as well as appropriate, e.g. dark green ink for poster: Two or three colours can be used with suitable combinations. Colour papers can also be used for giving interesting effects.

**Cover page:** The cover of illustrated literature has a function different from the page within. The cover should be attractive, colourful and tempting. The audience should feel an urge to look inside. A bulletin that never reaches the hands cannot possibly reach the brain where judgements and decisions are made.

### Presentation

There should be introduction, body and conclusion in the writing.

i. The introduction should be designed to attract the readers with simple and comprehensive language.

ii. The body should present or analyse the situation. The other factors to be considered are giving less statistics, emphasising the key points containing facts satisfying needs, bringing out the merits and demerits, winning the confidence of the reader, etc.

iii. The summary should contain all facts that create awareness for action. Finally the readers' view points must be kept in mind at all times.

### Evaluation

The written materials are evaluated based on reader's feedback.

### Advantages

1. It provides clear information.
2. To provide authentication of the information this is the best method.
3. Easy for retention and recall.
4. Information can reach large number of farmers in short time.
5. It can supplement the farm and home visit.

### Tips for Writing for Farmers

The writing should be in the spoken form, but slang should be removed and the language should not be too stylistic. Avoid words of other language. As far as possible use apt and commonly used words. Do not use the same words repeatedly. Write short sentences. There should be link between one sentence and the other. Write in active voice and never in passive voice. Do not use words or sentences which have double meaning or ambiguity. Do not use double negatives. Positive sentence followed by negative sentence would create interest. Paragraphs should be small. There should be continuity from one para to other. Where there is discontinuity between paragraphs, use sub-heading.

i. **Leaflet (flyer)** (Fig. 6.17): It is a single sheet of paper used to present information on only one topic in a concise manner and simple language.

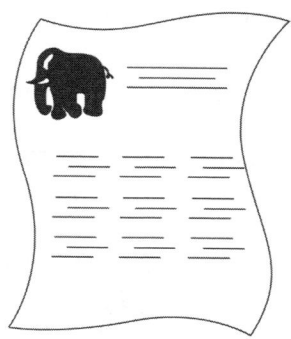

**Fig. 6.17:** Leaflet

### Preparation

1. Select a suitable topic based on farmers' felt need.
2. There should be only one idea, technique or practice.

3. Collect all relevant points and select only the most essential one.
4. Use short, simple and familiar words.
5. Include relevant pictures, illustrations, etc. in order to help the farmer's understanding.
6. Refer to local situations wherever possible.
7. Remember all the points for written materials. Give the sources for obtaining further information. Personal sentences, short paragraphs, less technical terms, illustrations, etc. are the desired characteristics of the leaflet.

*Printing*
a. Attractiveness can be increased by using different colour papers or inks and by illustrations or photographs.
b. Farmers with lower literacy prefer 16 point letters and those who have studied above fifth standard like 14-point letters.
c. Printing on pink or yellow paper is liked by the farmers.
d. The size of leaflet preferred by the farmer is 4" × 8".

*Advantages*
1. Reaches a large number of literate farmers.
2. Preserved and used for future reference.
3. Comparatively cheap.
4. Provides accurate information.
5. Easy to make.
6. Promotes literacy.

*Limitations*
1. Less useful in low literacy area.
2. Cannot be used in exclusion of other methods.
3. Will lose its significance if not carefully prepared and used.

ii. **Folder** (Fig. 6.18): Folder is a single piece of paper folded ones or twice. When it is opened the material presented are in sequence.

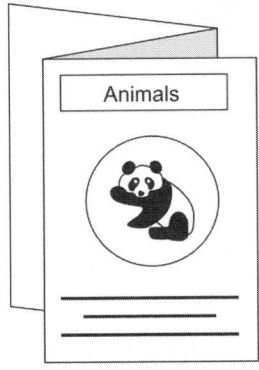

**Fig. 6.18:** Folder

*Preparation*
All the factors to be considered for the leaflet are to be considered for the folder also. In addition to that, the following factors may also be considered:
1. After deciding topic, based on the farmers' felt need, collect the relevant points. Arrange the facts collected in a logical order. Select the important points in 1-2-3 order (step by step).
2. While writing the folder there need not be complete sentences or paragraphs. The ideas and sub-ideas can be listed one below the other.
3. Folder will most suit to give 'how to do' a and b, package of practices to be followed in growing poultry, the steps to be followed in solving a farm or home problem, etc. Accurate and specific instructions are given.
4. Folder need not be complete, as it complements the other methods. However, the title, printing, etc. should be attractive otherwise, even if the folder is the only reading material available it may not be read at all.

*Printing*
a. Make the folder attractive by using photograph, line drawings and various colour papers and inks.
b. 1 : 1.5 ratio is more suitable width to length ratio.
c. 4" × 8" folder is found to be very attractive from the farmer's view point or make them of any convenient and attractive size.
d. Print the folder on heavier paper than the leaflet,
e. The front page of the folder is exclusively allotted for printing the design with title. Prepare a cover page design with two or three colours.

*Advantages and limitations:* Same as leaflet.

iii. **Pamphlet:** Pamphlet size varies from 2 to 12 pages. The first cover page should be printed in two or three colours with some action pictures. Full information about the selected topic is presented at greater length. When compared to a folder, pamphlet serves to the needs of farmers at different stages.

iv. **Bulletin:** A bulletin contains large amount of information. Its primary objective is to give information which the reader can apply to his own local situations. Its size varies from 12 to 20 pages.

*Types of bulletin*[1]
a. **Popular bulletin:** It is prepared for being given in the fields of extension agency and farmers.

---
1. R. Ratnakar, "Agricultural Journalism," EEI, APAU, Hyderabad.

b. **Technical bulletin:** It is designed primarily to present specific material to those working in specified fields.

Extension bulletins are for extension workers, progressive farmers, school teachers, extension training centres, etc.

*Preparation of bulletin:* Good 'eye appeal': It should be attractive to see and use direct style in writing. It should be simple, direct, clear and convincing. Choose words as you would with your friends. Select words and use them in proper relationship. Make sentences light. Be clear, precise and definite. Make sure you say what you have in mind. Check and recheck. Mention important information in the beginning. Have short paragraphs. Plan and prepare yourself about the facts, their coordination, adoption, interpretation and application.

Splash it with pictures: Have suitable and good pictures depicting action. These should have proportion and balance in size. Pen sketches and photos are to be prepared over graphs and tables. Write your own outlines, i.e. captions that explain photographs, sketches, etc. Figure it out yourself. Publications are printed in page multiples of 2–4, 8, 12, 16, etc. Decide on number of pages.

Your cover indicates: By your cover people know you. Make an appealing cover—colour, symbol, illustration should be appropriate to the subject discussed. Defend your title. Title of the bulletin should be given much thought. It should be concise and attractive.

Be brief: When a bulletin is short, the summary is necessary. When it is long, index of table of contents and summary are needed.

Give sub-heads: Use colour for attractiveness. Use suitable type of lettering. The chief function of type is to convey ideas and thought. It is achieved when it is read easily. In extension publications the suitable type size may be 10–12 points.

Prepare a dummy bulletin which should be printed on 'art' paper for longer use. Though more expensive than offset paper, art paper appears neater, type and photographs are more clearly reproduced.

v. **Booklet:** When the material is more and exceeds 20 pages and limited to 50 pages then it is called a booklet.

**Book:** When the number of pages exceeds 50 then we can call it a book.

vi. **News report/news article:** News reports appear in the newspapers. The newspapers vary greatly in their readers and coverage, from the huge urban daily newspaper to the small community paper. They are published by government and private organizations and can provide valuable channels for extension news.

All the information or reports received by the news office cannot be accepted and used in newspapers. Whether the news is going to appear or will be discarded depends on the news worthiness of information.

News is any timely information that interests a number of persons. Anything that makes people talk about it is known as news. If a dog bites a man, it is not news. If a man bites a dog it is news. The best news is that which has greatest interest for the greatest number of people.

News story attracts attention because it reports interesting day-to-day events or something new, different or unusual. News story is useful to develop farmers' interest inform the general public, communicate new information; create favourable attitude; and report the other methods like demonstration, meeting, etc.

**Kind of news stories**

1. *Before and after stories:* This is also known as advance event articles and follow-up event articles. These types of stories are meant to provide advance information on important meetings, demonstrations, and the like and follow-up of these events after they are over. Before stories include announcements of approaching extension meetings, tours, speeches, and other events. The after stories may be about recent meetings, tours, speeches or other extension events. Their main purposes are to report the results.

2. *Experience and success stories:* These types of stories highlight the experience and success of individuals, groups or institutions.

3. *New development stories:* These stories tell about a sudden outbreak of diseases, a new product that has come to the market or about some research findings.

4. *Subject matter stories:* A subject matter story is one which is timely and of interest to a large number of readers. It gives directions and is of practical value to the readers.

**Contents**

1. The event in a news report has to be recent.
2. It should contain who, when, what, where, why and how of an event.

3. Inverted pyramid form of presentation is the way of writing.
4. It begins with specifics and ends with generalities.
5. It is written in third person.

**Six keys of news[1]**

There are six key ingredients that newspaper editors often use to determine what key print and how they use it.

1. *Timeliness:* The more timely the information, the greater the news value.

2. *Nearness:* The closer the information seems to the reader (geographically and psychologically), the greater is its news value. That is why local newspapers prefer local area news.

3. *Consequence:* The more the readers are affected by the information, the greater is the news value.

4. *Prominence:* Prominent people, places, and things have more news value.

5. *Human interest:* Readers are attracted by human interest elements such as unusualness, conflict, progress, emotion, etc.

6. *Newspaper policy:* Newspapers have editorial policies that influence the kind and amount of information they publish. So, the use of various kinds of extension information may vary from paper to paper and period to period, based on editorial policies.

**Points to be considered while writing stories**

- News writing styles differ throughout the world. So, the best approach is to use the styles and formats that local news editors prefer and type the report with proper line space on the page. Editors prefer writing that is clear, simple, active and concise, because such writing permits easy reading. And they want copy that is accurate. One of your most successful techniques may be to keep readers in mind as you write.

- All the principles and guidance for mass writing material preparation should be considered, including all the principles of writing for the farmers, words, sentence, paragraphs inverted pyramid type, etc.

- The write-up tries to interest everyone, even general reader.

---

1. P. Mathialagan, Animal Husbandry Journalism, Mimeographed Lectures, Note for Veterinary Students, Dept. of Extension Education, VC & RI, Namakkal, 1994.

- The news should be fresh but not necessarily seasonable.

- Regardless of specific requirements, editors probably want news copy that is neat, readable. While writing news report, first write the body then lead and finally the title.

**Writing an article**

*Body:* The writing follows the principle of inverted pyramid form. All the information about the article collected. It is arranged in order of priority with the most important point at the top. The body is then is written by giving major details and minor details.

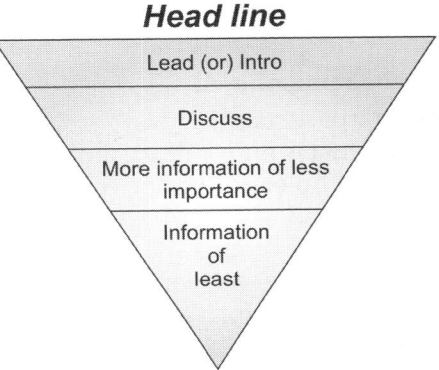

**Fig. 6.19:** Inverted pyramid pattern

*Lead:* The body should consist of different paragraphs with small sub-titles and a few sentences. If possible a photograph or drawing can be included to make the news more comprehensible. The body must have conclusion. It should contain what you wish the reader to do, i.e. the exact action you expect from the reader. Then the lead paragraph is written. It answers who, when, where, why and how. Lead should be confined to the facts for telling reader the story's content. It is the abstract or condensed form of the body. It must be in one or two sentences.

Example: "The State Government has allotted ₹ 2.5 crores to construct modernised carcass utilisation plant, the Chief Minister, said while laying the foundation stone here on Monday".

There are many types of leads, viz. summary lead, quotation lead, question lead and suspense lead. The summary lead is commonly written. Lead may form one or two paragraphs.

*Title:* Then the facts in the lead paragraph are condensed and the headline is written attractively, briefly and clearly so that the attention of the reader is compelled towards the article. It should be in one line. The special characteristics of this news story writing is that the same information will be repeated thrice in the article, viz. headline, lead and body.

vii. **Feature stories:** Feature articles are informative and sometimes involve news, but are distinct in several ways from the types of articles mentioned earlier. Feature articles often interpret the news and provide background for readers. Often they are intended to entertain or inspire as much as to inform. They may feature ideas, places, techniques, persons, organizations, challenges, and almost any other aspects of human activity. They often involve more human interest than news or information articles. The feature stories are published in periodicals like weeklies, monthlies, quarterlies, etc.

**Points to be remembered**

1. It aims at particular segment of the public. The audience that is highly educated and most of the people can be expected to welcome ideas and sentences of some complexity. It is designed to limited interest groups such as poultry farmers.
2. A feature story does not stop after presenting the facts as in news story. It goes beyond and explores the background, the birth and growth of ideas or events and provides a glance at the future too.
3. The articles appear less frequently, hardly once in a week. (Thus, there is more time to dig into the issue or situations, than the daily news stories.)
4. This is half way between newspaper and book.
5. The information given in feature article need not be new, but it should be of interest to the readers.
6. Seasonal information is given.
7. In articles the writer has more freedom than with other written methods.
8. Only undisputed truths are given.
9. There should be enough material to write the feature article.
10. Photographs fitting with the story may be published.

viii. **Wall newspapers:** Wall newspapers are similar in size and appearance to posters, and have more detailed current information and an illustration. They are similar in size and appearance to a poster, but they are different from posters usually attempt as they to communicate more than one fact or idea. They also have more illustrations and written materials.

*Preparation:* The normal size of the wall newspaper is 12" × 18". The letters are bold. Important points discussed for posters should be taken into consideration for wall newspapers. They are prepared in simple language, have a title. Information is printed in bold type along with illustration.

*Printing:* In most countries where wall newspapers are used in extension programmes, they are produced in quantity by a central office. Wall newspapers are normaly printed on letter press or offset, but silk screen printing also works.

*Distribution:* The printed wall newspapers are distributed by mail or through extension organization. Distribution varies according to the requirements. Mailing may be made directly to local leaders, school teachers, milk producers, sheep breeders' co-operative societies, religious leaders and others. Sometimes the local extension worker hand delivers, and even posts, issues of the paper.

*Application:* Wall newspapers have been used for a considerable time in rural areas to communicate news of political and social interests. Agricultural extension services in many countries have adopted the wall newspaper for educational programmers and it has become one of the most effective extension teaching tools. It is used not only to communicate news of extension activities but also to report results of research and to recommend new practices.

*Examples*

1. Announcing the appointment of a new livestock specialist.
2. Urging the use of IBD vaccine to prevent Gumbora in poultry flocks.

*Display:* Wall newspaper can be pasted on walls of buildings and at intersections. These can be pasted with great effect on village bulletin boards, at teaching centres, schools and public buildings. However, the place should be well protected from wind, rain, etc.

ix. **Circular letter:** Circular letter is a letter written by the extension worker and sent to many farmers periodically or on special occasion.

*Objectives*

1. To maintain regular contact with farmers.
2. To communicate some general information which could best be put in the form of a letter.

*Preparation*

1. Let the letters be brief and courteous.
2. Have a single purpose and write in simple language.
3. Give complete information.

4. Be clear in statements which should lead to action.
5. The letters should be a part of a programme or campaign.

*Application*

1. For dissemination of scientific information.
2. Can be used for organising village mela.

*Advantages*

1. Information can reach a large mass.
2. Preserved and used for future reference.
3. Comparatively cheap.
4. Provide accurate information.
5. Easy to make.
6. Promote literacy, develop goodwill and increase the tempo of work.

*Limitations*

1. Less useful in low literacy area.
2. Cannot be used in exclusion of other methods.

x. **Newsletter:** Newsletter can be an effective, low cost way to reach readers. The content of newsletter can be more localised and specialised than is possible with a general newspaper. Like the wall newspaper, the newsletter is well adapted to using local language and dialects. And a newsletter can include hand-written, type written or type-set copy. Duplication methods also can vary greatly.

A newsletter usually contains a larger share of reset-to-visual than does a wall newspaper, but not necessarily. Page size is smaller than of newspapers, so space is often limited and brevity is vital. In fact, brevity is one of the benefits that readers find in a newsletter. Newsletter writers try to get into each subject quickly and use short sentences and energetic words.

The newsletter can be directed more selectively than newspapers.

For example, a newsletter might be distributed only to poultry farmers in a village, hence, the content could provide news and advice about feed mixing and feeding of chicks. The newsletter can, therefore, be newsy, localized and specialised in what it covers.

Extension personnel might publish their own newsletter or they may submit news to newsletters published by other organizations, such as co-operatives that reach readers of interest to extension.

*Fact sheets:* Fact sheets are "boiled down" treatments of subject matter. They usually cover a single topic, and often they are limited to a single page.

Most fact sheets are illustrated with drawings or photographs, or both. The illustrations are used to show details or steps in a process, to make the information clearer and more understandable. One of the important uses of fact sheet is to provide current subject matter to field workers. Field workers often complain that the needed technical information is slow in reaching them. Much agricultural and animal husbandry information is carried in technical bulletins and other lengthy publications. These take considerable time in processing and distribution.

On the other hand, the essential facts can be put down and combined with drawings and/or photographs to make an effective summary which can be reproduced quickly and inexpensively in fact sheet form. This puts current information into the hands of local extension workers enabling them to give better service to farm families. Extension administrators, who are concerned with the problem of speeding up intra-staff communication of subject matter, should be aware of the advantages offered by fact sheets.

## Media Forum

A combination of mass media and interpersonal media has been found to be the most effective way of reaching farmers with new ideas, as the number of change agents are less. This media forum was originally developed in Canada among farm families and later spread to developing countries, including India.

Media forums are small organised groups of individuals (15–20) who meet regularly to receive messages through media (radio, TV or print) and discuss the contents. If radio, the forum members listen to the farm and home programme and discuss the subjects of broadcast. Their doubts are sent to the radio station, which of again gives the answers in the subsequent broadcasts. Indian radio forum is the largest one in the world. This was launched on a national basis in 1959.

Their members meet twice a week to listen to the half an hour programme from the network. Discussion usually lasts for about half an hour, after the completion of the network programme. A chairman leads the discussion and a secretary keeps a written record of decision and the questions which are to be mailed to radio station. All the media forum programmes have been found to be rather effective in creating knowledge, changing attitudes and in catalysing behavioural changes.

## EDGAR DALE'S CONE OF EXPERIENCE

We learn through experience. In a way experience is education. Education primarily involves transmission of ideas through communication. Many of our experiences are direct, whereas many are indirect. Similarly, many are concrete and many abstract. We gain all these experiences through our five sensory organs of seeing, hearing, touching, smelling and tasting. Using one for more of these organs we gain numerous experiences every day. Edgar Dale (1965) has summarised various sources of experiences in a pictorial device, called "Cone of Experience".

According to Dale, the cone of experience is merely a visual aid in explaining the inter-relationship of the various sources of experience. This individual "position" in the cone is most effective in terms of producing the desired quality and quantity of learning. The source of experience at the pinnacle of the cone is least effective, although most widely used. The more a particular source involves our sensory organs, the more effective it is for producing the desired learning. As we go up the cone, we find that the use of sensory organs is diminished. As such the bottom most and the top most sources represent the two extremes in the use of sensory organs. In order to present this proportion in its true perspective, Edgar Dale has selected the shape of a cone which has maximum space at the bottom and minimum at the top.

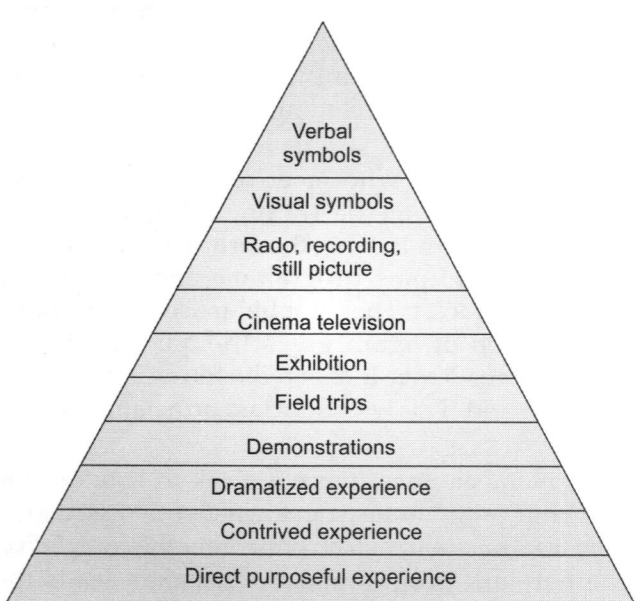

**Fig. 6.20:** Edgar Dale's cone of experience

A brief description of each of the sources of experience in the cone is given below.

1. **Direct purposeful experience:** This is the most effective experience in terms of producing the most desired learning among students. It involves maximum number of sensory organs. While a student is learning to operate a chop cutter, all his mental and sensory faculties are actively engaged in the process. Therefore, he is learning by doing which is the best type of learning. This type of learning tends to be permanent and is least likely to be forgotten.

2. **Contrived experience:** When it is not possible to see the reality, the reality is presented in a contrived form so that it may be meaningful to viewers. It may not be possible to see the whole 5,000 hectare livestock farm at one glance but it may be possible to represent it through a model so that one could get a comprehensive idea of where is what in the farm, its exact location and so on. Editing of the reality is called contrived experience.

3. **Dramatized experience:** Some past event is presented in the form of a drama to vividly bring back to the mind the actual happening. Dramatization will have much greater impact on the mind since many more faculties will be involved in seeing and hearing rather than merely mental images as in the case of reading.

4. **Demonstrations:** As said earlier, there are three types of demonstrations, viz. method, result and composite. In all of them not only seeing and hearing are involved but also doing with both hand and mind. This is why demonstrations are more effective in terms of producing desired learning than those sources where only seeing and/or hearing results in learning.

5. **Field trips:** In this case, the participants can only see and occasionally hear someone explain things. There is hardly any scope for the use of manipulative skill. This is the reason why field trips are supposedly less effective than demonstrations and, as such, are placed above them in the experience cone.

6. **Exhibits:** These are artificial representation of the reality. They can only be seen and thus employ only one sensory organ. This may account for exhibits being less effective than demonstrations and field trips and their placement above them in the cone of experience.

7. **Television:** There is greater participation in the case of television as the audience can both see as well as hear. Television has great potential as an educational medium as it can arouse and sustain interest and also leave lasting impression on the mind of viewers.

8. **Motion pictures:** Basically there is no difference between television and motion pictures. The reason for motion picture being placed above television in the cone of experience may be because of the easy and wide availability of television in homes and elsewhere, and therefore, its greater impact on the minds of larger number of viewers.

9. **Recordings, radio, still pictures:** All these employ only one sensory organ. One can only hear or see. This is the reason why they are less effective in terms of learning and as such placed above other sources in the cone of experience.

10. **Visual symbols:** These include the whole gamut of things that we can see with our eyes, e.g. posters, charts, flash cards, flannel graph, books, pamphlets, etc. In this case also only one sensory organ is employed and hence these are less effective than those where more than one sensory organs are employed.

11. **Verbal symbols:** At the pinnacle of the cone is located, the verbal symbols which are nothing but words and spoken language. Here all reality has been withdrawn and we are left with nothing but abstractions. Naturally they are least effective in terms of producing learning among students. Although it may sound paradoxical but in spite of this rather harsh reality verbal symbols are the most commonly used medium of communication not only outside but also inside the classroom.

## SELECTION AND COMBINATION OF EXTENSION METHODS

A wide range of extension teaching methods and techniques are in common use in India and other countries for promoting rural development by means of education. The teaching methods employed by teacher in extension work directly influence the effectiveness of the learners. In general, a combination of teaching methods are always effective in creating better understanding among learners.

The amount and quality of the learning resulting from the teaching effort is dependent on the selection of the most appropriate method for particular teaching situation and the skill with which the working tool is used.

### Methods and Tools

A single identifiable technique is called a tool, e.g. a lecture. A method, however, is a combination of tools (techniques) that are used to achieve the objective of a training session or teaching method.

### Factors to be Considered Before Teaching Activity

'Farm conditions' and 'Farm people' are the two main factors that should be considered in extension work before taking up of any teaching activities with the help of different teaching methods.

### Farm Conditions

i. Farms are in different conditions, e.g. climate, soil, size, sale of products, availability of farm labour, etc.

ii. Different extension teaching methods are most effective in varying situation. Differences and conditions not only exist between different regions but also between the farm within one region. No two farms work under exactly the same conditions. So, suitable teaching methods should be selected and applied.

### Farm People

Farm people learn best in different ways: Some by listening, some by seeing, some by doing and still others through discussion. Various extension teaching methods are most effective at different stages of adoption process. All people do not learn at the same speed, some may be at the stage of trying a new practice and want to know the details of how to do it when others are barely aware of the practice or are just becoming interested. For these reasons use a variety of teaching method that are most effective. Studies have shown that the more different extension teaching methods are used, the more people change their practice. The more exposures per individual to a new practice, the more likely the person will find his preferred method of learning.

Lack of proper selection and inefficient use leads to the following consequences:

a. The benefit of extension programme will not reach as many people as it should have.

b. There will be considerable delay in changing the behaviour of the people.

c. Many innovations might not be accepted by the people, since they will not be properly presented.

d. The extension worker might become frustrated by indifferent responses.

e. People might lose confidence in the extension programme.

f. Wastage of resources.

g. Extension of further development work becomes difficult.

## Selection of Methods

The selection of appropriate method is not an easy task. There is no single thumb-rule for its selection. In order to get more effective results the extension worker should:

i. select the appropriate methods;
ii. have a suitable combination of selected methods; and
iii. use them in proper sequence so as to have repetition in a variety of ways.

The following considerations should be taken into account in the selection of extension teaching methods:

### Factors Influencing the Selection

a. **Eduction level of audience**: For illiterates we select personal visits and for highly educated the written materials.
b. **Size of audience:** The group methods cannot be effectively used for the participant size exceeding thirty.
c. **The teaching objective:** If we want attitudinal change we go in for the group discussion and for skill change the demonstration method.
d. **The subject matter:** If simple technology which is new it should be told through the news article, whereas for complex one, face-to-face contact or audio-visual aids should be used.
e. **The state of development of extension organisation:** If the organisation is new and yet to gain the confidence of the people the result demonstration should be selected. The well established organisation can even use the circular letter.
f. **Size of the extension staff:** Large number of staff, more of direct contacts.
g. **Availability of media:** TV, radio, newspaper, etc. will also have an influence in selecting the method.
h. **Relative cost:** The cost involved in the method is also an important consideration in selection and use.
i. **Extension worker's familiarity:** The training of the extension worker for the proper handling of the selected method. The teacher should know his own capabilities while making selection.
j. **Needs:** Problems and technological needs of the people.
k. **The length of time:** The length of time the programme has been going on in the area.
l. **The significance of the programme:** Depending upon the importance of the programme the methods may be selected.
m. **General local conditions:** Such as seasonal work, weather conditions, availability of meeting places, organisations and leadership.
n. **Emergency:** The farmer can be advised during emergencies by phone call method.

## Combination of Methods

1. Each extension method has its own advantages and disadvantages. The face-to-face type of interpersonal communication is easy and effective for technology transfer. But this method cannot be used for technology transfer to large number of people. The mass media can help the extension worker to reach large number of people quickly. But only essential information can be conveyed by this method but giving the details of the technology is not possible. The mass method of radio has the limitation of appealing to ears only. The print media cannot reach the illiterates. So, it is recommended to combine different methods purposely. In other words, there is a best method for each purpose or function to be fulfilled.

2. Sometimes different media will be used at the same time. For example, a lecture is supported with audio-visual aids. Sometimes they will be used in succession. Written materials are used to prepare farmers for a group discussion.

3. Advertising research has shown that the person who receives the same message through different media will pay more attention because he recognises something familiar from another contact.

4. The value of combining media has been clearly demonstrated in studies of radio forum.

5. One method supplements and complements other methods. Hence, more than one method is necessary to bring about adoption by majority of farmers. The rate of increase in adoption of new methods by the farmer is very high when the exposure to new information is from 1–5 methods.

6. No one single method can reach all the people.

7. It is the cumulative effect, i.e. exposure to a unity of methods during a period of time that provides good results.

8. Skillful manipulation or handling of various methods by the extension worker will later determine the effectiveness of extension teaching.

9. Combination of mass media and group discussion can bring about considerable changes in behaviour, if well organised. The use of audio-visual aids to support talks and group discussion would also be thought of. Video cassettes are currently attracting considerable attention.

10. It is believed that combination of modern communication technology such as video, satellite communication, micro-computers, etc. with the rapid development of group discussion methods have not been explored adequately by many extension services.

11. It is desirable to use multi-media approach in the information communication programme.

The data on the overall effectiveness and cost benefit ratios of three media combinations are given below:[1]

## Effectiveness of Combination of Methods

| S.No. | Media | Ranking |
|-------|-------|---------|
| *Overall effectiveness* | | |
| 1. | Radio + slide show + field trip | 1 |
| 2. | Wall painting + slide show + field trip | 2 |
| 3. | Poster + slide show + demonstration | 3 |
| 4. | Exhibition + group discussion + demonstration | 4 |
| 5. | Film + group discussion + demonstration | 5 |
| 6. | Wall painting + demonstration | 6 |
| 7. | Radio + folder + demonstration | 7 |
| 8. | Film + folder + demonstration | 8 |
| 9. | Field trip + slide show + group discussion | 9 |
| 10. | Demonstration + group discussion + slide show | 10 |
| 11. | Field trip + group discussion + folder | 11 |
| *Cost benefit ratio* | | |
| 1. | Exhibition + group discussion + demonstration | 1 |
| 2. | Poster + slide show + demonstration | 2 |
| 3. | Wall painting + group discussion + demonstration | 3 |
| 4. | Radio + folder + demonstration | 4 |
| 5. | Folder + film + demonstration | 5 |
| 6. | Film + group discussion + demonstration | 6 |
| 7. | Demonstration + group discussion + slide show | 7 |
| 8. | Radio + slide show + field trip | 8 |
| 9. | Wall painting + slide show + group discussion | 9 |
| 10. | Field trip + slide show + group discussion | 10 |
| 11. | Field trip + group discussion + folder | 11 |

The above ranking of the three media combination reveals the effective methods. In another study it was found that combination of three media could give desirable impact in terms of knowledge gain. However, over and above three media combination there was no significant effect. Various studies have pointed to the effectiveness of different media depending on the situation, area, socio-personal and psychological characteristics of farmers. There is no generalisation regarding the effectiveness and combinations.

---

1. Adapted from H. Annamali, M. Manoharan, S. Somasundaram and K.M. Krishnakumar, "Extension Methods and their Principles". Palaniappa Printers, Tirunelveli.

## Suggested Method for Various Occasions

Based on the experiences and findings of various studies the extension methods that help most in including farmers in the process of change are as follows:

1. **Methods useful in getting attention:** Pictures related to the subject, news stories, demonstration, posters, radio talk, cartoons, displays, exhibits, radio announcement, leaflets, banner, wall painting, hoardings, tom-tom, personal contact, awareness campaign, etc.

2. **Methods useful in developing interest:** Meetings of various types, film strip and slide lectures, news, radio talk, bulletins and pamphlets, tours, result demonstration, VCR, photographs, charts, personal contact, etc.

3. **Methods useful in creating desire:** Object, circular letters, working models, sample and exhibits, success stories, charts, folders, field trips, etc.

4. **Methods useful in developing confidence:** Demonstration, field trips, discussion with scientists, success stories, etc.

5. **Methods useful in ensuring action:** Reminding circular letters, news stories, radio talks, personal contacts, campaign, leader contact, etc.

6. **Methods useful in maintaining satisfaction:** Individual contacts, news stories, success stories, personal and circular letters, etc.

### Methods used in different stages of adoption process

The extension methods that could be used in different stages of adoption process are:

1. **Awareness:** All printed materials, personal contacts, film-show, radio, TV, posters, local leaders, newspaper, campaign, leaflet, banners, tom-tom, circular letters, slide.

2. **Interest:** Personal contact, meetings, radio talk, leaflet, folder, bulletin, farm journal, film, slide, filmstrip, recorded cassettes, VCR/TV.

3. **Evaluation:** Demonstration followed by discussion, cassettes, field trips, farmers' experiences in any printed form, field day.

4. **Trial:** Personal contact, method demonstration, result demonstration, leaflet, folder, farm journals, field trips, field days, TV/VCR.

5. **Adoption:** Group discussion, method demonstration, result demonstration, field trips, slide, self-experiences, leaflets, folder, farm journals, training, campaign.

# Chapter 7

# Audio-Visual Aids

This chapter deals with audio-visual aids. An aid is an instructional device that assists the facilitators to teach the learners effectively. The aids can supplement the teachers' teaching effectiveness and help the learners to learn with greater understanding. But aids cannot supplant the teacher. An audio aid is any instructional device through which message can be heard but not seen. A visual aid is an instructional device through which a message can be seen but not heard. An audio-visual aid is an instructional device through which a message can be heard as well as seen.

## Significance of audio-visual aids

Audio-visual aids help to supplement the spoken word and convey the meaning clearly. Research and experience have shown that audio-visual aids can significantly capture audience attention, create and sustain interest, highlight the main points, make understanding easy, increase learning and impress ideas better by making teaching more realistic and facilities meeting of minds of the teacher and learners. Aids enhance the process of transfer of technology (cognitive process) and also the motivation to change (emotional process) which are the two important functions of aids.

## Classification of audio-visual Aids

The audio-visual aids can be classified as audio aids, visual aids and audio-visual aids.

## ▮AUDIO AIDS

### Public Address System (PA System) (Fig. 7.1)

PA system consists of microphone (mike), amplifier and loud speaker. It is used to amplify and reinforce sound. Mikes and speakers are connected to the amplifier. Again, the amplifier is connected to power source, which may be battery or alternating current (AC) or direct current (DC).

**Mike:** Mikes are of four types, namely unidimensional mike, multidimensional mike, collar mike and cordless mike. The mike has a diaphragm which vibrates to the sound produced in front of it. The sound energy is converted into alternating electric current and sent to the amplifier.

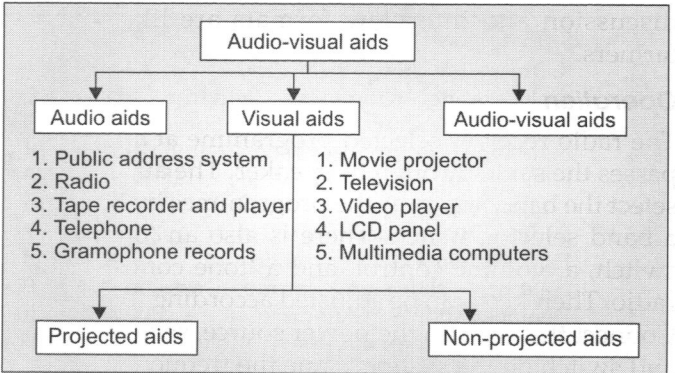

**Fig. 7.1:** Classification of audio-visual aids

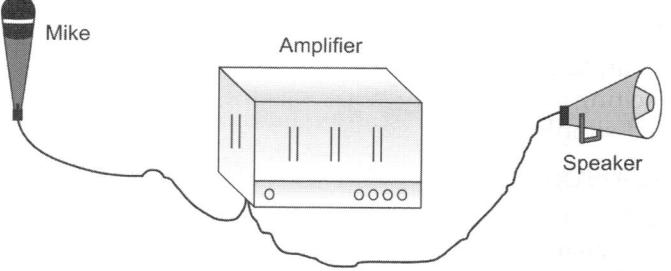

**Fig. 7.2:** Public address system

**Amplifier:** The amplifier is an electronic device to amplify the electric currents produced by the mike.

**Speaker:** The speakers are connected to the proper output terminals of the amplifier using wires taking into account the input capacity of the speakers. In connecting the speakers to the amplifier there are three methods, viz. direct, serial and traditional methods.

### Operation

1. Switch on the amplifier and observe that its pilot lamp glows.
2. Check the mike and adjust the volume.
3. Keep the mike at a distance of about 15 cm from the speaker.

## Radio

Radio is the most vital source of dissemination of animal husbandry and agricultural information to farmers. A separate division of Farm and Home section is functioning in All India Radio (AIR) for this purpose. Apart from the regular farm announcements, information on scientists, extension agents and experience of the farmers are broadcast in different formats. A special distance education programme known as "Farm Radio School" organized under the joint auspices of AIR and the State agricultural and veterinary universities. Radio forum is also functioning very well. Broadcasts of radio conferencing, songs, drama, group discussion and interview formats are liked by the farmers.

### Operation

The radio receives selected programme at a time, and passes the same through its speaker. The audience can select the band and hear the programmes by operating a band selector switch. There is also an 'on and off' switch, a 'volume control' and a 'tone control' to the radio. Their keys can be adjusted according to the need. Connect the radio to the power source, select the band and switch on the system. Tune the frequency knob to get the desired station. Advance the volume control and adjust the tone control.

### Use

As an audio aid, it can be popular, pleasing and even exciting and is used for broadcasting light information and simple technologies.

### Advantages

1. Fast medium
2. Cheap
3. Realism and authenticity
4. Emotional impact
5. Suitable to the illiterate
6. Handy and operated even with batteries.

### Limitations

1. Programme only for ears, so needs full attention.
2. One way communication.
3. As the broadcasts are 'one time' event, chance of missing the programme.
4. Farm broadcasts lose out in competition with entertainment. Needs talent to treat the technical message, to make the script and also for effective presentation.

## Audiio Recorder

The sound can be recorded in three ways: (i) Mechanical process, (ii) magnetic process, and (iii) optical process.

The audio records is done by the magnetic process on discs, on gramophone records by the mechanical process and in movie film recording by the optical process. The tape recorder offers wide scope for recording any sound, continuously use the matter, erase it and re-use the tape. The tape recorder and record player/CD player are the widely used audio aids, besides the radio (Fig. 7.3).

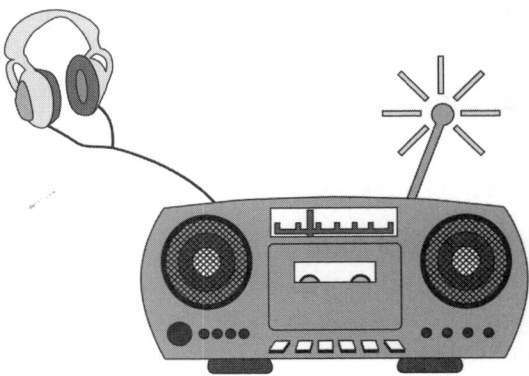

**Fig. 7.3:** Tape recorder

The tape recorder is an audio aid for recording sound on magnetic tape having a coating of magnetic oxide of iron. The tape is like a ribbon of ¼ cm width, usually made of plastic and in some cases of paper. The sound recordings are made by electromagnetic process and are played back when desired. These tapes are reeled in spools. The tape recorder automatically erases the old recording while making the new recording. Presently, the audio/sound recording devices are obsolete and replaced by modern electronic recording devices.

### Steps in Recording

1. Insert batteries in tape recorder/audio recorder or connect it with the power cord.
2. Load the cassette or recording discs.
3. Recording: (a) Recording from public address system—connect the audio recorder to the amplifier, adjust the controls and press the play and record button. (b) Recording from radio in two-in-one sets just load the cassettes, switch on the radio, press the play and record buttons.
4. Play back when recording is completed, press the stop button. Rewind the cassette, play back and check the recordings.

### Uses

1. It enables the extension worker to be in more than one place at a time.

2. It facilitates editing.
3. It helps to preserve recorded programme for future use.
4. It helps in transformation of sounds.
5. It can synchronise the commentaries for film strips, slide-talks, lectures and silent films.
6. It helps to rectify the defective speech. It can be used for recording the farm broadcasts which may not be at times convenient for the farmers.
7. It helps to record group discussion and meetings.
8. It is of immense help in various rehearsals.

## VISUAL AIDS

The visual aids can be classified into projected visual aids and non-projected visual aids.

### Projected Visual Aids

Any visual aid which is used for magnification of image on a screen in dark or semi-dark conditions can be called projected visual aid.

**Importance:** (1) The powerful illumination draws and holds full attention of the audience. (2) The projected visual aids are developed and produced by specialists and it convey exact meaning to the audience. (3) It saves the time of the teacher and the learner. (4) It is flexible in nature to meet the requirements of small and large groups by enlarging the projection on the screen.

**Principle:** The principle involved in projection is that when light falls on a transparent or translucent or opaque object, it passes through the object or is reflected by it, and then, if the light is made to pass through a convex lens and allowed to fall on a screen at a convenient distance, an inverted image of the object appears on the screen. If the object is initially kept inverted before the source of light, the image will be straight and comprehensible.

**Types of projection:** There are three important methods of projections in which three different patterns of light are made. These are (i) direct projection, e.g. motion picture projector, filmstrip projector and slide projector, (ii) indirect projection, e.g. overhead projector, and (iii) reflected projection, e.g. opaque projector.

1. *Film strip projector:* A film strip is a series of still photographs, diagrams, drawings or letterings on a strip of 35 mm film. It may be of two types, single frame 24 mm × 18 mm, and double frame 24 mm × 36 mm. The number of frames in a strip may range from 30 to 60. Perforated edges on the film fit over projector sprockets. Once adjusted to project the first frame, each succeeding image will be in focus and in proper position on screen.

*Uses*

1. Light, unbreakable, easily stored with information in condensed form.
2. Less cost, easy to produce, handle and transport.
3. Can keep the picture for long time on the screen.
4. Discussion possible, as projection can be stopped without breaking sequence.
5. Complete process of farm practices can be shown in one short projection.
6. Projection can be synchronised with commentary by a tape recorder.

*Limitations*

1. Commercially available film strips may not suit our requirements.
2. The surface of film strip may become scratched after prolonged use or may be burnt.
3. The sequence cannot be altered.

2. *Slide projector* (Fig. 7.4): Slide is a small film (35 mm) of glass or other transparent material of 2″ × 2″ or 2.5″ × 3.5″ size containing a single pictorial or graphic image which is projected by focusing light through it from electric bulb, petromax or lantern. It is one of the most popular and versatile visual media in education. The most commonly used slide today is made on 35 mm film for class room projection and 120 mm for theater projection.

**Types of slides**

1. Handmade slides
2. Photographic slides

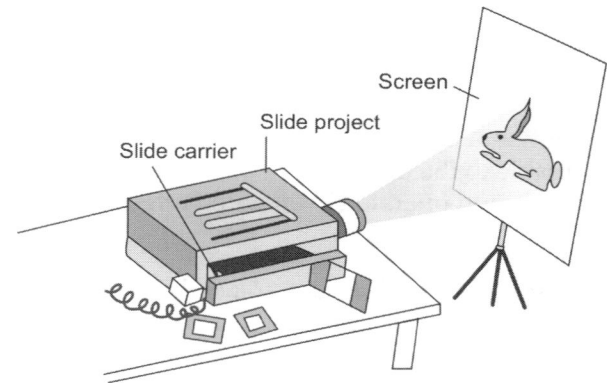

**Fig. 7.4:** Slide projector

*Operation*

1. Keep the slides in order and insert them in the slide carrier in an inverted position.
2. Set the projector and connect the cord.
3. Fix the screen.

4. Turn the switch first to 'fan' and then to 'lamp'. Similarly, at the end put off the lamp first and after the projector has cooled switch off the fan.
5. Focus and centre the image on the screen.
6. Turn the operating knob and adjust the objective lens to get a sharp image.
7. Now slide synchroniser is available. With this the slides are screened with the recorded commentary in the cassette player.

*Advantages*

1. A group of people can study the projected message simultaneously.
2. Magnification helps to put across the idea.
3. Low cost.
4. Colour slides can be made very easily.
5. Easy to handle and transport.
6. Slide sequences can easily be changed to keep them timely and localized.
7. Pertinent slides can attract attention, arouse interest, assist lesson development and learning process.
8. The audience can interact with the extension worker at any time to get their doubts clarified.
9. Complete process can be explained step by step.

*Limitations*

1. They do not show action.
2. A live narration is essential to be effective.
3. Overhead projector (OHP)

A projector which projects the image over the head of an instructor is called an overhead projector. The principle involved in this is indirect projection (vertical transparent projection).

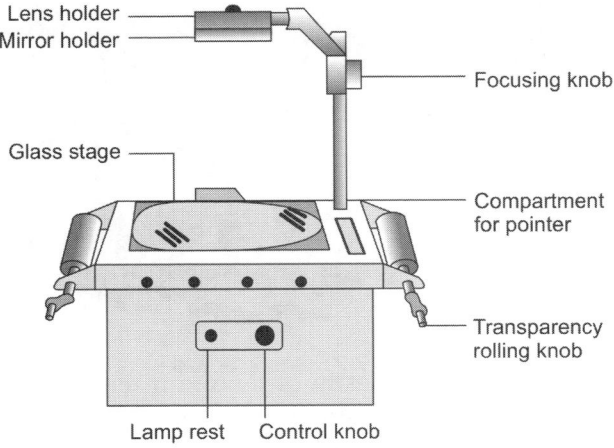

**Fig. 7.5:** Slide projector

**Setting the projector and screen:** Assemble and set up the projector on the table with the projector lens facing the wall or screen. Keep the screen at a suitable place so that no one's view is blocked. If the screen is high, the projected image may have a keystone effect in that the base of the projected image will be smaller than the tope of the picture on the screen. To avoid this keystone effect raise the front of the overhead or slant the screen with the bottom if the screen placed some 18 inches further back than the top of the screen.

**Operation of OHPL:** It is very simple and easy to operate (1) Plug in the power cord. (2) Turn on the switch. (3) Place the transparency over the aperture (on the glass top) with the bottom of the image towards the screen. (4) Raising or lowering the image on the screen may be accomplished either by tilting the front surface mirror by means of a lever on some models or raising the front of the projector by means of adjustable legs on other models. 5. To get a clear image on the screen, focusing is done by turning a focus knob which raises or lowers the projection head.

**Suggestions for effective utilization of OHP**

1. Arrange and keep all the prepared transparency in the required order.
2. Stand at one side of the projector and ensure that you are not obstructing the view of the students.
3. Place the visual on the OHP table (aperture), switch on the projector.
4. Do not leave the light of the projector with projected materials on for long periods of time after you have made a point. Students will have the tendency to see the image on the screen and ignore what the teacher says. Shift the audience's attention back to you by switching off the projector during changes of transparencies and especially, when you have finished referring to a particular transparency.
5. Plan ways to add meaningful details to the transparency during projection; this infuses an element of spontaneity.
6. Use a pencil as a pointer while pointing to specific portions on the transparency. Lay a pencil directly on the transparency. Avoid pointing to the screen.
7. If a visual consists of several lines or items of materials, project only one line of the visual at a time by using masking techniques with opaque

sheet. Move the opaque material down one line at a time when the desired projectual is ready for use.

8. When writing on the transparency which is on the OHP, don not obstruct the view by your hand.

9. After the class session, remove all markings on the transparency with clear cloth if it is not required for further use.

*Advantages*

1. Projector is positioned in front of the class.
2. Bright image in fully-illuminated room.
3. Teacher controls presentation.
4. It is the most versatile projection medium.
5. Teacher can make his own transparencies.
6. Transparencies eliminate repetitive chalk board work.
7. Complex subjects can be presented in comprehensible units.
8. Colour can be used effectively and economically.
9. The presenter can change the sequence of transparencies or return to one previously shown.
10. By superimposing overlays a gradual build up of a situation can be done.
11. The overhead offers the "best" advantages of visual media by focusing the attention of the students, facilitating comprehension of abstract and complex subject, and improving retention.

3. **Opaque projector** (Fig. 7.6): Opaque projector is also known as epidioscope/director projector. It works on the principle of reflecting light from an opaque surface to the screen. This projection allows on-the-spot projection of readily available classroom materials, such as maps, newspapers, photographs and illustrations from books and magazines. Three-dimensional objects, especially relatively flat ones such as coins, plant leaves and insect specimens can be magnified for close inspection.

**Operation:** (a)Place the epidioscope on stand or table and connect the power cord. Keep material on platen. Since the operator faces the screen, materials are placed on the platen face up, with the bottom of the picture towards the screen. Turn on the fan and then the lamp. The screen image is normally less clear than in the case of a slide or OHP where light passes directly through the picture. Bring image to sharp focus by raising or lowering the legs and moving the projector

towards or away from the screen. After showing the visuals turn off the lamp and then fan.

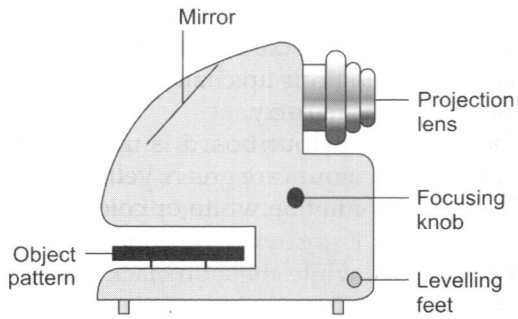

**Fig. 7.6:** Opaque projector

*Advantages*

1. Handling of equipment is simple
2. It projects a wide range of opaque material.
3. The actual colour of the materials is also transmitted to screen.
4. Rare figures and pictures can be projected from books.

**Non-projected Visual Aids**

1. **Chalk board** (Fig. 7.7): The chalk board, popularly known as black board, is the most universally used teaching aid. It is one of the oldest, cheapest, most effective, most versatile and easiest to use of all the visual aids. Little skill or training is needed to make use of this popular teaching device.

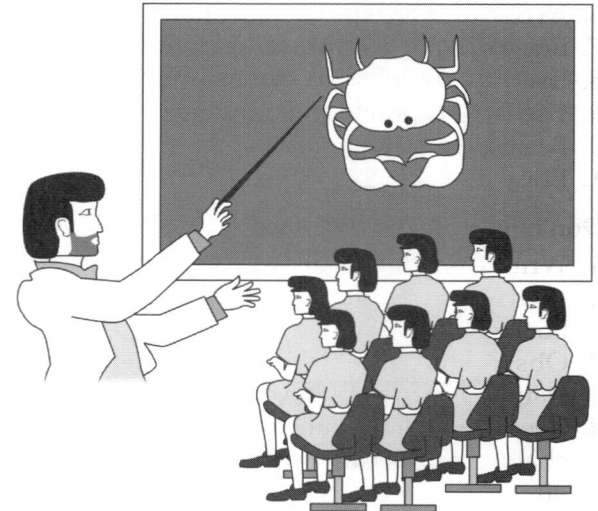

**Fig. 7.7:** Chalk board

a. *Varieties*: There are many varieties of chalk boards available. They are: (1) Fixed, (2) Suspended (3) Roll-up, (4) Foldable, and (5) Magnetic.

b. *Materials*: Rigid boards may be prepared from ordinary thick wood, plywood, metal, fibre board or even heavy cardboard. Rigid type is more durable. Linoleum or rexin cloth can be used in making roll-up chalk board. This type is compact, easy to carry.

c. *Colour*: Black colour board is most commonly used. Other colours are green, yellow and white.

d. *Chalks*: They may be white or coloured. Yellow chalk on olive green background is pleasing to the eyes than white chalk on black paint. In dark rooms fluorescent chalk can be used.

e. *Combinations*: They may be chalk-cum-bulletin board and chalk-cum-felt board.

f. *Placement*: Place chalk board so that the lower edge of the board is at the level of the viewers' eyes. The distance between the board and first row of the seat should be about three metres.

g. *Letter size*: ¼ inch visible from 8 feet, ½ inch visible from 16 feet, 1 inch visible from 32 feet, and 2 inch visible from 64 feet. Thickness of the letter should be 1/5 of the height of the letter.

**Suggestions for better use**

1. Clean the chalk board properly before starting writing.
2. Write slowly and keep even pressure of the chalk on the board.
3. Consider word, sentence and paragraph spacing for good arrangement.
4. Avoid overcrowding.
5. Write in a straight line.
6. Avoid glare and ensure adequate lighting.
7. Erase all unrelated writings on the chalk board.
8. Use colour chalk for emphasis.
9. Use large captions and drawings.
10. Be brief in writing.
11. Erase from top to bottom.

**Don'ts in using chalk board**

1. Writing on the corner of the chalk board.
2. Writing in blank spaces of already written board.
3. Obstructing the writing on the board by standing in front of the board.
4. Keeping other teaching aid, in front or beside the chalk board because they distract the viewers' attention.
5. Speaking to the board. Do not talk as you write.
6. Going out without erasing the board.

2. **Flannel board** (Fig. 7.8): Flannel board, also known as felt board, consists of a stiff backing covered with felt material on one side. Flannel graph or flannel strip is any graphic or written material used on a flannel board. The flannel graph works on the principle that one piece of rough textured cloth will adhere or stick to another. When flannel graphs are backed with rough textured cloth, or sandpaper they adhere to the flannel board. The drawings, photographs, printed illustrations or other instructional materials can be cut and pasted with a piece of rough cloth or coarse sandpaper glued to their backs. Sandpaper strip 1" or so wide should be struck at intervals. A medium or coarse grain sandpaper will work best. If sandpaper is not available, spread some glue on the back of the cardboard. Before the glue dries, sprinkle it with sand. The flannel graph is well utilized for teaching different kinds of educational stories. Intelligent extension worker can handle the flannel strip on the board and attract attention and stimulate interest. The flannel graph can be of particular use with illiterates.

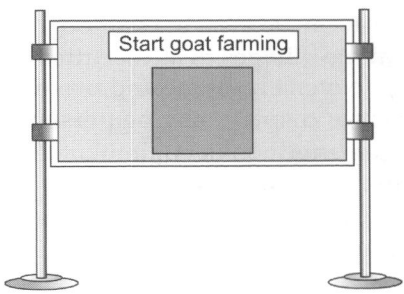

**Fig. 7.8:** Flannel board

**Suggestions for use**

1. The title of the story should be in large letters at the top of the board.
2. Keep the story simple enough to be understood by the audience.
3. Use large, bold illustrations and consider legibility.
4. Use of arrows, cartoons, etc. adds interest.
5. Before using the board, slightly tilt it so that the flannel strips do not fall down.
6. Keep the flannel board out of the windy locations to avoid the flannel strips being blown off.

**Presentation**

1. Carefully plan the steps of the presentation.
2. Arrange each part in the order it will be added to the board.
3. These parts may be numbered on the back and stored in folders.

4. Rehearse the presentation in advance. This provides you time to make sufficient changes.

5. Stand beside the board, not in front of it. The audience should be able to see the board at all times.

6. While placing a flannel graph on the board, apply it with slight downward movement, accompanied by firm pressure to avoid the material sliding off the surface.

7. Leave the materials on the board only as long as they are needed.

8. Avoid excessive handling. It distracts the audience.

9. After classroom presentation, a flannel board can be displayed in another part of the room to serve as a reminder of the lesson.

3. **Bulletin board** (Fig. 7.9): Bulletin board, also known as "tack board", is a device specifically set aside for displaying many items of interest and educational value to the intended learners or audience. It can be used in the modern classroom as well as in the villages to attract attention, stimulate interest, deliver a message and produce action. The materials for display may be personal news, local announcements, booklets, circular letters, bulletins, cartoons, maps, charts, graphs, newspaper clippings, posters, drawings, specimens, models, photographs, etc.

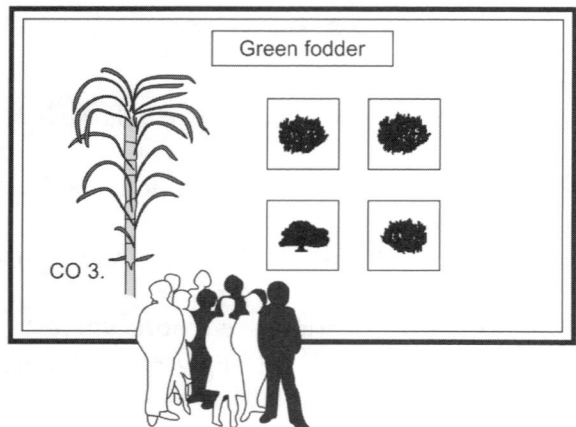

**Fig. 7.9:** Bulletin board

Fixed, folding, and movable or suspended the types of bulletin boards are available. The material like softwood, plywood or cardboard, pegboard (given a three-dimensional effect), a blanket, a banana leaf or a coconut mat, grass mat tacked to a wall, heavy corrugated cardboard wire screening, and the wall of the building can be used as a bulletin board.

The bulletin board will be chosen depending upon the availability and nature of display. A banana leaf may be good for a temporary display, but in a classroom something more permanent is needed. A sheet of wall board is ideal. The background may be khadi cloth, bamboo mat or sugarcane stalks with bamboo or wooden frame for use in villages. It may be of and width, though the ideal dimensiar is 30" × 40", or 36" × 48" depending on the situation. Portable bulletin boards may be of smaller size.

**Display:** The following steps make displays effective:

1. Collect, classify and select materials pertaining to the subject. Remove all old displays, dust and clear bulletin board.

2. Arrange all materials according to good form of composition. Prepare neat titles and brief descriptions. Use colour harmony and balance. Observe variety and sequence when a number of materials are used. Do not overload the board—keep to related ideas and one theme. Change the material on the bulletin board regularly and keep timely information. Use a few but large materials to create title with a few and large sized words that can be seen from a distance. Fix the materials to the board without damaging them.

3. The thumb tacks, push pins, bamboo splinters, thorns, staples, glue, tape or straight pins can be used to fasten the material to a bulletin board.

4. A bulletin board may be placed indoors or outdoors. If it is to be placed outdoors protect it from sun and rain by a covering of clear plastics. Choose a location where the board will be seen. It should be fixed at eye-level.

4. **Magnetic board:** Magnetic board is of recent origin. This board is made of steel on which magnets can be fixed. The teacher can promptly fix pictures, charts, letters, etc. on it with the help of a magnet.

Magnetic boards serve the same function as flannel boards. The only difference between the two is the adherence method. But it has certain advantages over flannel board. It can be very useful where display items are heavy or when presentations must be given in windy places. Its construction permits the use of a more complicated special background and symbols can be moved while still adhering to the board.

5. **Poster** (Fig. 7.10): A poster is designed to make a public announcement of a special idea, and timely information. It usually includes only a few words

with an illustration to catch the attention of the viewers and to pass a simple message at a glance. It should be attractive, brief and clear. It is called the ABC of poster.

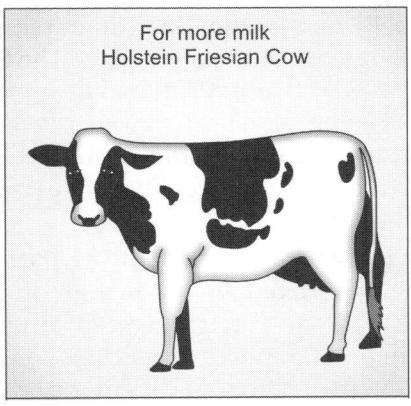

**Fig. 7.10:** Poster (Extension Department, Veterinary College, Namakkal)

1. *Caption:* It should be as small as possible. A caption having not more than five words is the best one. Never write the caption vertically as it creates difficulty in reading. Do not break the caption. The words selected should be arresting words, in slogan form, and printed in plain and bolder letters.

2. *Illustration or picture:* It should be bold and bring out the message clearly. Avoid unnecessary details in the illustration. It should be prepared based on the audience experience and objects familiar to them should be used. Dramatic illustrations would stop people and make them to look.

3. *Colour:* Use bright attractive colours to print picture and words. Highlight the main prominent message with a more prominent colour. Do not use more than three colours. Avoid odd combinations of colours. Background colours preferred by the villagers are yellow, green, light blue and dark blue.

4. *Space:* Plenty of space must be given between letters, words, lines and illustrations.

5. *Layout:* It should be well balanced so that viewer's eye can smoothly travel. It should hold his attention and clearly bring out the message to the viewer. Make rough layout of your poster on a small scale 1/8 or ¼ of actual size. After the rough layout is completed it should be shown to a few people at the level of the target group. Misconception or ambiguity, if any, should be removed. Then final picture may be made by an artist.

6. *Size:* Must be large enough to be easily seen from a distance. It has been found by recent studies, a poster of 28″ × 44″ size is more effective with 2″ size for plain letters for caption in slogan form.

7. *Lettering:* Use plain, bold lettering and lines.

8. *Display:* Place posters where people pass or where people gather.

6. **Charts:** A chart is a visual symbol summarizing or comparing or contrasting or performing other helpful services in explaining subject matter.

**Points to be considered while printing a chart:** Chart should be with bold and simple lettering, brief words, simple design, colourful (not more than 3 colours) and large enough to be seen.

a. **Types of charts**

*Flip chart* (Fig. 7.11): Flips carry a series of ideas arranged sequentially. Individually charts are tagged (or) bound to some support. During teaching, these flips are turned one by one in a sequence.

1. The top of chart is concealed with one or more blank sheets until the person is ready to take the topic.

2. The sheets should be rolled smoothly over the top to avoid wrinkling which will become increasingly annoying as more and more sheets are turned over.

3. The person must stand to one side while displaying and turning the chart.

4. Each heading is covered by a strip of white paper attached by paper clips and they are removed at the appropriate moment. This process creates a certain amount of suspense and adds attention.

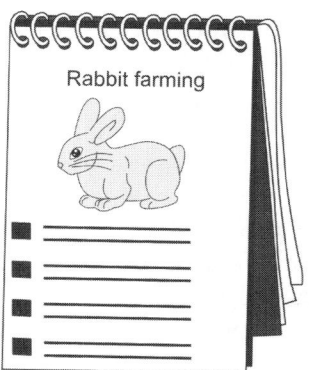

**Fig. 7.11:** Flip chart

5. If it is necessary to refer to special pages, mark them in some way such as folded corners, paper clips, etc.
6. Drawings can be prepared invisibly in light yellow pencil.

It can be used as chalk board or as previously prepared sheets. It is suitable for telling consecutive story with a number of points which need to be emphasized in outline fashion. Less expensive. If sheets are just flipped over and not turned off, material is available for reconsideration and review.

*Tabular chart*: Anything that is recorded or presented in a tabular form is a tabular chart.

*Flow chart*: These are made by lines, arrows, rectangles, etc. They show the structure of an organization, institution, association, etc. It can also be used to show the story of a product as to how it has been obtained through a series of processes.

*Overlay chart*: This consists of a number of sheets which can be placed one over the other conveniently and form a part of the whole picture. This enables the viewer to see not only the different parts but also how they appear when one is placed over the other. After the final overlay is placed, it shows the ultimate product. This type of presentation is dramatic and effective.

*Pull chart*: The content of the chart is put fully in suspense by placing another sheet of paper of the same size on it with the help of two paper clips.

*Strip teaser chart*: This chart is similar to pull chart. In this, the message is concealed by placing strips on each line. The strips are prepared using thin paper. The ends of thin paper strips are pinned or pasted at both ends of the message. Whenever the message is to be exposed, one end of the strip is set free. This has the advantage of creating anticipation and surprise.

*Tree chart*: These are used to show development or growth of things. In this, the origin is a single line. The various developments are shown as branches.

*Strip roll-up chart*: In this type of chart, the points are recorded on series of strips, rolled up in sequences and displayed in order on a large of paper. This type of chart leads to dramatic effect. It helps the trainer to develop lesson systematically.

*Window chart*: The information is put concurrently at the chart and is released through the window at the required time.

b. **Types of graphs:** A graph is more or less an accurate representation of quantitative data and is widely used in showing comparisons, trends, developments and relationships. The function of a graph is to present somewhat confusing and discouraging statistical data clearly and interestingly. An interesting graph will arrest attention. A good graph requires little explanation and tells the story at a glance.

*Bar graph*: These are made up of a series of bars arranged horizontally or vertically from a 'zero base'. The distance between the bars and thickness of the bars should be constant. The size, length or colour of bars represents different values. These are helpful in comparing and contrasting many subjects.

*Pie graph*: It is very helpful where a breakdown or distribution of values is important. These are in the shape of circles and used to show how several parts make up the whole. Each section should have its own colour and the size is based on the section's proportion.

*Line graph*: These are useful in showing the trends and relationships. A single continuous line may represent growth or expansion. Multiple lines will show the relationship.

*Pictorial graph*: They give the viewer a vivid picture and create rapid association with the use of graphic messages like cartoons, illustrations, etc. The number and size of picture conveys the proportionate amount.

7. **Flash cards** (Fig. 7.12): Flash cards are a series of illustrated cards flashed (turned over at short intervals) before the learners in proper sequence to emphasize important points in a presentation.

**Preparation**

1. *Cards*: Select white or light-coloured thick paper cardboard. Even that can be prepared on a paper and pasted to a cardboard.
2. *Size*: It should be large enough for everyone to see. For a group of 30 to 50, it should be of 36"× 48" size. For small groups, 22"× 28" size is adequate.
3. *Number*: It is best to limit the cards to 10 or 12 for a talk.
4. *Content*: Each set should have a title card. The story should be divided into a number of scenes

which are to be presented in a number of individual cards. In order to prepare more effective cards, study the talk, pick the main ideas that learners want to remember and prepare picture for each idea, which will give visual impact to the idea. Each card must have message presented in simple line drawings, photographs, cartoons, and cutouts with a few words.

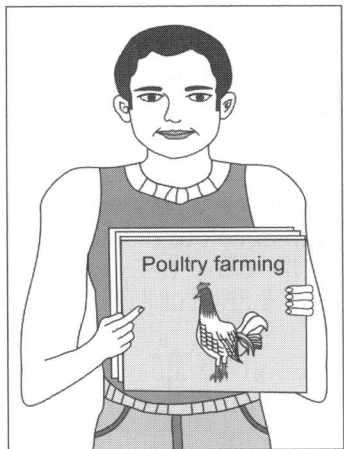

**Fig. 7.12:** Flash card

5. *Design*: Make rough sketch on plain paper. Draw a guideline for needed lettering, mark off area for illustrative materials. Draw with pencil and then trace with crayon, paint, or ink. Use pen with a thick point or brush.

6. *Lettering*: Have letters that are large enough for the group to read, at least 1″ high.

7. *Colours*: Use dark colours. But not more than three colours.

8. *Words*: Use minimum wording - not more than 10 to 12 word per card.

**Presentation**

1. The speaker must be familiar with the story for each card.

2. He should use simple words and local expressions.

3. Stack the cards in their proper order.

4. If the cards are small, hold them in such a way that the audience can see it clearly, ideally against the body (chest). If they are large, they may be placed on an easel.

5. The teacher should turn the body as he turns the cards towards different parts of the group to show them to all members of the group.

6. As one card is finished, slip the front card to the back of the set.

7. Some important points may be jotted on the back side of the previous cards to help in telling the story. At the time of presentation glance at these points as you tell the story.

8. After the story is completed, display the cards on a bulletin board or pass them onto interested persons, if needed.

9. Use this teaching aid along with other teaching tools.

10. It will be effective for a small group of not more than 30.

**Advantages**

1. Flash cards can be made quickly from inexpensive local materials.

2. Easy to carry and use.

3. Help speaker emphasise main points of his talk.

8. **Photographs:** A photograph or picture is more than 1000 words; they speak for themselves. They are faithful representation of reality and exact visual recording of things. They have no language barrier and they speak a universal language. They are suited to teaching illiterates. Pictures are useful for recollecting and reinforcing the memory. They may be actual photo prints or printed in book, newspaper or magazine. They may be in black and white or colour, and used in personal teaching situations or as display in exhibitions. To be an effective teaching aid a photograph must tell a story, illustrate only one point, show action and emotion, have plain and simple background and easily understood.

9. **Pictures (illustrations):** Illustrations are non-photographic representation of reality, e.g. drawings, paintings, etc. They are used as teaching aids like photographs.

10. **Exhibits and displays:** Exhibits and displays have the common characteristics of posters. There is difference between exhibits and displays. The exhibits are more of 3-dimensional materials, while displays are mostly 2-dimensional. The most effective exhibits are built around a single idea with a minimum of supporting information. Make it simple, understandable, portable, and impressive in size. Make it duarble, and attractive having. Label legibly and briefly. Use local materials as far as possible since specimens from locality will have greater significance.

11. **Models** (Fig. 7.13): Models are replicas of real objects and can be used in any teaching situation. They may be of life size, smaller or larger than the things they represent. They are often called three

dimensional visuals. When real things are not available or are too complex or too small for study, models are used. Models improve the efficiency of teaching because they have the capacity to bring into play all the five senses. Scale models, cross sectional models, working models (mock-up) and simplified models are the different types of models. Mock-up is functional device. It shows the operations of essential parts of real objects, e.g. milking machine.

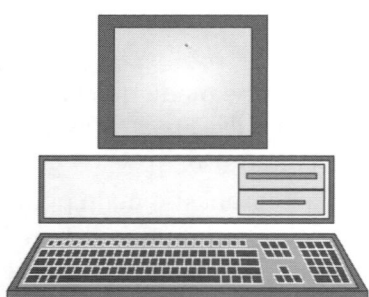

**Fig. 7.13:** Models

12. **Specimen** (Fig. 7.14): A specimen may be a part of an object or be one of a group or class taken to represent the whole group. The objects are usually mounted in a special way as specimen. The methods of preservation of specimens are: (1) Dry preservation method e.g. insects, bones, (2) wet preservation method, e.g. worms, mummified foetus, etc. (preserved in formaldehyde), and (3) live preservation method, e.g. birds, fish, tick, etc. The specimen are real and hence appeal to senses and they offer better scope for study.

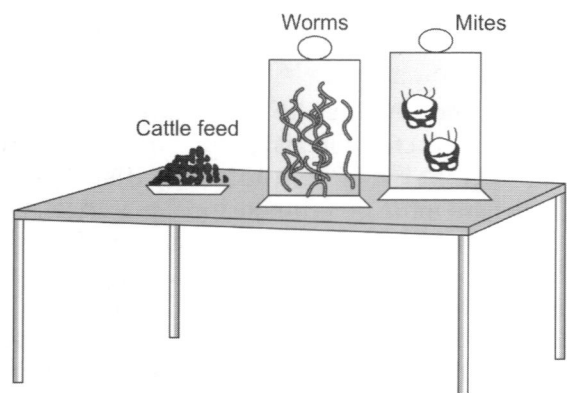

**Fig. 7.14:** Specimen

13. **Real objects** (Fig. 7.15): Real objects are the best visual aids as the learners recognise them. The learners can be taken to the field situation to show them the real objects like pasture, fodder plots and livestock.

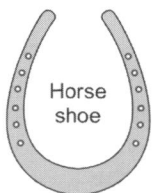

**Fig. 7.15:** Real objects

14. **Dust and mud sketching:** If an extension worker does not possess any aid and wants to explain with illustrations, he can draw many on sand, dust or mud. This can help to visualise the message, especially during farm visits.

## AUDIO-VISUAL AIDS

### Movie Projector (Fig. 7.16)

The movie projector is an audio-visual aid through which motion pictures are projected. Different types of motion picture projectors are available based on the size (width) of the film, classified as 70 mm, 35 mm, 16 mm and 8 mm. The 16 mm projector is used for classroom purposes. The motion picture film is divided into two parts, i.e. the picture track and sound track.

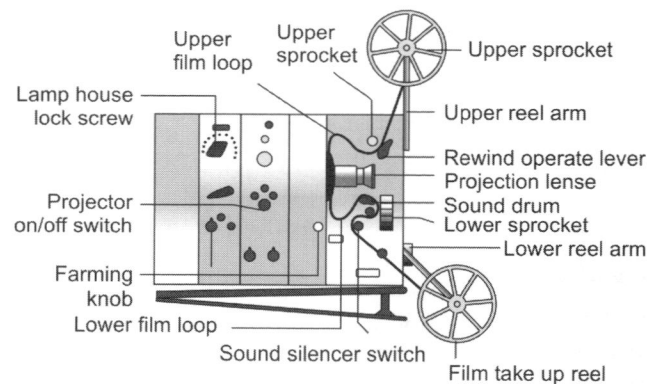

**Fig. 7.16:** Movie projector

The sound picture camera rapidly snaps 24 still pictures or frames per second (16 frames for silent motion pictures). When these still frames are projected in a sequence on a screen the impression of life and motion is apparent to the viewer. Sound is recorded on the photographic film. As the film moves through the sound motion picture projector the recorded sound is reproduced.

### Setting up the Projector

1. Keep the projector on the table so that light passes above the head of the audience.

2. Remove cover.
3. Attach reel arms.
4. Put spring belts.
5. Give connections to the power source and to the speaker.
6. Switch on the projector lamp.
7. Initial adjustments focusing the picture on the screen by adjusting the lens are made.
8. Adjust the distance between projector and screen, until the middle of the lighted area is slightly greater than the middle of written portion of screen, centre the light vertically.

### Threading the Film

1. Fix empty reel on lower arm and full reel on upper arm.
2. Take the lead film, examine for beginning.
3. Check if rewind/operate lever is in operate position.
4. Take 4 feet lead film, attach the end to the take up reel.
5. Follow the white guideline.
6. Bring the film through upper sprocket.
7. Open the picture gate by pulling the lens.
8. Push the lens to its original distance to close the aperture plate.
9. Run the film over the guide roller, under the pressure roller, around the sound drum and over tension roller.
10. Thread the film under the lower sprocket.
11. Finally thread under snubber roller to the lower (take off spool) reel.

### Types of Screens

Screen is to provide maximum possible visibility of the image with minimum glare or strain on the eyes. Different screens are used for different purposes.

1. **Beaded screen:** Which will reflect the rays so sharply to the tune of 20°. So, these screens are more suited for long and narrow halls.

2. **Matte screen:** These screens will reflect rays to a wider angle of 30°. These screens are suited to for rays rooms like auditoriums.

3. **Silver or aluminum screen:** Used for asfero - pictures, colour slides or films.

4. **Lenticular screen:** Useful for semi-darkened rooms.

5. **Improvised screen:** A rectangular piece of white cloth is fixed on the wall or a white washed wall is used as a screen.

### Screen Arrangement (Fig. 7.17)

The screen should be fixed at a height of 4 feet from the floor to bottom of screen or at a height of one foot above the heads of the front row of the audience so that all the audience is able to see easily the bottom of the picture. Adopt 20° angle for beaded screen, and 30° angle for matte screen.

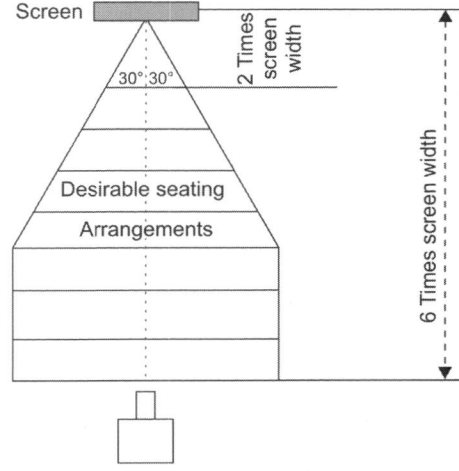

**Fig. 7.17:** Screen arrangement

### Seating Arrangement

Adopt 2″ and 6″ formula, i.e. the front row should be two screen widths away from the screen, and the hind row six screen widths away from the screen.

### Operation

1. After threading the film in the projector, test its operation by hand before, turning the motor. Place the sound box or speaker near the screen.
2. Turn switch to 'ON' position.
3. Turn the volume control to 'O' position.
4. Rotate the project-lamp switch to the projection position and finally to lamp position.
5. Adjust the focusing by turning the lens to get sharp image.
6. Adjust the volume control for requisite sound, after starting the picture. Adjust the tone control to obtain clear sound.

**Principles of operation:** The film unwinds from the feed reel goes through the picture head where it is illuminated by the light source, and is then projected on the screen by the field lens.

The film then is passes through the sound head. Here the tack on the film is illuminated by the exciter lamp.

The sound's image is turned into electrical signals by a photo cell assembly, then amplified and heard through the amplifier and speaker assembly.

A standard reel of sound film of length 400 feet takes 10 minutes' time at the rate 24 frames per second. Stop the projector as soon as the last picture appears. Rewind the film on the take up spools and remove the film from the projector after the audience has disbursed.

### Points to be remembered

1. Have thorough knowledge of the subject you plan to teach.
2. Preview the film.
3. Before projection, explain the subject, stimulate viewers to look for certain things in the film.
4. At the end of the show, have forum.
5. Follow-up.
6. Technical details—be familiar in handling the aid, ensure adequate power supply. See the availability of darkroom without cutting off ventilation. Have spare projection lamp. Load the projection and keep it ready before audience arrives. Check the screen and seating arrangements.

### Advantages

1. They enable the teacher to recreate events, action, and time.
2. Real experience can be shared by the teacher and the learner.
3. Compells attention.
4. They overcome physical limitations, elements of time, size of the object and distance.
5. They help to overcome barriers of illiteracy.

### Limitations

1. High cost of film projector.
2. Non-availability of uninterrupted electricity in villages.
3. Lack of experience in handling projector.
4. Scarcity of appropriate films.
5. Difficulty in transporting and maintaining projector and film.

### Television (Fig. 7.18)

Television is an audio-visual aid used for mass teaching. It is more personal than radio by virtue of the fact that people can retain the matter 50% or more when both hearing and seeing are employed. So, it is nowadays widely used as an important audio-visual aid. Television is variously referred to as the small screen (monitor) and the idiot box. The word television comes from a Greek word meaning 'far' and a Latin word meaning 'to see'. Hence, it is 'to see what is far'.

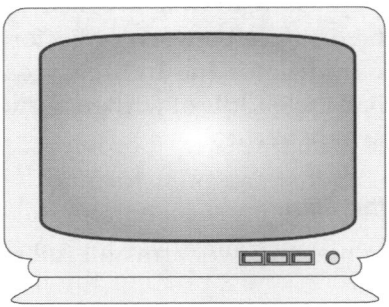

**Fig. 7.18:** Television

The programme is telecast in air by converting the audio and video waves into electromagnetic waves which are then rectified in the antenna and converted to audio–video waves in the TV set. Among all the aids available TV occupies a special status because of its profound influence on the audience. A live transmission of an event is possible only through this medium with its unique potential to communicate to the two most important sense organs, simultaneously to an exceedingly large number of audience. TV can hopefully meet the new challenge of quick transfer of the rapidly changing farm technology.

### Advantages

It attracts attention, increases interest, develops desire, creates conviction, promotes action and builds up satisfaction. TV, video, film and plays can achieve a mixed goal of providing information in an entertaining way.

### Limitations

1. Intense competition with entertainment.
2. Expensive.
3. If editing is not done properly, programmes become ambiguous.
4. It requires certain showmanship.
5. It cannot be used where there is no electricity.
6. The entertainment aspects will dominate and the information content may be missed.

## Video

The term 'Video' is used to denote pictures which have been converted into electronic signals. The video produced can be telecast through TV station to reach the masses. Video lessons produced can also be used for teaching of small group of farmers with the help of video projector or LCD panel.

### *Advantages*

This will immediately attract the attention of the learners. This will be useful when the presentation has to be repeated at many places. It provides an interactive and consistent instructional format. Learners can perform and learn, practise laboratory exercises within short period of time. It improves the teaching quality. Deletion, addition and updating the lesson and the content can be made instantaneously.

### *Disadvantages*

It involves much cost, time and technical skill in production.

## Puppetry

Puppetry is most suitable for villagers. It is an expensive activity and an easily acquired art. The puppets can hold an audience, provided they are played with a lively sense of drama. The puppets are of four types; Glove or hand puppets, string puppets, rod puppets, and shadow puppets. Out of various types the glove puppet is the simple and easy to work with.

## Folk Songs and Drama

The villagers have a great fascination for folk songs, dance and dramas. These are very good sources for conveying information in a better way.

## ▌COMPUTER-ASSISTED ELECTRONIC AIDS

The development of computers and improvements in telecommunication aids offer farmers many new opportunities to obtain technical information like research findings, markets, data on growth and management process quickly. He can select and apply the most productive, labour-saving, low cost and profitable technology. Previously, the TV, radio and newspapers gave generalised advice to farmers, but with modern aids extension can provide custom-built advice for each farm and farmer without visiting the farm personally.

## Microcomputer

Computer is one of the powerful tools which can aid in processing of information and communication. It can store and display all kinds of information. Microcomputer is the smallest general purpose processing system. Modern computers have become much more user-friendly.

## Videotext

It is computerized information storage and retrieval system. It transmits information from a central computer by cable to the screen of a home TV with a modified receiver or a computer. The amount of information the system can store is limited only by the capacity of its computers.

## Teletext

It is a system somewhat like videotext in which printed information is telecast through television rather than transmitted through a telephonic line. It has no interactive capacity and it has a very much smaller database. Teletext is information oriented rather than entertainment oriented. It is less expensive than videotext.

## Teleconferencing

It is the interaction between individuals or groups through satellite television.

## Computer Multimedia

It is a multifaceted instructional strategy that brings together text, graphics, animation, video, still images, audio and motion video. Understanding the vast capabilities of the multimedia several software packages have been developed which are used as teaching tools by the instructors. It is a strong teaching tool since it facilitates more complete use of learners' senses in learning. It enables all the learners to actually hear and see what is actually happening in a given problem situation. Those who are accustomed to making slides and transparencies of OHP and presentations will find their task much more simplified. Teachers can create the entire lesson and presentation with a running commentary through multimedia.

## Interactive Video Disc

This system consists of a video disc player, microcomputer and monitor. The monitor accepts signals from both computer and disc player. This capability enables simultaneous presentation of video images, texts and computer graphics on the screen. It can be useful where there is shortage of trained teachers and large number of students are to be trained. It helps in updating farmers' training materials and also in location-specific training.

## Internet

Internet is a network for information. It is an acronym for International Network and it is a network of networks. A network is anything that connects two or more people. And a network can be two computers connected by a wire. If X types a message in his computer, he does not have to print it out, as the office clerk can route it to anyone. This network of computers is called Local Area Network (LAN). Wide Area Network (WAN): If your branch office was hooked with a few more branches, then the LAN could be part of an even greater network, such as a WAN. Then an information could travel between different departments of one branch on several computers. Similarly, there can be networks of other organizations. If all these networks are joined into a giant network, then this can be called big Internet Work or Internet. The Internet can be defined as a global collection of computers and computer networks that exchange information. So, the Internet is an information system. It can be used as an effective teaching aid.

## Electronic Mail

Electronic mail is an electronic aid. It allows to send and receive messages to and from other Internet users. Whether you are using electronic mail on a local area network or the Internet, the transmission of the electronic mail is the same. You identify to whom you want the message to go to, and give the command to send it over the network. After you have acquired an Internet server and established an Internet address, you can begin sending and receiving electronic mail. Berkeley mail is the most widely available mail programme.

## Advanced Information/Communication Technologies

Some of the advanced information/communication technologies are as follows:

1. **Radio trunking:** It is a two-way communication system which uses radio frequencies to transmit voice and data. Further, it allows point to multi-point mobile radio communication, which means more than two users can talk to one another simultaneously. This is a distinct edge over the cellular phone systems. Unlike ordinary phone, the user does not need to punch in numbers to make a call. As the system has a facility of programme keys, merely pressing a key would suffice. This, of course, adds to user convenience.

2. **Radio data system (RDS) paging:** This has been introduced in India in 1999 with All India Radio launching FM based paging services. Thus, the AIR became the first public broadcaster in Asia to adopt paging for providing public information. RDS paging has only a 2% share of the global market.

3. **Cyber space:** 'Cyber' means 'to steer, guide or control'. It originates from the Greek term 'kubeman'. Cyber space was first used in science fiction. It means the global pool of information held on computer network connected together by sophisticated transmission based on technology that can be accessed by any one. The information that can be accessed includes moving images and animated graphics.

4. **Virtual reality technology:** It is a major break-through in the way humans interact with computers. Computer generated images displayed in the head sets and sound from built-in head-phones along with data. It has various applications in education, business, entertainment, etc.

5. **Video phone:** Novel series for taking picture along with the sound.

6. **Satellite based agricultural communication system:** It is also called farm data info system. It has recently been developed by several US and Canadian agricultural groups. The system uses a computer keyboard and a colour or monochrome monitor to display signals received through a satellite dish mounted on a roof or patio. This information is available in both printed and pictured formats.

7. **Teledon:** Using a television set, equipped with a special decoding, as the users' terminal, the sector is connected via a telephone system, to a large central computer in which is stored a vast data base of information. The user can select the desired content from a menu. A keypad resembling a remote TV channel selector is used to go through the menu and select an item and the information appears on the TV screen in colour graphics and text.

8. **View data:** This transmits information from a central computer by telephone line to the screen of a home television set or a computer. The amount of information which the system can store is limited

only by the capacity of its computer. The farmer can search for information stored in the database and can request the computer to make certain calculation by combining information from his own farm.

9. **Video disc:** The video disc provides many advantages for storing large amount of information, both visual and textual, and can be connected to a computer to provide a very powerful interaction in training and teaching systems. Thus, video disc is likely to become a major player in the training and extension fields in the future.

## Hybrid Communication Tools

### Webinars

The web-based seminars/interactive presentations using a telephone and the internet are increasingly becoming popular in developed countries, where a broad audience of attendees can participate in a seminar without having to leave their desks. These are as effective as on-site presentations without the travel expense.

### Personal Digital Assistant

PDA is the ultimate hybrid communication tool to empower farmers. Also known as Palmtop computer is a mobile device that functions as a personal information manager. PDAs are rapidly being replaced by the widespread adoption of smart phones. These devices have the ability to connect to the Internet. A PDA has an electronic visual display, enabling it to include a web browser, audio capabilities enabling use as a portable media player, and also enabling most of them to be used as mobile phones. Most PDAs can access the Internet, intranets or extranets via Wi-Fi or Wireless Wide Area Networks. Most PDAs employ touch screen technology.

### Videoconferencing System

Videoconferencing may be described as a method of conferencing between two or more locations where both sound and vision are transmitted and received so as to enable simultaneous interactive communication. Videoconferencing can save significant amounts of money in terms of both travel costs and time leading to open up new methods of communication, e.g. linking several schools together to enhance the learning experience. All videoconferences must have these three basic elements: Environment, equipment and network. It is even possible for a PC application running at one

site to be shared with another site so that either site can annotate and take control of the software. When PC documents are shared in this way it is termed "Data Sharing". Videoconferencing can be applied in meetings, Interviews, teaching, management and diagnosis.

### Type of videoconferencing session

- One-to-one conferencing from PC desktops.
- A teacher by him or herself teaching remotely to a group of students.
- A teacher in a classroom teaching his own and students in another school.
- A teacher with both local and remote students but with the added dimension of full interaction from both student groups.

### Component of videoconferencing system

1. The display—for example a plasma screen
2. Cameras
3. Microphones
4. Sound mixers
5. Speakers
6. Echo cancellation
7. The networks used to carry videoconference traffic
8. The user interfaces—for example the remote control and the web interface cables.
9. Peripheral equipment—for example a laptop or second camera and the Codec which is the main brain of the system.

### Information System

Information system or web-based information system uses Internet web technologies to deliver information and services. It is a software system whose main purpose is to publish and maintain data by using hypertext-based principles.

### Component of Information System

**Hardware:** Examples are physical computers, networks, communication equipment, scanners, digital drives, and so on.

**Software:** Information system can be designed by using commercially available software such as Adobe Creative Suite, Microsoft FrontPage, Microsoft Visual Studio, etc. and using open source software such as Joomla, Zope, Plone, Drupal, Moodle, eFront, etc.

**Data:** Information is an organized, meaningful and useful interpretation of data, such as animals' breed, health, production, etc. Information systems can change data into useful and meaningful information to its users.

**Process:** Process is a guide consisting of orderly steps, which need to be followed and implemented in order to get a certain decision on a certain matter.

**Human:** The main objective of an information system is to provide invaluable information to managers and users, whether inside or outside the company. Users can be broken up into three categories as: End users, internal users, external users.

### Types of Information System

1. **Transaction Processing System:** Commonly known as TPS and is one of the first systems to be automated. It can access and record information about all transactions related to the organization. TPS now uses the latest technology for e-commerce concept which is a new challenge in the field of transaction processing for shifting to online transaction processing system.

2. **Management Information System:** This system will take the information that has been extracted from TPS and generate reports which are required by the management for planning and controlling a company's business.

3. **Executive Information System:** A decision support system specifically used by the executive management in making strategic decisions. It is a tool that provides online access directly to the relevant information, in the format that is useful and can be browsed.

4. **Decision Support System:** The main focus of this information system is for the effectiveness of the manager in analyzing the information and making a decision. It is used for handling decisions that are not structured, i.e. decisions which are made in case of an emergency.

5. **Expert System:** It is a programme that produces a decision which is almost similar to decisions made by an expert in a certain discipline. This information system can imitate the way humans think and consider in making a decision.

6. **E-Learning System:** A new breed of Information Systems (ISs) known as Learning Management Systems (LMSs) are evolving to enable learning in organizations. Most web based system includes three major components which will be relied upon to differing levels depending on the nature of the systems tasks. They are web client, web server and web scripting.

### Open Technologies

In "open technologies" approach, there is a scope for farmers to adapt, adopt and innovate and use them for their farming. This approach can significantly contribute to satisfying need for customized solutions. The term "open technology" is considered to have emerged in the context of information technology. In the context of agricultural technology, "open" can be described as allowing innovation at all levels by all who can use it and not just at one place. It also means that the technology must be valued as judged by the community and that the control of technology is with the user. This does not mean that technology or its related information is not patentable. It is, but the patent is not locked and its value is realized through rapid innovation it triggers for better products.

## SELECTION OF AUDIO-VISUAL AIDS

Audio-visual aids will not automatically increase teaching effectiveness. While preparing the aids the structure of the message must be carefully planned, treated and designed so as to support the lesson. Synchronising the audio and visual channels is a must, otherwise confusion will result in. The planning and preparation of such aids require time, thought and imagination. Audience nearly always picks up much irrelevant information, so the visual aid producer must try to restrict this by using appropriate forms of presentation. It is perhaps even more important to always pretest audio-visual materials while using them.

The teacher should choose the aid which is best suited for a particular situation. There is no best teaching aid suitable for all situations. The teacher can select the audio-visual aids based on the following points:

**Teaching objective:** Film and video can be useful in the emotional process because they can arouse farmers, emotional involvement in the problems the extension agent wishes to discuss. Puppet show, drama and other folk aids can also serve this purpose effectively.

**Subject matter:** Based on the subject matter to be taught the extension workers can select the aids, e.g. to teach the breed characters of a cattle, a colour photograph can be used.

**Nature of the learner:** According to the age, education, interest, experience, knowledge and intelligence of the learner the extension workers can select the aids, e.g. TV for illiterates.

**Cost of the aid:** According to the availability of the financial resources one can select the aids. When there is a tight budget, low-cost teaching aids like charts can be used.

**Effectiveness of the aid:** To carry information to masses within a short period of time, radio and TV can be used.

**Experience of the teacher:** The extension agent, and his familiarity and skill in handling the aid are also important in selection. One who does not appreciate the importance of classroom chalk should not be encouraged to use an advanced aid.

**Availability:** An effective extension agent makes use of indigenous materials. When the teaching aid he would like to use is not available with the extension agent and if there is no power supply in the remote village then he has to choose the non-projected visual aids.

### Effective Use of Audio-Visual Aids

1. Planning ahead will help to solve anticipated problems.
2. Make sure that the aids are suitable for the audience size and the learner at the last row of the class must be able to see the aid. All aids are in good working condition before the presentation is started.
3. Use of a variety of well composed visual aids will hold audience interest.
4. Make the place where the presentation is to be made convenient and comfortable.
5. Do rehearse in order to make a smooth presentation.
6. Arrange your visuals in sequence and keep aids out of sight until ready for it.
7. Stand beside the aid, not in front of it. Present aids at the crucial moment. Remove all unrelated material.
8. Speak to the audience, not to the aids.
9. Avoid any misunderstanding by discussion and application. Sometimes the method of presentation attracts so much attention that it detracts from the message itself, e.g. flannel board. Hence, it may be necessary to explain first how a flannel board works and how flannel strips adhere to it so the talk is not interrupted.

There are a number of audio-visual aids used widely to increase extension effectiveness. To get the expected result the aids should be properly prepared, aptly chosen and appropriately presented. It is essential to pretest audio-visual materials before distributing them for general use. Technical development of these devices is increasing much rapidly than research into their optimal use. More research attention must be paid to study the effectiveness of aids.

### SATELLITE INSTRUCTIONAL TELEVISION EXPERIMENT (SITE)

National Aeronautics and Space Administration (NASA) and the Indian Space Research Organization (ISRO) jointly experimented an innovative satellite project named as SITE in India for a span of one year from 1975 to 1976 under India–US partnership. The main objective of the project is to educate rural people on various issues through satellite broadcast in order to address the grassroot level problems of the country.

The objectives behind this project were to educate the rural population on health and social issues through satellite programmes and also to gain expertise in technical features of satellite broadcast. The television programmes were produced by All India Radio and broadcast by NASA's ATS-6 satellite stationed above India for the duration of the project. The project got assistance from various international agencies such as the UNDP, UNESCO, UNICEF and ITU. Twenty backward districts from six states, namely Bihar, Odisha, Madhya Pradesh, Andhra Pradesh, Karnataka and Rajasthan were selected and TV sets were set up in schools or Panchayat centres in the selected villages. SITE broadcasted health, agriculture, development, education programmes and also organised special training programmes for school teachers. At the end of the project NASA shifted its satellite away from India on July 1976. SITE had a significant impact on Indian villages especially in the field of agriculture and family planning. Through the experience learnt from SITE, ISRO launched "Indian National Satellite System" (INSAT) in 1982.

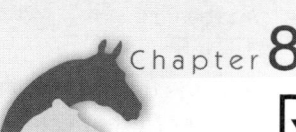

# Chapter 8

# Rural Sociology as Applied to Extension Education

## INTRODUCTORY SOCIOLOGY

### Sociology

It was in the year 1893 that French philosopher August Comte, who is also considered to be the father of science of Sociology, coined the term Sociology. The term Sociology is derived from the Latin word, *socius* meaning 'Companion' or 'Associates' and the Greek word *logos* meaning 'the Study' or 'Science'. The etymological meaning of Sociology is the Science of Society.

Sociology, according to August Comte, is the science of society and social orders and progress subject to natural and invariable laws, the discovery of which is the object of investigation.

### Rural Sociology

Rural sociology is that branch of sociology which attempts a comprehensive and systematic study of rural communities so as to arrive at an objective understanding of the existing conditions and formulate the principles of changes in the rural societies.

According to F. Stuart, rural sociology is the study of rural life, rural population, rural social organizations, the social processes operative in rural society and of social relationship of interactions, or in other words, rural sociology is the study of all the social phenomena of rural life.

According to A.R. Desai, rural sociology is the science of rural society. The law of the structure and development of rural society in general can aid as in discovering the special laws governing a particular society.

According to O.P. Dahama, it is the study of sociology of life in rural environment which systematically studies rural communities to discover their conditions and tendencies and to formulate principles of progress.

### Importance of Rural Sociology for Animal Husbandry Extension Worker

It is well known that the majority of the world population lives in rural areas. The pivot of rural sociology is amelioration of living standards and welfare of the rural society. Hence, the subject demands a thorough knowledge of the village under study.

A large share of India's population lives in rural areas. Hence, the overall growth of the nation depends upon the collective well-being of the rural people along with their livestock population.

Extension worker's prime objective is to bring constructive changes through a variety of extension education programmes. Herein the success of a rural welfare programme largely depends upon the rural population's support, co-operation and participation in the programmes. Therefore the extension worker needs to understand and always remain conscious about the culture, laws, structure, customs, beliefs, etc. of farming community because these factors remarkably affect the attitude, approach, behaviour, etc. of the rural people.

The following points will highlight the importance of rural sociology for animal husbandry extension worker.

### To Understand the Beliefs of Livestock Farmers

Farmers, almost a large majority of them in our country, undergo no formal or scientific training in livestock farming. Mostly all their knowledge of livestock farming is based on traditional pratices, religious orientations, idiosyncratic experiences, superstition and so on. Such is the rural environment in which the extension worker comes to offer his service. Extension worker, for the reasons given above, faces a high degree of resistance and challenge from the farmers when he adopts scientific and hi-tech methods in farming and treating the animals. The resistance is at times so strong that the farmers even hesitate to permit vaccination against certain fatal diseases.

Some of the superstitious beliefs of the rural population are that death of the animal is due to the anger of God, some do not prefer one's sheep delivering two lambs and farmers consider it as inauspicious (bad for family) when their cows calve on Fridays. Hence, to be a successful extension worker, a thorough knowledge of the rural community vis-à-vis its customs, beliefs, structure, folkways, etc. is absolutely necessary.

### Rural Reformation

The prime objective of the rural sociology is primarily meant to bring about welfare in the rural society. To achieve this objective adequate knowledge of the rural society is essential. The following points dwell on the relevance of rural sociology to an animal husbandry extension worker.

a. **Village reorganization:** Rural sociology helps the extension worker to identify the disorganized units in the village and reorganize them.

b. **Institutional co-ordination:** The knowledge of the subject enables the extension worker to understand the importance of co-ordination between the vital institutions, viz. economic, political, social, health, religious, etc. This understanding is necessary for improving the standard of living of the rural people.

c. **Economic status:** Rural sociology lays stress in improving the economic status of the people. Hence, the knowledge in the subject helps to devise programmes to increase the yield in farming and animal husbandry with the help of technology comprising scientific and systematic formulae.

d. **Educational status:** Education makes the people less dependent (on others) who otherwise rely on others to satisfy even their rudimentary needs. Further, education helps the people to solve rural problems, in case they arise. Rural sociology lays a great deal of importance to improve the educational status of the people.

### Formulation of Successful Development Programmes

Many social welfare programmes have been launched so far. But all have not been successful because the programmes that met with failures were not in accordance with either principles underlying rural sociology or cultural background of the place where they were launched. Hence, to formulate a successful development programme, the extension worker needs to have a thorough knowledge of the culture in relation to customs, beliefs, tradition, folkways, mores, etc. of the place where he/she wants to implement the programme. It is only after getting a thorough description about the place, that the extension worker sees light in his way, that is where to go, how to go and so on. Rural sociology helps the extension worker to acquire all the necessary knowledge needed for the formulation of the development programmes.

### For Effective Implementation of the Rural Programmes

The extension worker, who goes for the implementation of the rural programmes, needs a thorough knowledge of the place where he is going to implement the programme. Especially he is required to know the resources available in that region. So, that he may utilize the already existing benefits and facilities vis-à-vis infrastructure, youth clubs, associations, etc. in the place. This will not only make his programme implementation effective but also minimise unnecessary wastage of time in mobilising groups, looking for place and other aids and so on. Further and the extension worker should know the economic motivation, risk orientation, credit orientation and cultural factors that directly or indirectly affect the implementation. Rural sociology helps the extension worker to gain knowledge about various groups (operational in rural societies), rural institutions, cultural background, economic motivation, risk orientation, etc. of rural people.

### To Establish Rural Institution

To establish rural institutions and ensure successful functioning of sheep breeders, poultry producers, milk producers co-operative society, youth club, farmers club, etc., the change agent requires complete knowledge of the rural society. Especially the knowledge of the groups and rural leaders and leadership is important. That is available in the science of rural sociology.

The first unit of development in a country is village. It is the centre of culture in any country. 80% of the rural people are engaged in food production and they are the source, the urban people rely on for food. Based on this fact, studying the majority's interests, problems, their way of life, doing research and developing plan for their welfare study of sociology indispensable.

### Importance of Rural Sociology for a Veterinary Practitioner

a. **To become successful veterinary practitioner:** The veterinary practitioners who work in rural areas need to bear in their minds that the expectations of the rural clients vary to a large extent from that of the urban clients. Farmers are largely dependent upon their livestock that happens to be their main source of livelihood. Hence, they become highly anxious and desperate when their animals fall sick. As a result they expect an immediate cure in the animals when their state of health is impaired. Such being the mindset of the rural clients, for a veterinarian to be successful, he needs to familiarize with the feeding habits, cultural beliefs, festivals ceremonies (involving animals). It is only when the practitioner is familiar with these he would be in a position to identify the cause of the disease and provide immediate cure.

For example 'payasam' (semisolid sweet) is one of the main dishes in Tamil Nadu that is prepared during marriages, festivals, etc. There have been cases where this dish (the left over) is fed in excess amount to cattle on the next day of the function. The ruminants immediately develop ruminal acidosis (tympany). Like the example given above there are several other cases where the veterinarian needs to relate the disease and its possible cause in relation to the feeding habits, festivals and ceremonies (involving animals), etc. which might enable the veterinarian to diagnose the disease with proper interpretation.

b. **Employment opportunities:** In a country with a population of one billion plus, it is highly difficult for the government to provide employment opportunities to all the veterinary graduates. This being the case, veterinarians have been seen in large numbers working in a number of hatcheries, feed companies, veterinary pharmaceuticals.

The veterinarians who work in these establishments need to have a regular and close contact with the rural clients (farmers) to boost their business.

It is the knowledge of rural sociology that plays a crucial role in strengthening the veterinarians with a comprehensive knowledge about the rural society that happens to be their main source of livelihood. Rural sociology helps veterinarians develop a scientific outlook, critical thinking and objectivity with precision.

### Importance of Urban Sociology to the Veterinarians

'Urbs' is a Latin word. The Romans used this word to refer to a city. Urban sociology studies interaction and inter-relationship among urban population. In other words, the interaction among individuals in an urban setting is the subject matter of urban sociology.

No urban society is seen without animals for human beings, in general, have a special liking for rearing pet animals. In rural societies, it is only the farming communities that are seen with cattle, sheep, etc. On the other hand, in urban communities people from all walks of life rear pets animals like dog, cat, etc. As a result the role of a veterinarian in urban society is multifaceted and highly challenging because he needs

to adjust and adapt himself to the varying expectations of his clients. In general, attitude, customs, and behaviour of urban clients is quite different from that of the rural clients. To be successful in his work, the veterinarian needs a thorough understanding about the urban society.

In rural societies, farmers rear animals mainly to fulfil their economic needs. But the urban people bring up pets mainly to satisfy their emotional needs. The veterinarian would be causing a great displeasure to himself and his clients if he ignores the feelings and sentiments that clients have towards their pets. Urban people, in general, possess a good educational background that makes them ask pertinent questions on animals' health. Hence, extension worker should have the willingness, knowledge and patience to answer the questions raised by the clients. Urban sociology helps the veterinarian in imbibing the traits that are necessary for the veterinary practice.

### Comparison between Rural Sociology and Extension

| Rural sociology | Extension |
|---|---|
| 1. It is a scientific study of the laws of structure and development of rural society | It is the education given to the rural people to enable rural society. They extract and benefits out of resources available. |
| 2. It is an objective study of the rural people: It studies the behavioural patterns of the rural people as they are. | Extension is relatively prescriptive, i.e. it seeks to bring in changes in the attitudes, behaviour patterns of the rural population with the view that those changes pave way for their prosperity. |
| 3. It attempts to identify the needs and spheres of interest of rural people. | Extension attempts to identify the problems and design programmes that educate the rural people in terms of their impending problems and solutions to those problems. |
| 4. It analyses the rural–social relationships, in local organizations, rural areas. | It endeavours to empower all the leadership in village organizations so as to achieve its objective of community development. |
| 5. It studies existing social situations and assembles facts of rural communities. | The assimilated facts assume significance here for depending on the social data, extension programmes are designed for rural development. |
| 6. It studies the social, cultural, of political and religious problems, rural society with the view of comprehending the problems of rural societies. | Here those problems are studied vis-à-vis their importance in extension work in villages. |

## Characteristics of Rural Society

An individual's milieu (social environment) has a direct bearing on his life. Human beings live in two types of environment, viz. rural and urban. One can observe remarkable differences between the rural and urban societies that are embedded in their respective cultural and sub-cultural patterns.

As such there is no important differences in intelligence and understanding levels between rural and urban people. Here it is necessary to mention that urban centres provide more opportunities to its people vis-à-vis exercising one's innate and latent skills. This is because division of labour is one of the essential features of urban societies.

The characteristics of rural society can be better understood in relation to those of a urban society.

1. **Contact with nature:** The life of rural people, owing to their occupational requirements (agriculture) is more or less blended with nature which makes them evolve beliefs and convictions about nature that are quite different from those of urbanites who live away from the nature. The close contact that rural masses have with nature more often than not puts the rural lot in deep miseries for it is they who predominantly fall prey to the bitter and terrific manifestations of nature, viz. cyclone, drought, flood, etc.

2. **Occupation:** Agriculture is the fundamental occupation in the rural society. Animal husbandry is the backbone of rural agriculture. Agriculture and animal husbandry operate largely as a way of life, a family occupation. In the face of uncertainties in agriculture, livestock production has been found to provide economic stability to the farmers. Livestock and backyard poultry production provide much more stable economic base than crop production in rural areas. These are non-agricultural occupations in rural areas, but they are secondary in economic importance.

   In urban areas, there is a high degree of division of labour. On the other hand, an agriculturalist has to be a jack of all trades (carpentry, blacksmith, plant pathologist, veterinarian, etc.).

3. **Size of the community:** The village communities are smaller in size in comparison with urban communities. Agriculture demands a higher land man ratio than industry does. Agricultural lands may vary in size depending upon the farming practised.

4. **Density of population:** In rural communities, density of population is low. Due to the low density of population, the inhabitants of the community have intimate relations.

5. **Homogeneity of population:** The population in villages is homogeneous because the people more or less practise similar culture, customs, etc. besides being united closely to each other in terms of occupation which is mostly agriculture or livestock production. On the other hand, urban societies are highly heterogeneous due to high degree of division of labour.

6. **Social differentiation and stratification:** Rural societies are characterized by low degree of social differentiation and stratification due to their homogeneous nature, whereas in urban societies there is high degree of social differentiation and stratification for such societies make way for quite a lot of divisions in terms of occupations which determine an individual's domestic and social conditions.

7. **Social mobility:** Due to low degree of division of labour, individual differences are hardly appreciated in rural areas. Hence, social mobility, as far as rural societies are concerned, is something that these societies hardly seek for. In urban centres, it is a different case as individual differences are rewarded and encouraged with special social status. There is a constant urge among the people to move up in the social hierarchy.

   Here a mention needs to be made how certain types of rural agriculture introduce migration habits among groups of people referred to as 'migrating labour'. The social status of the people who migrate from one place to another depends on the place where these migrants wish to settle themselves.

8. **Social interaction:** Rural people have fewer contacts per person because the density of population is less. However, the rural masses have primary contacts, i.e. their interaction is plain and diffused than being manipulative, impersonal, cursory, formal, which is the case in urban centres even though the people here come to interact frequently.

9. **Social control:** In rural communities, submission to the collective will is paramount. Any deviation is dealt with strict punishments, for instance the deviant may be ostracised from the rural community, in urban societies social control means are formal and impersonal and the deviants are considered for reformation and rehabilitation.

10. **Social solidarity:** Social solidarity is more pronounced in rural societies for a large number of

their members trace similar ancestry, share a common set of beliefs, customs, folkways and more importantly similar occupation. But in urban centres, they are breeding grounds of individualities and diversities that form people from different walks of life. Hence, it is unlikely that people will show high level of social solidarity here.

11. **Leadership pattern:** Choice of leadership in rural areas tends to be more on the basis of the known personal qualities of the individual. And it has been found in some cases that a person is chosen as a leader considering his father's or forefather's performance as leader. When it comes to the urban centres, a position of leader purely depends on an individual's capabilities vis-à-vis his leadership traits.

12. **Standard of living:** It is well known that rural areas are not provided with sufficient provisions in terms of educational institutions, health services, housing facilities, domestic appliances, transport facilities, recreational facilities, etc.

Need one tell how the standard of living in urban centres is with all the latest gadgets and technology that make life easier than ever before.

## Differences between Rural, Tribal, Urban Communities

Even a superficial observation of rural, tribal and urban communities would reveal that there exist explicit differences among the three vis-à-vis their dress habits, dialect, accent, customs, folkways so on and so forth. And a close analysis will bring to light the implicit differences in relation to their behavioural patterns, beliefs, attitudes among them. It should be borne in mind that the differences in their attitudes, beliefs, customs, etc. make for their differences in other spheres of lives. But with rapid advancement in communication technology and tribal transition, the differences among these communities are getting lesser and lesser. Therefore the differences existing between rural, tribal and urban communities are more of a theoretical concept than based upon the facts of community life.

| Rural community | Tribal community | Urban community |
|---|---|---|
| 1. **Nature of environment**<br>Here the members of the community are in close association with nature. | In tribal community, the members live quite away from the civilized world; their dwellings are mostly remote and inaccessible, i.e. forest and hilly regions. | In urban community, the members live in a more complex and man-made environment. |
| 2. **Homogeneity**<br>Rural communities are homogeneous in nature for the members more or less subscribe to common culture, beliefs and pursue similar kind of occupation. | Here the degree of homogeneity is more than that of rural communities, for there is a hardly any difference among the members of tribal community, for members, almost all, trace common ancestry. | Due to high degree of differentiation and specialization, urban societies are heterogeneous in nature. |
| 3. **Occupation**<br>Here people are predominantly engaged in agriculture and animal husbandry.<br>The occupation in these societies is often determined by tradition and customs. | Primitive occupation such as hunting and gathering of forest products are pursued by the tribals. Nomadic tribe's chief occupation is rearing of animals. | Here the members pursue a wide range of occupations depending on their specialisation like banking, engineering, managerial, medicine, catering, health, hospitality, etc. Cities' physical featuers give no scope for agriculture |
| 4. **Size of community**<br>Communities are smaller than those of urban. | Tribal communities are smaller than rural and urban. | Size of urban community is larger than that of the rural and urban. |
| 5. **Density of population**<br>Lower than in urban community. | Lower than rural and urban communities. | Here the density of population is more when compared with the other two. |
| 6. **Social stratification**<br>In rural communities, the society is stratified based on its people's ascribed status, viz. caste, creed, sex, etc. | In tribal societies one hardly observes any remarkable social stratification. | The urban society is stratified on the basis its members' achieved status, viz. educational qualification, technical skills, etc. |
| 7. **Social mobility**<br>Since individuals in rural communities are stratified based on castes, birth, etc. people are put to remain in their same positions (that they got by virtue of birth) even if they exhibit outstanding talents, skills, etc. Further, less degree of specialisation does not make way for social mobility. | Social mobility is something these communities hardly ask for, because sustenance of *status quo* is paramount in these communities. | In urban communities individuals are appraised based on their achieved attributes than on the ascribed ones, hence upward mobility and downward mobility are quite possible in urban centres. |

*Contd...*

| Rural community | Tribal community | Urban community |
|---|---|---|
| **8. Social interaction**<br>In rural communities, the members are less in number, will mingle with each other easily and their nature of interaction is plain, informal and diffused. | In tribal communities, the interaction of its members is limited within the members of the same tribe, hence there is little the members share in this interaction | Here one can observe a great deal of interaction among the members. However, the social interaction here is formal manipulative, restrictive, impersonal and so on. |
| **9. Social control**<br>Here social control laws are repressive and rigid. The village's collective interest precedes the individuals. Social deviation is dealt with stringent punishments.<br>Examples: ostricism from social intercourse. | In tribal community, the tribe as a whole must submit itself before the unchallenging supremacy of the tribal head. Social deviance is regarded as disrespect to the tribal god (totem). | In urban community, individual's interest precedes the collective interest. Social control laws are formal and impersonal. However, they are reformative and rehabilitative |

## Difference between Tribal, Rural and Urban Farming

| Sl.No | Characteristics | Tribal | Rural | Urban |
|---|---|---|---|---|
| 1. | Structure | Unorganised | Unorganised | Majority of the farms are organised |
| 2. | Land holdings | Majority of the farmers are landless or marginal farmers | Majority of the farmers are landless to small farmers | varies from landless to small farmers |
| 3. | Farming system | Subsistence farming | Semi intensive farming | Intensive farming |
| 4. | Market accessibility | Poor facilities | Medium level | High |
| 5. | Type of farming | Organic mixed farming | Mixed farming | Commercial farming |
| 6. | Contacts with extension agents | Less | Medium | High |
| 7. | Cattle breeds | Dual purpose | Dual purpose | Milch animals |
| 8. | Adoption of modern technologies | Negligible | Poor | Medium to high |
| 9. | Draught animal population | High | Medium | Low |
| 10. | Industrial pollution | Very low | Low | Very high |
| 11. | Infrastructural facilities | Very poor public amenities | Poor public amenities | Very good public amenities |
| 12. | Bondage towards livestock | Very high | High | Low |
| 13. | Ethno veterinary practices | High | Medium | Low |
| 14. | Adoption of preventive vaccination practices | Low | Medium | High |
| 15. | Production capacity of the animals | Low | Medium | High |
| 16. | Type of sheds | Kutcha | Kutcha | Pucca |
| 17. | Disease resistance in animals | high | Medium | Low |
| 18. | Value addition of farm products | Poor | Poor | Medium |
| 19. | Grazing pattern | Open grazing | Grazing supplemented with concentrates | Stall fed and supplemented with fodder and concentrates |

## PRIMARY CONCEPTS OF RURAL SOCIOLOGY

### Society

Society is a group of people living together, sharing common values and general interests, long enough to be considered by others and by themselves as a unit. It has also been defined as 'a group of people who have lived together long enough to become organized and consider themselves as a unit more or less distinct from other human units. A society may include many communities and even more neighbourhoods (a smaller entity than the community can be a village).

### Community

Community refers to a group of mutually dependent people living in a more or less compact and continuous geographical area, having a sense of belonging and sharing common values, norms and interests and acting collectively in an organized manner to satisfy their needs through a common set of organization and institution. The community has both territorial dimension and social dimension, the former being its geographical area and the latter being the group themselves. There can be larger communities like nations and smaller communities like neighbourhoods. The larger community provides pleasure and friendship. Community exists within larger communities, it consists of group of individuals where as society it is the web of social relationship.

### Association

A group of people organizing themselves for the purpose of fulfilling common interests is known as association. There can be a number of associations functioning in a community. Associations emerge for some specific purpose, e.g. dairy farmers' association for the purpose of sale of milk. Thus, associations fulfil the common needs of their members. Elected/nominated office-bearers lead the association.

### Institution

Institutions are 'crystallised mechanisms' that clearly define ways through which society meets its needs that have existed long enough to become embedded in the social structure. According to Hoton (1964) 'an institution is an organized system of social relationships which embodies certain common values and procedures and meets certain basic needs of society'.

In other words, associations or organizations, which have set of rules and regulations, are known as institutions, e.g. a veterinary college is an association of students and employees but an educational system is an institution.

### Informal Institutions in Rural Society

There are five major institutions in both rural and urban societies, viz. family, religious economic, political and educational institutions.

a. **Village:** Village is the oldest permanent community of human beings. Animal husbandry and agriculture helped man acquire knowledge and skill gradually. Then he went to lead a settled life and human communities became stationary. The nomadic man started to lead to a settled mode of life due to the formation of village.

#### Classification of village

*Migratory village:* In this type of villages, people migrate from a village when food and other resources get exhausted.

*Semi-permanent village:* In this kind of villages, the villagers live relatively for a longer period of time when compared to the period that the people of the migratory villages spend in their villages, and migrate from the villages only after knowing that there is no scope for food and other essential resources.

*Permanent village:* In permanent villages, people live permanently and build up all social relations with other members of community. This kind of villages are far more organised with relatively increased amenities than the migratory or semi-organized villages as the members live here permanently.

*Grouped or nucleated village:* Here, people reside in clusters. Their farms are spread around the village.

*Dispersed or non-nucleated village:* In this type of villages, the people have their dwellings alongside of their farms. Hence, the distance between their houses is more when compared to the distance in grouped or nucleated villages.

*Co-operative village:* In co-operative villages, people receive their common services from co-operative bodies.

*Semi-collective village:* In semi-collective villages, the lands belong to collective body of village, people work in the farm and receive their share in kind or cash.

*Collective village:* The villages in Israel are examples of this type of villages. The properties are collectively owned. There are common dining halls, stores, etc. Individual houses are provided. The population feels a great deal of security for all the members of the village.

b. **Family:** Family is the most multifunctional of all institutions in society and is a social system of organized relationships involving workable and dependable ways of meeting basic social needs.

**Specific functions of family**

1. Sex regulation.
2. Production and rearing of children.
3. Socialization.
4. Maintenance of economic and religious life.
5. Provision of love, affection and security.
6. Provision of social status to the individual of the family.

Burgess and Locke have defined family as "a group of persons united by ties of marriage, blood or adoption, constituting a single household, interacting and communicating with each other in respective social roles of husband and wife, mother and father, son and daughter, brother and sister; and creating and maintaining a common culture".

**Classification** (Fig. 8.1): Family is classified based on membership, structure, residence, marriage and ancestry.

**Nuclear family and joint family**

*Nuclear family:* It is composed of a husband, his wife and their children. Nuclear families are the consequence of rapid industrialisation and modernisation wherein newly married men and women move away from their traditional joint families and establish their own near their places of employment.

*Joint family:* Joint family is one of the essential features of Indian society. However, this joint family system is fast declining owing to factors like industrialisation, urbanisation, modernisation etc. Family can be further classified into:

*Patriarchal family:* The elder-most male member in the family wields the authority.

*Matriarchal family:* The elder-most female member in the family is the head of the family.

*Matrilocal:* When the husband goes to live in his wife's house, it is called matrilocal family.

*Patrilocal:* When the wife goes to live in her husband's house, it is called patrilocal family. A majority of families in Indian society are patrilocal.

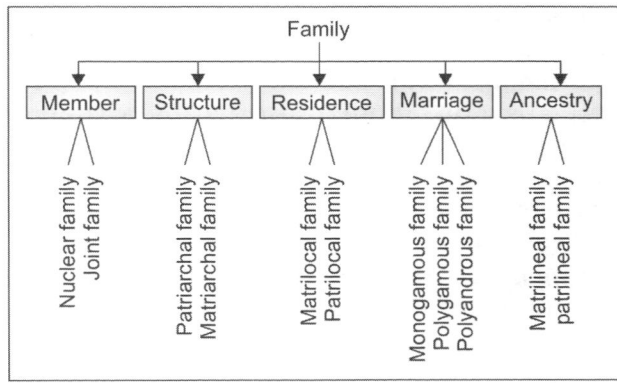

**Fig. 8.1:** Classification of family

*Monogamous:* It is a family constituted by one man to one woman.

*Polygamous:* Here one man marries more than one woman.

*Polyandrous:* Here a woman marries more than one man, and lives with all of them or with each one of them alternatively.

*Matrilineal:* In matrilineal families the lineage is traced through the mother and the elder-most woman in the mother's lineage is believed to be the prime ancestor.

*Patrilineal:* In patrilineal families, the lineage is traced through the father and the elder-most male in the father's lineage is believed to the prime ancestor.

**Functions**

The following are the functions of the family:

*Satisfies sex needs:* Family provides legitimacy for sexual relationship whereby it satisfies the urge for sex in human beings.

*Procreation and child rearing:* One of the important aims of family is procreation (reproduction). Family plays a pivotal role in rearing of the children. It is in the family that the child is taught all the essential traits vis-à-vis attitude, mannerisms, behaviour, discipline and other capabilities that the child needs to be an accepted and active member of the society.

*Provision for home:* Family provides home for its members. It is in this home that children are brought up with food, love and care. And for the grown-ups, home is a place where they rest and spend their free time peacefully leaving behind all the stress and strain of their hectic work life.

*Education:* A child is not born with the social qualities but he/she learns them being a member of the family in which he/she is born. The process of socialisation, though affected by a couple of agencies, it is the family that takes the leading role in socialising the child by teaching the culture, customs, beliefs, habits, folkways, etc. of the society to which the child belongs.

*Economic benefits:* Family looks after the economic needs of its members, i.e. the members who have acquired the skill and potential to earn, voluntarily support those family members who are in the stage of infancy, childhood or those who are not fully capable of earning by working outside.

*Provides status:* It is well founded that an individual is assessed primarily on the family he/she comes from. The status or position enjoyed by the senior members of the family, i.e. grandfather, father, etc. directly or indirectly affects the status of those members of the family who are in the process of establishing their positions in the society.

*Provides recreation:* Family by its nature is a primary group wherein members come into contact and rejoice with one another, leaving behind all their egoistic propensities, inhibitions, etc. and amuse together instilling happiness and peace in the minds of the young and the old.

*Transmission of culture:* Family plays a key role in preserving and practising the culture handed over to it by the ancestors and passing it to its next immediate generation. This way the traditional culture and heritage of the family passes from one generation to the next without becoming disintegrated or decayed.

c. **Religious institutions:** The religious beliefs, worship patterns, objects of worship, rituals, ceremonies of the people are varied and numerous. However, the bedrock of every religion is its hold on the individuals, groups of a society in almost every aspect of life vis-à-vis beliefs, attitudes, morals, etc. Secondary institutions within the major institution of religion include temples, churches, mosques and organised groups for propagating religions.

### Formal Rural Institutions

The school, panchayat and co-operative society are the basic formal institutions in every village. There has to be organic link between each of these institutions to bring about integrated approach to solve rural problems.

a. **Educational institutions:** Educational institutions, besides providing intellectual development, serve to socialize individuals in a society vis-à-vis the beliefs, customs, norms, folkways, etc. of that society.

This process is referred to as socialisation. Socialisation informally starts at home and then formally at school. Educational institutions have emerged from the background of homes, temples, mosques, churches or ashrams to the formal village schools, colleges and universities.

Many village schools are the first formal institutions. It is the integral part of the community. School teachers are not only involved in teaching but also act as the member of the community. School as community centre performs the following activities:

1. Leadership education.
2. Training students against leadership qualities through students' association, school co-operatives, etc.
3. Developing discipline through scouting, red cross and other social movements.
4. Developing a sense of cohesiveness and co-operation by organizing science exhibitions and educational tours.
5. School acts as a community centre for all community development programmes that are organized by government and voluntary organizations.
6. Teacher acts as a friend and guide to the villagers and introducer and coordinator to extension workers.

b. **Economic institutions:** Economic institutions provide physical subsistence, viz. food, shelter, clothing and other necessities. It includes economic institutions of agriculture, industry, exchange and consumption of commodities. Secondary institutions included within the major economic institutions are credit and banking systems, advertising, co-operations, etc. (Co-operatives dealt in detail in Chapter 5.)

c. **Youth club:** Today's youths are tomorrow's leaders of the nation. All the aspirations of a country rest on the hidden potentialities of our youths. One of the most effective way of moulding and channelising the potentials of youth towards overall development is through the medium of youth club. The training of youths in club work will mould them for future responsibilities. Besides individual development, youth clubs also contribute substantially towards the development of the society and the country. Since the very inception of Community Development Programme, youth clubs were organised on the pattern of 4-H clubs of USA. There was a lot of enthusiasm in the early years and youth clubs were formed in almost every village under a targeted programme.

1. **4-H Club:** It was Mr. Beson who was instrumental and a source of inspiration for the name "4-H", the motto and plan of organisation, much of which is adopted and followed now. In 1959, it was from a generous grant from the Ford Foundation, 4-H club that was established in the USA.

4-H signifies the four broad objectives of the organisation, namely:

1. Head—pledged to clearer thinking, intelligent understanding and appreciation of the environment in which we live and development of scientific attitude towards the problems of the farm and the home.
2. Heart—pledged to greater loyalty, to the development of desirable ideals and standards for farming, home making, community life and citizenship.
3. Hands—pledged to larger service, to learn by doing, to the acquisition of technical skills in farming and home making establishing suitable farm or home enterprises and their demonstration.
4. Health—pledged to efficient working, the intelligent use of leisure and to better the way of living.

**The Motto of 4-H clubs is "To make the best better":** The projects that boys and girls may take up are purely based on their individual interests and profit, and may or may not be an objective of the project.

The 4-H clubs are organized on completely democratic lines, that is, under the supervision of county agriculture agents, and voluntary leadership is provided by citizens—farmers, teachers, businessmen, clergymen.

Club work provides the missing element in much of school instruction—a close and personal relationship between book knowledge and actual life relationships and problems. 4-H club boys and girls are awarded prizes in country-wide shows and contests when they surpass even their seniors (in terms of age) in terms of achievement.

**Recreation:** The programme of the 4-H clubs are designed in such a way that they are inspirational, entertaining and thought-provoking.

The 4-H movement, founded out of a noble resolve and based on ideals of self-help, co-operation and progressive citizenship, has gained considerable momentum cutting across national boundaries. The movement's contribution to international understanding and goodwill is indeed commendable.

2. **Indian rural youth clubs**

*Rural youth:* The Ministry of Human Resource Development (1985), considers 'youth group' in India as persons between 15 and 35 years of age.

**Social profile of youth:** According to the Ministry of Human Resource Development (1985), youth is a very special period with special challenges and it is during this period that an individual sees his/her body, personality, intellect, social attitudes developing independent of one another frequently and explosively. It is during youth, that an individual is full of potential and problems. The social structure of Indian society affects the life and growth of Indian youth.

**Basic needs of young people:** Some of the basic needs of the youth as identified by Singh and Prasad (1967) are (1) need for a good physique (2) need for security and belonging, (3) need for love and sympathy, (4) need for fun and fellowship, (5) need for achievement and competition, (6) need for recognition and appreciation, (7) need for new experience, (8) need for the feeling of personal worth, (9) need for spiritual development and, (10) need for sense of continuing learning.

**Need for youth club**

1. Effective implementation of any development programme needs competent leadership. Youth clubs develop such leadership, so that the youths are latus also to shoulder responsibilities for their community's development.
2. Youths are much more energetic, enthusiastic and receptive to new ideas and to work on new programmes. They have great influence on their parents in the acceptance of the practice at their own farm.
3. For providing proper scientific outlook to make them solve their problems by themselves.

4. Since the youths are the future leaders of the country, to have good youth club is important for shaping future leaders. Youth club works have gained significant importance in extension education programmes.

**Objectives**

1. To develop desirable values, ideas and standards for family and community life.
2. To bring change in knowledge, skill and attitude of the sound rural people through training and group projects.
3. To develop leadership qualities in the youth
4. To build co-operative and democratic principles in their young mind.
5. To cultivate the habits of healthy living.
6. To develop human resources and conserve nature's resources.
7. To impart ability in solving their own problems themselves through learning by doing, creative thinking, discussions, holding organised meetings and thus to enable them develop a consciousness of their responsibilities and the duties of a good citizen.
8. To help the rural young people lead a wholesome life comprising spiritual and moral values.
9. To make the rural youth appreciate dignity of labour, i.e. attach equal worth and reverence to any labour be it agriculture or software development.
10. To make the rural youth act as agents of change that guarantees prosperity to the community.
11. To train the rural youth in a way that their leisure time activities are entertaining and useful to the community.
12. To induce the importance of continuous learning among the rural folk.

Role of extension worker in youth work:
1. Study the interest of the people.
2. Identify the needs of the rural youth.
3. Explain to youths the benefits and opportunities they get in club and influence them for action.
4. Secure the support from parents and local leaders by explaining the importance of the club.
5. Guide and supervise the youths in organising the club.
6. Motivate them for voluntary participation in regular club meetings.
7. Plan the club activities.
8. Guide the members of youth club to select their project with the acceptance of their parents.
9. Recognise the good work by giving prizes and rewards.
10. Help them in getting outside agencies' assistance.
11. Help them to measure their achievement.

**Starting a youth club**

The extension worker should analyse the situation and identify the needs of the youths and interests of their parents. He must seek the co-operation of the local leaders, progressive farmers and others by explaining the importance of youth club.

The extension worker needs to invite the youths, local people, village level worker, local leaders and club members from the neighbouring villages for the meeting and explain what the members should do, what their parents, roles are and duties of the office-leaders and other citizens.

Enrol the members, hold election of office-bearers, briefly review youth organisation and the activities, explain how the club forms its standing committees to perform various activities. Many more members of the club will be able share the responsibility when they serve on committees. Distribute some reading materials to members on the projects. Fix the date of the next meeting and conclude the meeting with songs, etc.

Success of any club lies in the regularity in conducting meeting and the intensity of participation of members. The meetings should begin and end in time. Each meeting should have three parts.

1. Business: Issues or ceremonies.
2. Programme: Talk, demonstration, project instruction, etc.
3. Recreation: Songs and games—not only to hold the interest of the group but to teach them how to work together.

**Organisation of club work**

*Membership:* The membership of the club is voluntary. All rural youths, who have achieved the age of 15 years, can, with their parents' approval become member of the youth club. Each club should have twenty members. Any number of clubs can be started in the same village.

*Role of the member:* He should select a project in animal husbandry or agriculture or industry or craft. He must be ready to learn by doing. He should maintain his project record.

*Meeting:* Every member should attend meetings. The meetings should be held twice a month. Each meeting should have an agenda.

*Office-bearers:* The elected president, vice-president, secretary, treasurer and captain are the office-bearers. The president usually presides over the meeting. In his absence the vice-president will perform his job. The secretary will prepare the meeting agenda and record the minutes of the meeting. The treasurer will maintain the club accounts. The captain will lead the games and recreational activities.

*Projects:* Economic, cultural, social and recreational projects can be selected based on the members' needs, interests, abilities, family situations, availability of resources, local demands, availability of capable volunteers, etc.

*Youth advisory committees:* If there are two or more village youth clubs, to establish co-operation and co-ordination in club activities, youth advisory committees should be formed. The local leader, one member from each youth club, members of Project Advisory Committee, extension teachers or school principals and village level workers are the members of the committee. The Youth Advisory Committee will meet at least once in each quarter to review club and advise on plans and programmes for the rest quarter. The committee also guides to conduct tours, exhibition, contests, camps, etc.

### Youth work in India

Youth work in India is not well organised. Some of the youth work is done by a few organisations like 1. Young Farmers' Association, India; 2. Bharat Sevak Samaj; 3. Bharat Sevak Dal; 4. Bharat Scouts and Guides; 5. National and Auxiliary Cadet Corps; 6. National Service Scheme; 7. YMCA; 8. YWCA.

### Goals of Indian youth programme

According to the Ministry of Human Resource Development (1985), the basic goals of Indian Youth Programmes are:

1. Enabling young people to become better and responsible citizens, and better individuals through self-improvement and social service.
2. Promoting awareness among young people of the variety, diversity and richness of India's culture and traditions and the need to preserve and promote the same as it is unique in its basic unity and apparent diversity.
3. Restructuring educational system to relate it meaningfully to employment opportunities especially for youth.
4. Training is given to the youth vis-à-vis use of new technology in fields of immediate concern, for example agriculture, animal husbandry, etc.
5. Stress is laid on empowerment of women wherein measures are taken to ensure equal access (for women) to education, equal wages, maternity and child benefits, etc.

   The overall condition of young women in India is looked into with due concern.
6. Youths are educated so that they could effectively tackle the situations that challenge their physical, mental and social being.
7. Helping the youth realize their duties and responsibilities and make them good citizens of this country.

### National Service Scheme

The National Service Scheme envisages involvement of the university students, on voluntary and selective basis, in programmes of social service and national development.

NSS saw its dawn in 1969 and today it is spread in all our states and universities. Its organizational set-up is a three-tier system comprising the central, state and university/college level advisory committees. It is the college unit that plays the central role in NSS operation and guides the execution of regular and camping programmes.

The following are the objectives of NSS:

1. Serve the society within their (students) possible limits while they are undergoing instruction in the educational institution.
2. Kindle and arouse social consciousness among students.
3. Provide the students opportunities that would enable them to come out with creative and constructive ideas in relation to community development.
4. To derive optimum benefit out of education by its application for the cause of a healthy society.

The activities of NSS are broadly of two categories, viz. regular or concurrent programmes and special camping programmes.

A student, under regular activities, is expected to work as a volunteer for a continuous period of two years and render community service for a minimum of 120 hours per annum.

Some of the activities of the NSS are:

- Planting saplings.
- Improvement of campuses.
- Blood donation.
- Constructive work in villages and slums.
- Service at welfare institutions.
- Adult and non-formal education.
- Programmes revolving around health, family welfare, etc.

## GROUP ORGANISATION

Man is a social animal. He is born and brought up in a social group. One cannot imagine life without groups. Right from the very birth, the individual is seen amidst one group or other. Primarily it is the family with father, mother, siblings, grandparents, from which the child learns the basic habits, gestures, etc. by imitation. Later it is school, peer groups, neighbourhoods, being a member of which, the individual learns a variety of habits, customs, folkways, etc. that are approved by the society. The influence of teachers, friends, peers is indeed very important so much so the attitudes, values, behaviour, etc. of the individual is the outcome of this influence.

Thus, it needs to be said that man becomes what he is called to be only because of the influence of quite a number of groups around which he moves about in the course of his life. This learning that the individual undergoes from birth to the end of his life is called socialisation.

### Group

Group is a unit of two or more individuals who are in reciprocal communication and interaction with each other. In the widest sense the word 'group' is used to designate a collection of items. The consideration of the following terms will give a clear understanding of what we generally mean by 'social group'.

i. **Category:** Means collection of items that have at least one common characteristic that distinguishes them from other items which have other characteristics in common. Individuals between 15 and 20 years of age, for instance, are referred to as an 'age group'.

ii. **Aggregation:** It is a collection of individuals in physical proximity of one another like cinema audience, spectators at a football stadium. There may be some interaction between the individuals in an aggregation but it is generally of a temporary nature and lacks definite pattern of organisation. Interaction will normally be lacking.

iii. **Potential group:** It is a group made up of number of people having some characteristics common but does not possess any recognisable structure. A potential group may become a real group, if it becomes organized and comes to have a union or organisation. Students form a potential group as long as they have no union but once they become organised, they form a social group.

iv. **Social group:** It is a collection of two or more individuals in which there are psychological interactions and reciprocal roles based upon durable contacts, shared norms and interests, distinctive patterns of collective behaviour and structure, organization of leadership and followership.

### Definition of social group

MacIver states that "any collection of human beings who are brought into social relationships with one another is a social group".

According to Williams, "a social group is a given aggregate of people playing inter-related roles and recognised by themselves and others as a unit of interaction".

### Concept of Group Formation

A minimum of two individuals can form a group when they are able to share their thoughts. However, a mere coming together of people does not form a group. There should be interaction or communication among them. Interaction means exchanging of ideas by meaningful paralanguages (or) artifacts, or facial expressions, or kinesis (body movement) or words and communication means sharing of common experiences.

Two persons sitting physically close to each other (e.g. in a bus without speaking with others) may not form a group when they do not interact. On the other hand, two persons talking over telephone or wireless phone or through satellites or letters form a group as they communicate with each other. The communication and interaction should not be one way but it should be reciprocal.

Common interests, shared values and norms are the essential part of the social group. This may not be true for all the groups. Members with different views may come together for some time and interact for agreement or disagreement. They may not share a common purpose and yet may engage in strenuous reciprocal interaction on a psychological plane.

## Characteristics of Social Group

1. **Relationship:** Members of group are inter-related to one another. Reciprocal relationship forms an essential feature of a group.
2. **Sense of solidarity:** The members of the group are united by a sense of solidarity and a feeling of sympathy.
3. **We-feeling:** The members of a group help one another and defend their interests collectively.
4. **Common interest:** The interests and ideals of the group are common. It is for the realisation of common interests that they have formed a group.
5. **Similar behaviour:** The members of a group behave in a similar way for the pursuit of common interest.
6. **Group norms:** Every group has its own rules or norms which the members are supposed to follow. One must remember that social group is dynamic and not static. It changes its form and expands its activities from time to time. Sometimes the changes may be sudden, while at other they may occur so gradually that members are not conscious of them.

## Classification of Group

Social groups have been classified in various ways by different authors. No single classification is applicable to all social groups. Major social groups as classified by renowned sociologists, are as given below:

1. Primary and secondary group (CH Cooley)
2. In-group and out-group (Summer)
3. Involuntary, voluntary and delegate group (Dwight Sanderson)
4. Communities and associations (Tonnies)
5. Genetic, congregate, disjunctive and overlapping group (Giddings)
6. Unsocial, pseudo-social, anti-social, pro-social group (George Hasen)
7. Temporary and permanent group (Charles A. Ellwood). The characteristics of these groups are studied here.
1. **Primary and secondary groups:** They are distingui-shed from each other by their type of social contact and degree of formal organisation. In the primary group there is face-to-face association, contacts are personal, individuals live close to one another socially and do not need the formal framework of a constitution to achieve their purpose. Members of a family, a neighbourhood, friends' circle are good examples of primary group. In this type of group members are loyal to one another because of personal regards and the sharing of many interests. The secondary group is larger, relationships are more formal, secondary, specific and indirect in its contact such as political party.

### Characteristics of primary group

*Physical proximity:* Face-to-face relationship is an essential feature of a primary group.

*Small in size:* A primary group is small in size and this facilitates physical proximity, convergence of interests, etc.

*Stability:* A primary group exists for the group's collective good than for individuals. Further, for intimacy to prevail in the group, it requires to be stable.

*Similarity of background:* Members of a primary group come from a more or less similar background in terms of culture, socialisation, etc.

*Self-interest:* In a primary group individual member's self-interest is subordinated against the group's collective interest.

*Intensity of shared interests:* All the members of a primary group voluntarily come forward to work for the overall benefits of all its members.

*Association:* Though there are not any explicit rules of conduct for the members of a primary group they fall in line on their volition as it is in association.

The face-to-face contact does not mean that it exerts a compelling influence over its members.

### Difference between primary and secondary groups

| Characteristic | Primary group | Secondary group |
| --- | --- | --- |
| 1. Size | Small | Widespread |
| 2. Kind of co-operation | Co-operation with other members is direct. Members sit together | Co-operation is indirect and less. Members co-operate to achieve common goal and objectives |
| 3. Type of structure | Informal structure. There is spontaneous adjustment in working of the group. No formal or detailed rules. The structure is simple | Formal structure. Regulated by formal authority. Secondary group is, therefore, carefully worked out |
| 4. Relationship | Direct, intimate and personal (face-to-face) | Indirect, less intimate and impersonal. Need not have face-to-face contact |

2. **In-group and out-group**

   *In-group:* It is the group with which the individual identifies himself, his family, tribe, sex, college, occupation, religion, etc. by virtue of his awareness of likeness. It has inclusion of some persons and exclusion of others. It has collective pronoun 'we'. It has some sympathy and a sense of attachment to other members of the group.

   *Out-group:* It is defined as contract between 'they' and 'we' like we are democrats and they are communities. We are Hindus and they are Muslims. Such attitudes that "these are my people" and that "those are not my people" the produce a sense of attachment to other members of in-group while a sense of indifference and even antagonism to the members of out-group.

3. **Involuntary, voluntary and delegate groups**

   *Involuntary group:* The group evolves out of kinship ties. A man has no choice to what family he will belong.

   *Voluntary group:* It is one that a man joins of his own volition. He agrees to be a member of it and is free to withdraw his membership at any time.

   *Delegate group:* It is one that a man joins as a representative of a number of people either elected by them or nominated by some power. Parliament is a delegate group.

4. **Communities and associations**

   *Community:* It is a social group with some degree of "we-feeling" and living in a given area.

   *Association:* It is a group of social beings related to one another who have instituted a common organisation with a view to secure a specific end.

5. **Genetic, congregate, disjunctive and overlapping groups**

   *Genetic group:* It is a family in which a man is born involuntarily.

   *Congregate group:* It is the voluntary group into which one moves or joins voluntarily.

   *Disjunctive group:* It is one which does not allow a person to be a member of other groups at the same time, e.g. college or nation which does not allow their members to be members of other colleges or nations at the same time.

   *Overlapping group:* It is one whose members also belong to other groups of the same type such as members of Indian Political Science Association.

6. **Unsocial, pseudo-social, anti-social, pro-social groups**

   *Unsocial group:* It is one which largely lives to itself and for itself and does not participate in the larger society of which it is a part. It does not mix up with other groups and remains aloof from them.

   *Pseudo-social group:* Participates in the larger social group but mainly for its gain and not for the greater good.

   *Anti-social group:* It is one that acts against the interest of society. A group of students that destroys public property is anti-social group. Similarly, a political party that plans to over-throw a popular government is anti-social.

   *Pro-social group:* It is the reverse of anti-social group. It works for the larger interests of the society. It is engaged in constructive tasks and concerned with increasing the welfare of all the people.

7. **Temporary and permanent groups**

   The groups assembled for short period are called temporary groups, e.g. crowd, mob, herd, etc. The groups living in a geographical area for a longer period are called permanent groups, e.g community, state, region, tribe, etc.

8. **Other groups**

   *Reference group:* Every person in society has his reference group. It is a group of persons whom an individual consults before taking an important decision. A reference group, therefore, may contain members from primary group, informal group or formal group. In complex societies, a person can be a member of different reference groups. But in communities like a village, a person has a specific reference group. The decisions taken in consultation with a reference group naturally influence the behaviours of the member. Sometimes a person may not be a so-called member of any reference group but he may consult a group as it might comprise experienced and respected persons in society and take decisions according to their advice.

   *Horizontal groups:* They are large, inclusive groups such as nations, religious organisations, political parties, etc.

   *Vertical group:* They are small divisions such as economic classes. Since the vertical group is a part of the horizontal group (the larger group) an individual is member of both.

   *Cultural interest group:* These groups are created for the development of special interests. They are formed on account of factors such as economic interest, aesthetic interest, political interest, educational interest or recreational interest.

*Crowd:* It is a temporary group interacting in physical proximity with relation to some common interest or focus of attention.

*Mob:* It is a gathering of persons mostly in a state of disorder and whose behaviour is uncertain.

## Methods of Approach to Different Groups

In rural India, a number of social groups and institutions are found which determine the pattern of individual's life in the community. The development workers or extension officers are mainly concerned with the groups and their mobilisation. Therefore, they need to understand the fundamental differences of different groups and their functioning. According to Dahama and Bhatnagar (1985), the household, neighbourhood, informal group, family group and religious group are the commonly found rural groups of India.

Information on each of these groups is given below.

### Household

This group includes members of family and other persons who may reside there to assist in farming and other household activities. There will be greater degree of interaction among the members. The decision to adopt or reject an innovation will involve the entire group. Therefore, involving a large household for an adoption would be difficult because of the individual differences. The best way is to start the work with smaller household.

### Neighbourhood

The households of rural India exist in clusters. The proximity of the families binds them into a strong group. Several neighbourhoods constitute a village. The interaction and dependence on each other in a neighbourhood is greater as they have to share many things like water, roads, electricity drainage, bathing pools, sports, security, etc. As the neighbourhood has a large number of individuals, there will be key persons. To start the work in a neighbourhood, it is better to start with the help of the influential key persons.

### Informal group

The informal groups like friends' group, mutual aid groups, etc. are normally formed in rural India based on caste, age, income and other factors. These groups remain for a longer time. The relationship between the members is personal and there will be frequent meetings. These groups are to be observed intensively to identify the most frequently and intensively involved members in counselling, joy, gossip, casual conversation, etc. Development worker has to approach such members and get their approval which amounts to the approval of the entire group.

### Formal Group

As the name indicates, the formal groups have procedures of functioning. These groups have a name or title, selected and titled officers, a written purpose, definite rule of operation and a regular, common, meeting time and place. Formal groups like panchayat, co-operative, school, etc. are commonly found in villages. The development worker has to work through the office-bearers of these groups.

### Family Group

It is a basic social unit. The eldest member, who is generally the head of the family, normally decides on matters related to the family and his decisions are final. Any change brought out in family requires his consent. Before any change could be brought about, his consent for the change is essential.

### Religious Group

Villages are structured around the religious institutions like temples, churches, mosques, etc. Development worker has to identify the influential religious persons whose words have value. The religious festivals can be best utilised for welfare programmes (street plays, puppet shows, etc. on the extension programmes).

## Procedure for Formation or Organisation of Groups

It is individuals who are the units or elements of groups.

Human needs and interests are to be satisfied. Man seeks to fulfil his needs either by working alone or forming group, i.e. joining with others in his society.

As already said it is not for the fulfilment of all his needs, that a person wants the help of others. For example, to lift a burden of 10 kg, he may not seek the help of others but if he has to lift a burden of 25 kg, he may seek the assistance of others.

In the same way if an individual wants to practice for a race, he can practise all alone without anyone's participation or co-operation. But, a cricketer preparing for the game, needs the involvement and participation of a few others to practice well.

### Self-centred and Group Centred

It needs to be seen whether the group members are self-centred or group-centred, i.e. when members of a recreation club join together, it is primarily for the fulfilment of each other's individual interest, that the members come together. On the other hand, in the case ∫ a students' union or factory workers' union, the members come together keeping in view the group's collective interest than that of any individual member. No individual is completetly free from his own self-interest, hence it is not proper to say that in a group-centred unit, the members do not seek or mind their individual interests. Therefore it would be good if the group is formed for the furtherance of both individual and group interests. But if the group members are predominantly self-centred then the group's strength and endurance would be grossly challenged.

Further, organising a group-centred unit is far more easy than organising a self-centered group for it is quite difficult to bring together members who are more concerned about their own good than the collective interest of the group.

### Organization of a Group

When it comes to organising the group the specific situation in the community needs to be borne in mind. It is important to take into account the potential members of the group their characteristics, etc. If the potential members show tolerance, compromise the differences that they may see in others and co-operate with neighbours, the group has indeed a lot of favourable factors. On the contrary, if the potential members are critical, suspicious, slow to compromise and lack co-operation then these are indeed unfavourable factors for the formation and stability of the group.

### When a Group can be Formed

Now the question arises when to form/organize a group. In this regard there is as such no rule of thumb that calls for the formation of a group. The basic principle is as follows:

A group may be organised at any time. There are individuals who have a need or think they have a need that cannot be satisfied individually and there is no group already in existence to meet that need. But the members need to look whether there already exists any group (for the same purpose). This is to avoid useless duplication. If a group already exits for the same purpose, then the aspirants for the new group could very well join it instead of forming a new group but if the entry of new members outnumber the optimum number of the group already existing group, then the new group aspirants may as well form a new one.

### Stimulation for the Group Formation

The stimulation for the members to form a group is initially provided by the mass gatherings or meetings of the members where the members become conscious of their plight and resolve to take a concerted action for the fulfilment of their needs and interests. Further stimulation is also induced by the members who are connected with other outside programmes and local administration. However, the direct stimulation is from the very purpose of the potential group, its explanations and its ways of accomplishing their needs.

### Factors that Determine the Formation of the Group

The following factors determine the members who are to be the group members. The conditions for the membership, types of members, financial programmes, and whether the new group is affiliated to any already established local or central body whereby it could receive the help and support of the parent group so as to further the cause of the newly-formed group.

## ▌SOCIAL STRATIFICATION

Society is heterogeneous in nature. There are rich and poor, industrialists and peasants, rulers and sweepers, etc. Everywhere society is divided into various classes based on economic, social, political and religious factors.

The process by which individuals and groups are ranked in a more or less enduring hierarchy of status is known as stratification. Every society is divided into more or less distinct groups. No society is unstratified. Where there is social stratification, there is social inequality. Since social stratification means division of society into social classes, examination of social classes is important. In India, there is a special type of social stratification in the form of castes. Therefore, it becomes important to know the castes. There is also a separate territorial group, comprising of blood relations, called tribes.

### Social Class

#### Definition

Social classes are defined as abstract categories of persons arranged in levels according to the social status they possess. There are no firm lines separating one category from another. Classes are loosely organised groupings, whose members behave towards each other as social equals. Social class is a culturally defined group that is accorded a particular position of status within the population as a whole, i.e. a social status in a given society.

Each social class has its own particular social behaviour, its standards and occupations. The relative positions of the classes in their society arise from the degrees of prestige attached to their status. Status is the basic criterion of social class, or in other words, class is a status group.

## Meaning and Nature of Social Class

In a social class, there is, firstly, a feeling of equality which is exemplified in its members' behaviour, standard of life, occupation, etc. Secondly, there is a feeling of inferiority in relation to those who stand above in the social class. Thirdly, there is a feeling of superiority to those below in the social hierarchy. Thus, the fundamental attribute of a social class is its social position or relative inferiority or superiority to other social classes. In Rome, for instance, there were the slaves, plebeians, and five superior classes.

## Element of Stability

Every class has its own distinctive ways of life. A social class is distinguished from other classes by certain customary modes of behaviour that are taken to be characteristic of that class and may be concerned with such things as mode of dress, the type of conveyance, the way of recreation and expenditure. Thus, the upper class members are masters rather than servants.

## Class and Group

There is a clear cut distinction between a class and a group. Many a times, while referring to age class it is wrongly spoken as age group. Actually it is not a group but a statistical category. It sometimes assumes a class significance. This distinction will become more clear from the types of social classes described hereunder:

### Development of social classes

According to CH Cooley, there are three principles conditioning or favouring the growth of social classes, They are:

1. Marked differences in the constituent parts of the population—Negroes form a separate class.
2. Little communication and enlightenment.
3. A slow rate of social change when the population is composed of different races.

Indian society remained static for about three thousand years with the result, that the untouchables were not permitted to use public wells, enter temples, etc. Industrialisation and growth of cities loosened these class restrictions.

In the earliest stages of civilisation, i.e. in the age of primitive barbaric tribes, there were no social classes. There was no superiority over neighbours because they were always engaged in the struggle for existence and lived from hand to mouth. When these tribes grew in culture and especially in military strength, the first result was that the conquered enemies were eaten, tortured or in any case put to death. After developing a soft attitude the captured were not eaten or killed but spared and enslaved. Thus, a class of slaves was formed. A slave could be flogged, sold, pawned exchanged or put to death.

## Guild System

Modern classes are the ones that have gradually taken shape rather developed where feudal lords (or) landed gentry were at the top and the serfs at the bottom of the society, there was another class: Lawyers, doctors, financiers, etc. who were considered to be the higher class in the town.

## Bourgeoisie System

The industrial revolution divided the society into two distinct classes, viz. the capitalists and the proletariats. Apart from these two, there was a new class called the middle class. This present day middle class is a heterogeneous group consisting of doctors, lawyers, engineers, teachers, architects and many other white collared workers whose number is on increase. Based on income and standard of living, the present middle and lower middle classes are stratified.

## Different Classes

The classes may be based on power, prestige, wealth or a combination of these and other factors.

1. **Tribal classes:** These are culturally defined groups recognised as such by society, e.g. tribal and non-tribal.
2. **Cultural classes:** Cultural class has further social strata that have developed sub-cultural patterns of behaviour. The patterns are distinguished from each other, e.g. Hindu and Mohammedan cultural classes.
3. **Economic classes:** There are groups engaged in different economic activities or standing in different relationships to the means of production in a society, e.g. business, service, farmer and other classes.

4. **Political classes:** These are groups formed on the basis of political power, e.g. DMK, BJP, Congress, Janata Dal, etc.

5. **Self-identific classes:** These are conceived in terms of the identification of their members, e.g. NEEC, Farms Radio Club, etc.

6. **Participation classes:** These are described in terms of the identification of social ties between the members. These social ties are sociable contacts, marriages and similar relationships in which the class as a whole participates, e.g. village people's participation in Mattupongal vizha (harvest festival) or any religious function.

## Caste

The word caste has originated from the Spanish word 'casta', which means breed, race, strain of a complex of hereditary characteristics. Caste is a social category whose members are assigned a permanent status within a given social hierarchy and whose contacts are restricted accordingly. It is mostly referred to as the extreme form of a closed class system. A man born into the caste of his parent, lives being a member of the same caste, all through his life. With few exceptions he cannot fall to a lower caste or he may be expelled from his caste group. Personal qualities or abilities have no part whatsoever in determining the caste of an individual, with lineage being the only criterion.

### Definition

Caste, according to Herbert Risely, is "a collection of families or group of families bearing a common name; claiming a common descent from a mythical ancestor, human or divine, professing to follow the same hereditary calling and are regarded by those who are competent to give an opinion, as forming single homogeneous community".

Lundberg says that "a caste is merely a rigid social class into which members are born and from which they can withdraw or escape only with extreme difficulty."

As per Blunt, caste is "an endogamous or a collection of endogamous group bearing a common name, membership of which is hereditary, imposing on its members certain restrictions in the matters of social intercourse, claiming a common origin and regarded as a single homogeneous group".

According to C.H. Cooley, "when a class is somewhat strictly hereditary, it may be called caste".

When status is wholly predetermined, so that men are made to bear their lot without any hope of changing it, then class takes the extreme form of caste, according to MacIver.

Hentry Maine is of the view that caste started without occupational classes. After receiving the religious sanction, they have become solidified into the existing caste system.

### Characteristics of Caste System

The following are some of the important features of the Indian caste system, according to N.K. Datha:

1. Member of a particular caste is not permitted to marry outside his or her caste.

2. Every caste lays down certain restrictions vis-à-vis its members, food habits, social intercourse and so on.

3. In general, there is common occupation that almost all the members of a caste pursue.

4. Castes are stratified based on the social status they enjoy in a society, this social status is largely based on the occupation that the members of a caste pursue.

5. One's caste position is always an individual's ascribed status rather than an achieved one.

6. The prestige that the Brahmin class enjoys is the highlight of the whole caste organisation.

**Differences between class and caste**

| Class | Caste |
|---|---|
| 1. The stratification system based on class is open. Either entry into or exit from a class is quite possible for anyone who meets/fails to meet the requirements of the given class. | Stratification is quite rigid: Neither entry into nor exit is easy here. Only those individuals who are born into a caste can be the members of that caste and not anyone else. |
| 2. Class is more or less oriented with an individual's achieved statues, i.e. by hard work, initiative and enterprises a man can change his social status. For example, lorry driver becoming a lorry owner, a teacher becoming a principal, etc. | It is impossible to change one's caste status. |
| 3. Classes are secular in origin. | Caste in divinely ordained |
| 4. They are not founded on religious dogmas. | Religious beliefs with its supernatural explanations is the basis for caste. |
| 5. The selection of spouses is according to the likes and dislikes of an individual. No restriction in this regard exists in the stratification system based on class. | Endogamy (marriage within the caste). Here if anyone marries a person form a different caste, he is more often than not ostracised from that caste. |

*Contd...*

| Class | Caste |
|---|---|
| 6. The feeling of class consciousness is necessary to constitute a class. In the absence of this class consciousness the class loses its strength and begins to disintegrate. | There is no need for any subjective consciousness within the members of caste. Since the caste is evolved from some common ancestry, caste consciousness is generation to another with ease. |
| 7. There is no rigidly fixed order of prestige. For example, a group of political leaders or a group of cine actors do not always enjoy the same status. Their social status depends on public opinion. | Status given by the caste to the individual of that caste is constant and unchangeable, no matter what his social or economic status is, i.e. even if an individual becomes economically bankrupt, his caste status is intact. |

### Influence of Caste on the Society

1. **Segmentation:** Primarily caste system has segmented the society into quite a number of divisions which adversely affects the 'we feeling' in the community.
2. **Hierarchy:** Stratification based on caste is almost a rigid one where those at the top fringe continue to remain in their positions permanently. However in the recent times, education, Western influence have made the caste system lose its original rigidity.
3. **Restriction:** Restriction on feeding, drinking and social intercourse is laid down by the caste on its members.
4. **Restriction on marriage:** A member of a caste cannot marry outside his or her caste. When this restriction is violated, the member who has violated this restriction is often ostracised from the community.
5. **Disparities:** Caste system perpetuates differences among the members of a society wherein the so-called upper castes enjoy a number of privileges. On the other hand, the castes that are deemed as lower or backward are put to bear untold exploitation and ill treatment at the hands of the upper castes.
6. **Non-traditional caste occupation:** In India, rural society structure and community are traditionally well-defined. Caste and sub-caste occupations clearly distinguished exchange of services within the system. The carpenter, blacksmith and other performed job of making farm equipment for the farmer, and in return received grain at the time of harvest. The system traditionally operated with clearly defined roles and role expectations, with various castes and sub-castes. However, with advanced technology, mechanisation of agriculture, industrialisation, and modern communication, 'disruption' of the system and increasing conflict in traditional roles have occurred. Caste occupation and consequent roles are replaced by more remunerative occupations, perhaps in nearby, factories. Some of the rurel people become engaged in business, and other occupations disrupting their traditional caste occupation system.

## LEADERS AND LEADERSHIP

The main purpose of identification, development and utilisation of rural leadership is to make available large number of teachers to teach the farming community. It is impossible for any country to provide enough number of veterinarians/extension workers to carry information to each and every doorstep in the farm community. A local leader who has acquired the knowledge of improved practice extends the same to neighbours, friends and relatives. In any society and in every group in a community there are a few individuals who can influence others in the group and make decisions on behalf of others. They are the local leaders. Most of the time the veterinarian is an outsider to the villagers. The people and their sociocultural patterns prevalent in that area may be new to him. Hence, the local leaders form the vital link between the veterinarian and the livestock farmers. Common man has much faith in local leaders.

Good extension work results from joint efforts of the technically trained extension staff and the local leaders of a village. Hence, it is essential to identify and develop leadership that will facilitate and enhance effective working relationship with the rural people.

### Definition of Leader and Leadership

#### Leader

- Leader is a person who effectively influences a group to co-operate in setting and achieving goals.
- According to Sprott, "Anyone who acts as a model to others is often called a leader".
- According to Dahama and Bhatnagar, leader is a person who has been spontaneously considered or chosen as being influential."

#### Leadership

Leadership is the process of influencing people to strive willingly for mutual objectives. It is the ability of a leader to induce his group members to work with confidence and zeal to achieve the goals and objectives.

Leadership is defined as a process by which an individual directs, guides and influences the thoughts, feelings and impressions of others.

According to Dahama and Bhatnagar, "Leadership is the process of influencing the behaviour of the individuals in a given situation or situations".

## Qualities of Leaders

1. Leader understands and adheres to democratic principles.
2. He respects the rights and dignity of the others.
3. He is committed to work and readily accepts responsibility and work for the group.
4. He has the knowledge of basic needs and interests of the group.
5. He is unbiased.
6. He will recognise and praise where it is ought to be.
7. He is optimistic, enthusiastic and realistic.
8. He possesses integrity and also enjoys the trust and confidence for his group.
9. He makes decisions only after understanding the problems thoroughly.
10. He has the power to influence the group.

## Styles of Leadership

Leadership style refers to a leader's behaviour. The behavioural pattern that a leader adopts in influencing his followers is called style of leadership.

1. **Autocratic or authoritarian leadership:** An autocratic leader is one who likes to run the show himself. He takes all decisions himself without consulting the followers. He gives orders and insists on implicit obedience. Subordinates are expected to do what he dictates. Thus, under this style the decision making power is vested in the leader. He holds out threats of punishment on the assumption that people are lazy and will avoid work and shirk responsibility.

   *Advantages*
   1. Autocratic leadership permits quick decision as a single person takes decisions.
   2. It provides strong motivation and satisfaction to the leader.
   3. Many subordinates prefer to work under centralised authority and strict discipline.

   *Disadvantages*
   1. People dislike this style especially when the motivation is absent.

2. It leads to frustration, low morale and conflict which affect organisational efficiency.
3. There is resistance to change as workers feel harassed and disturbed.

2. **Participative/democratic leadership:** A democratic leader makes decision in consultation with his followers. He decentralises authority and allows the group to share his power. Instead of taking unilateral decisions, he allows the group to discuss the problem at length and express their opinions freely.

   *Advantages*
   1. It reduces resistance to change and increases acceptance of new ideas.
   2. It improves the attitudes of the group members.
   3. It increases co-operation.
   4. It facilitates the development of future leaders.

   *Disadvantages*
   1. It may be dilatory in arriving at decisions.
   2. It may be used covertly to manipulate members.
   3. It may not be liked by people who want minimum interaction with superiors and colleagues.

3. **Free-rein or laissez-faire leadership:** A free-rein leader gives complete freedom to his followers to establish their own goals and policies. He does not lead and avoids power. He lets the group to operate on its own.

   *Advantages*
   1. Complete freedom to members.
   2. There is maximum opportunity for the development of the members.

   *Disadvantages*
   1. As there is abdication of formal leadership role, informal leader emerges to fill the void.
   2. The government does not get the benefit of leader's inspired motivation, guidance and socioemotional support.

4. **Paternalistic leadership:** A paternalistic leader serves as the head of the family and treats his followers like his family members. He assumes a paternal or fatherly role to help guide and protect the followers. He provides them with good working conditions, fringe benefits and welfare facilities and services. Paternalistic leadership has been quite successful in Japan because of its cultural background.

## Classification of Leadership

There are several classifications of leaders, depending on the chief interest in the study of leadership.

1. **Origin of leadership**

   (a) Leader appointed by executive, (b) leader appointed by group, (c) self-appointed leader.

2. **Purpose of leadership**

   (a) Intellectual leader, (b) artistic leader, (c) executive leader

3. **Nature of leadership**

   (a) Autocratic leader, (b) democratic leader

4. **Nature of relationship**

   (a) Institutional leader, (b) dominant leader, (c) expert leader, (d) persuasive leader.

### Other Classifications

**Whyte's classification**

a. Operational leader

b. Popularity leader

c. Assumed representative

d. Prominent talent

e. Elected, selected or nominated

**Dharma and Bhatnagar's classification**

a. Democratic, autocratic and laissez-faire

b. Formal and informal leaders

c. Professional and lay leaders

d. Political, religious, social and academic

An Animal Husbandry Extension Worker/ Veterinarian is a professional leader and also a formal leader. He needs the help of other formal leaders and local lay leaders for effective implementation of the programmes. These lay leaders may be traditional, political or religious leaders. A few of the types of leaders who are important in livestock extension are as follows.

### Formal and Informal Leaders

**Formal leaders:** People who hold recognised positions of authority are called formal leaders. Once the pattern of leadership in a society is understood it is easy to identify these leaders. Some inherit their positions, others are elected and some others are appointed by higher authority. There may be numerous formal leaders functioning in a village and they vary from village to village. Some examples are panchyat president, village headman, co-operative society president, religious leaders, etc. Extension programmes should be worked out through formal leaders. The veterinarian should identify the right person to approach for a specific issue. The influence of leaders may vary with place and time. The veterinarian need to get the support of the traditional formal leaders for success of any programme.

**Informal leaders:** These are people who are not holding any particular position of authority. They are respected by others because of an attractive and forceful personality and because they seem to know the best action to restore to in any situation.

### Professional and Lay Leaders

**Professional leader:** Leaders who have received specialised training in specific field of their work are called professional leaders. They are engaged full time in an occupation and are paid for their work. The degree of involvement in extension work may vary between different professional leaders, e.g. veterinarian and agricultural officer.

**Lay leaders:** They may or may not have received special training and are not paid for their work. They need not be full time workers and may be associated with local group or organisation. They are also called local leaders or natural leaders, volunteer leaders. These local leaders may be either formal or informal leaders depending upon the recognised position of authority they hold. Usually in a village the lay, informal or formal leaders will also be the opinion leaders.

**Traditional leaders:** The traditional type of leaders assume their role based on the assumption that some people are born leaders. Leadership is thought to be a characteristic handed down from one person to another chiefly through heredity. Traditional leader plays an important role in rural life, because he is characterised by the possession of sound economic and social status rooted in the past and outside contacts. The significance of traditional leaders is becoming less due to the influence of social change and a new pattern of leadership is evolving. However, for extension work in the Indian villages the co-operation of the traditional leaders is always needed.

**Political leaders:** All political parties have their own grassroot leaders at village level. It is very important that the veterinarian gains the support of these local leaders for all developmental efforts irrespective of the political party they are affiliated to. Once the local political leaders find the veterinarian to be a politically neutral figure, the programmes may be applauded as non-controversial, at all stages.

## Identification and Selection of Leaders

There is no scarcity of local leaders. It is said that there are one-tenth leaders and nine-tenths followers. When the villagers gain experience in self-help development new leaders will emerge out of new situations. Distinction is required between professional and lay leaders because the problems of selection and the methods of training will vary greatly in terms of whether or not one is training professional leader or lay leader. Various sociologists, for identification and selection of leaders, have used various methods.

### Selection of Professional Leaders

1. **Interview and records:** The most commonly used method of selection of professional leaders is based on an interview, and perusal of academic records, previous experience and occupational records of the individual.

   *Advantages:* Large number of professionals can be screened through this method within a short period of time.

   *Limitations:* The main constraint is that one can observe and evaluate the person who appears for the interview only while he is interviewed, which is indeed a very short period to know about the candidate.

2. **Tests:** Sometimes in addition to the interview of the applicant may be subjected to written test or a battery of tests. While selecting professional leaders in industry and management, to measure the ability, aptitudes, attitudes and interests, these battery of tests may be conducted.

   *Advantages*

   1. The use of a battery of tests along with interview provides a better basis for selection.
   2. These tests will measure academic training and practical experience and especially, the candidate's personality.

   *Limitations*

   1. To conduct these tests a thorogh knowledge of psychology is required. Only well-trained experts alone can conduct these tests.

3. **Performance tests:** There are two types of performance tests: "Leaderless group tests" and "leader appointed tests", that form the basis for selection of professional leaders.

   a. *Leaderless group tests:* In this test, 7 or 8 persons are given a common problem to solve and it is left up to them to select their own leader.

Observations are made during the tests to determine who could be the leader.

   b. *Leader appointed tests:* A person is appointed as leader and then it is observed how well he directs the activities of the group.

*Advantages*

The functional ability of the professional leader in a real life situation as the leader of the group can be observed.

### Selection of Lay Leaders

Selection of a right leader is a vital process. As wrong selection of local leader will affect the development of the programmes as well as the credibility of the extension worker.

1. **Sociometric test:** An extension worker visits his project area and requests all the members of the community, group or organisation to indicate whom they usually consult for advice on farming. The person named by the maximum farmers is accepted as the possible leader. In this method every member of the group has to mention his choice. Assumption is that a person liked by majority of the people is the most influential or natural leader in the group and is capable of leading the group. Figure 8.2 illustrates this type of test. As in the diagram when 'C' is interviewed, he may indicate that he generally goes to 'X' for getting opinion on farming. 'D', 'E', 'F' and 'G' may also say that 'X' is the person whose suggestion they accept on farming. Then 'X' is the natural or local or informal or operational or potential leader of this group. He may not even think of himself as a leader and may say that he is not a leader. But for the group he is the operational leader in relation to farming practices.

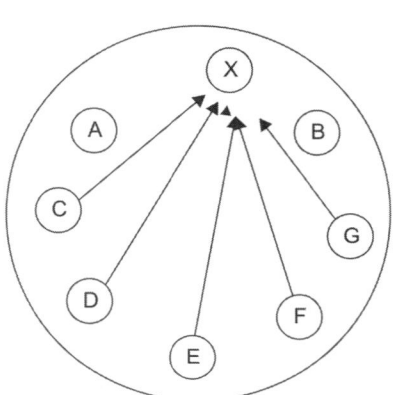

**Fig. 8.2:** Sociometry

*Advantages*

1. This is simple and valid method.
2. Suitable to most of the situations.
3. This method is very useful to the extension worker in finding out the natural or local or informal leaders in the villages, who are the highly influential persons that help in the introduction and popularisation of new or improved technologies in the group.
4. By this method we can also identify the second leaders (occupying second and third positions as opinion leaders) and they can be utilised for different functions simultaneously.
5. This method can be applied for selecting even the professional leader though it is highly suitable to select lay leaders.

*Limitations*

1. It is difficult to contact all the members.
2. Identified individual may not be ready to shoulder responsibilities.
3. He may not be a neutral person.
4. Statistical analysis of this method is complex and time consuming.

2. **Election:** In this method the group members elect the leader. In the process of identification and right selection, the extension agent can help the people by explaining what sort of person is required to lead the group.

*Advantages*

1. Highly democratic method.
2. It can be used for selecting individuals to receive leadership training.

*Limitations*

After election is over, the defeated persons and his supporters may not co-operate in group activities.

3. **Discussion method:** Through observations of discussions, the person with sound knowledge and ability is soon recognised and a mere talker easily is spotted.
4. **The workshop method:** Through this method, where the large group breaks up into smaller groups and the responsibility of the programme and decision-making rests upon the smaller unit, leadership emerges in each group. The extension worker or professional leader in the workshop has the position of consultant-observer, discussion group leader, etc.
5. **Informal dialogue method:** The veterinarian will have good background information on potential influential people from his office staff like stock-men, flock men, field assistant and inseminators. He can also open up dialogues with clients bringing animals to veterinary dispensary for treatment. By this way he can identify local leaders.

6. **Construction with predecessors:** The extension worker can interact with his colleagues who have already worked in that area and easily identify the leaders. Further he will get a background information about his present area, people, sociocultural pattern, etc.
7. **Group observation method:** The veterinarian should observe a group in action which will enable him to spot a potential leader. He can observe the community in any type of situation like gatherings and meetings. For getting reliable results, the group should not be aware of this.
8. **Key informant technique:** The veterinarian, during his village visits, can meet the key informants in a community and ask them to indicate the opinion of leaders in their village.
9. **Active participants:** They can also be located in the community meetings. Active participation is an indication of their leadership ability. These are the persons who are taking initiative to make or lead in making decisions relative to the events or actions selected.
10. **Social participations:** Higher the social participation of a person the more is the promise in him of becoming a leader. It is assumed that a person already in active participation in the existing organisations will be useful to provide leadership in the new situation.
11. **Self-rating technique:** In this technique each respondent is asked to evaluate his own abilities to act as a leader. How far others think him as influential. The success of this method depends upon frankness and boldness of a person to express his true feelings.

## Training of Leaders

The basic idea of training leaders assumes leadership as something that can be taught and learned. This incidentally brings up to the two general theories of the origin of leaders, i.e. the biological theory and psychological theory.

**Biological theory:** It assumes that some individuals are born to be leaders, i.e. the children of great leaders, who also become leader.

**Psychological theory:** This theory stresses that only the situation and not just the person makes a leader.

The biological theory may be true that heredity may produce leaders but it does not always follow that all their children will be leaders. No amount of training can make a leader out of a person if he has limited inherent talents. It must be recognised that heredity and training of potential leader are both subject to the situation in which this individual finds himself. Careful selection of person is essential for successful leadership development. It is not enough to select potential leaders for training, merely on the basis of ability. They need to exhibit a genuine interest in leadership and be motivated to work with people.

### Training of Professional Leaders

1. **Pre-service training:** It is a basic training for professional leaders in preparing them to take up a new job. It is usually college and institutional study of subject matter, extension principles, methods, psychology and sociology.

2. **Induction training:** It is given soon after the professional leader is introduced to the new position. During this period, he will get apprentice-ship experience and gain full understanding of the new job to be done and greater confidence in his capabilities to perform extension work. It also develops desirable attitudes, work habits, skills and techniques. It also permits the trainee to determine whether the selected professional leader is fit for the work and gives an opportunity to administrators to assess the trainee for regularising his job as permanent one.

3. **In-service training:** This training begins after the professional leader enters service and often continues until the time of his retirement. It may be interpreted as the process of keeping the employes informed of changing problems and situations as they arise and suggesting ways and means of solving those problems, e.g. refresher training to Veterinary Assistant Surgeons and Extension Officer of Animal Husbandry.

4. **Graduate training:** It refers to highly formal training in an institution beyond the bachelor's degree level, e.g. doctorate or post-graduate. diploma in formal education in veterinary universities, agriculture universities, etc.

5. **Orientation training:** It refers to carefully planned, scientific and effective introduction of the new worker to his job. It is a shorter training course.

### Training of Lay Leaders

Either formal or informal method can be used.

**Informal methods**

It may be:

i. *Observation:* This is done by closely observing how others have performed.

ii. *Reading:* By studying the printed literature, circular letters, etc. from community development workers.

iii. *Dialogue:* Talking with other leaders or progressive farmers or others in the field of interest.

**Formal methods**

1. Lecture: It may be supplemented with other formal methods.
2. Group methods like discussion, workshop, forum, panel, symposium, buzz, etc.
3. Audio and video lessons.
4. Field trips.
5. Apprenticeship.
6. Formal leaders' training camps.
7. Direct assistance from experts.

Giving responsibility to local leaders so that they develop self-confidence.

### Leadership Phenomena

After selection and training, the leader must be properly utilised for doing extension work by the extension worker. Hence, regular follow-up by periodical contacts should be made by the extension worker. It is especially important to keep watching young leaders, helping them into the leadership responsibilities as they develop. The leaders should adopt any practice first in their own farm and make others to follow. Their participation should be tendered through the programme. If the leaders are duly recognised they will work with more zeal. For this, they should be kept in forefront.

### Advantages and Limitations of Leadership in Extension

#### Advantages

1. More numbers of teachers will be available to educate the farming community.
2. Information will reach large number of people in short period with less expenditure.
3. Since leaders adopt the new idea first, neighbours and group members will quickly adopt the technology without resistance. They believe more

readily the idea coming from (local leader) than the third person (extension worker).

4. The rate of social change will be rapid.

5. Build up confidence over the extension programmes.

### Limitations

1. It is not very easy to locate and train a suitable person required for the extension work.

2. Selected leader may not have adequate followers in the group.

3. He may not have sustained interest and may not show much involvement in extension work.

4. Local leaders may try to use prestige connected with position for personal benefit.

5. Sometimes leaders may misuse their powers, popularity and publicity gained.

### Roles of Leadership (Hepple)

1. **Group spokesman:** The leader has responsibility of speaking for the group and representing the group's interests and position faithfully and accurately.

2. **Group harmonizer:** The leader is responsible for pointing out the group, when political conflict situations arise, that the common purpose is sufficiently worthy of co-operation, that the differences should be resolved peacefully. But it should be remembered that the role of the group harmonizer is to promote harmony in line with the basic purpose of the group and not to promote it simply for harmony's sake.

3. **Group planner:** The group expects its leader to have new ideas for initiating activities. To meet this expectation the leader must be able to plan, to visualize in his imagination the ways by which the group can satisfy its needs.

4. **Group executive:** As a group executive the leader is responsible for seeing that the business of the organisation is carried on according to democratic principles. He is responsible for seeing that individuals and sub-groups carry out work.

5. **Group educator or teacher:** The leader must share with the followers his knowledge and experience. Such sharing of experience and insight is teaching. It is possible that the best way to play the role of group planner is by playing the role of group teachers. Good leadership depends largely upon teaching because the good teacher is not a director.

6. **Symbol of group ideal:** All social groups have implicit or explicit norms or ideas. As a rule, persons accepted as leaders are those who have adopted these norms and live by them. The group expects his leadership to embody the ideas of the group. If a person cannot accept the ideas of the group and consistently makes an effort to alter them, he should decline to accept the role of leadership for the organisation.

7. **Group discussion chairman:** Generally a group meets for a panel discussion or a forum or a group thinking conference as something apart from the routine business of the organisation. In view of the increased use that is being made of various types of discussions, leaders would do well to have some training along this line.

8. **Group supervisor:** Professional leaders such as extension officers, in addition to serving as leaders of social groups also devote a portion of their time working with lay leaders and group organizations like youth clubs, co-operativies, farmers' associations, etc. These organisations have their own lay leaders. The extension officers' role is not to take over the work of the lay leaders, but rather to serve in the capacity of advisory personnel.

## CULTURAL FACTORS IN SOCIETY

The word 'Culture' has been derived from the Latin word 'Cultura'. Culture is a sum total of various social practices and traditions. Culture is a way of doing things that is acceptable to society. It is nothing but a kind of acquired behaviour of human beings. In a sense culture is abstract for it is manifested in behaviour. Culture is that we come to know about when we observe how the people (of a particular society) dress, their marriage, family life, livestock farming, method of cultivation, pattern of religious ceremonies, leisure pursuits and so on. Cultural behaviour is acquired behaviour and not original of man. Culture is transmitted to an individual by others such as his parents, friends, teachers, etc. It is a product of human experience. Hence, culture is man-made.

The following definition of culture by Edward B. Tylor is the most famous and it helps us have a comprehensive understanding of culture: "Culture is that complex whole which includes knowledge, beliefs, art, morals, law, customs and other capabilities and habits acquired by man as a member of society."

According to Sargent et al: "Culture is a pattern of learned behaviour shared by the members of a society.

It includes not only the way of making things and doing things but the pattern of relationship of many people, the attitudes they foster, the beliefs and ideas they have and even the feelings with which they respond".

## Society and Culture

The basic difference between society and culture is that society is people, culture is their behaviour. Members of a society share to some extent at least a common culture, live within it, alter it, and transfer it to the next generation, e.g. three villages in Tamil Nadu, Goundampatti, Malapalayam and Lurdhupuram may have many common characteristics but may represent three different societies, each with its own culture.

In general sense, these villages might also be grouped together and referred to a belonging to an overall Indian culture which includes such diversity.

## Different Orders of Culture

Culture may be thought in terms of three different orders as meant by Raiph Linton.

1. Material—industrial products such as syringe, artificial insemination gun, Bard Parker blade, etc.
2. Overt behaviour—outward behaviour patterns of persons like customs, folkways, mores, etc.
3. Psychological, i.e. attitudes, values, beliefs, etc.

Can we classify material and overt behaviour as overt culture and psychological under covert culture.

## Organisational Structure of Culture

Culture has a structure that is made up of various units i.e. cultural trait, cultural complex and cultural pattern.

a. **Cultural trait:** Cultural trait is the small unit of culture, i.e. irreducible unit of learned behaviour. These are material and non-material traits.

*Material traits*, e.g. Bullock cart, dhoti, sari are all traits of material culture of Indian village society.

*Non-material traits*, e.g. (1) Vannakkam, Namaskar, i.e. pressing the palm together and bowing slightly in respectful greeting to an elder, (2) pulling the ham of sari over the head to cover a woman's face in the presence of outsider.

Linton has presented an analysis of participation in culture in terms of three categories of cultural traits, i.e. universal, specialists and alternatives with a fourth category of individual peculiarities.

**Universal**: Certain cultural traits are essential to all and are known as universal, e.g. young people show extreme respect and obedience to the elders.

**Alternatives:** Culture in which the individual has a choice among several forms of behaviour, e.g. when a cow comes to heat the farmer can get his animal inseminated taking it either to veterinary dispensaries or to sub-centre or milk produces' co-operative society which, ever he chooses, as the most convenient or beneficial for him.

**Specialities:** These are elements of culture shared by some groups but not by all groups in a society, e.g. cart occupation.

**Individual peculiarities:** Individual peculiarities are fears, prejudices, or capacities. The greatest amount of uniformity occurs in the participation in universals, followed by that in participation in the specialities. These two form a core of culture that is surrounded by the alternatives.

b. **Cultural complex:** It is a group of cluster of related cultural traits like:

1. Mattupongal festival in livestock farmers' community.
2. Thread ceremony in Brahmin community.
3. "Girl coming to age" function (attaining puberty) in Hindu family.

These are some of the examples of clustering of a large number of related cultural traits to form a cultural complex.

c. **Cultural pattern:** It is a group of cultural complexes, e.g. cultural pattern of rural Hindu society.

*Customs:* Customs are socially prescribed forms of behaviour, transmitted by tradition and enforced by society and their violation tantamount to social disapproval.

Customs are the accepted ways of doing things (by people) together in personal contacts.

Customs are interwoven with our social life, and are part and parcel of our society. Customs are usually well established and difficult to change. Various types of behaviour, if they are organised or repetitive, have generally been called customs.

*Classification of customs:* Customs can be classified into unidentified acts, convention, mores, taboos and rituals.

*Unidentified acts:* Certain personal habits and patterns of behaviour that require no social approval are called unidentified acts, e.g. (a) a farmer prefers goat's milk, (b) using a particular brand of toothpaste.

*Folkways:* Folkways are the customary ways of behaving in a society over which society exerts some force for conformity. Folkways are the ways by which rural folk do things, e.g. (a) removal of shoes before entering into house, (b) vanakkam (greeting others with folded hands).

Folkways are the expected forms of behaviour but are not rigidly enforced. Violations of folkways are not punished. But people do develop bad opinion of such persons. For example, showing respect to the superiors by saying *vanakkam* with folded hands is a folkway in Tamil Nadu. If a subordinate fails or ignores this custom he may not be punished but he will not be in the good books of the superior. Folkways arise from experience and develop due to frequent repetitions of petty acts, often by large members acting in the same way when faced with the same situations. Some of the folkways represent a successful routine that was invented for doing something and then was followed by others who desired to get similar results.

For example, in a culture where dairying was primary occupation, animals suffered due to nasal schistosomiasis (snoring diseases caused by cauliflower-like growth inside the cattle's nose). Even after getting treatment, the cauliflower-like growth did not subside immediately and snoring sound persisted. An individual just cut and took a finger size branch of Erukku (*Calotropis gigantea*), removed all the leaves and inserted into the nose and then moved it in and out a few times and scrapped all the growth. Within a few days, his animal became all right. People were eager to find out what he did and how he did it. Other farmers also followed that practice. As a veterinary surgeon in that area the author has tried the above method in a few cases and got good results. Now it has become the usual pattern.

*Superstition:* An irrational belief in supernatural influences is known as superstition. Sometimes folkways are based upon false inferences; people may assume a casual relationship between two things that really does not exist. For example, in a farm, a cow delivered a male calf on Friday and later, the farmer fell ill and died. The farm women explained that the death was due to the birth of male calf on Friday and therefore, one must avoid keeping such cows (though it was a heavy yielder) in future unless she wants to take the chance of misfortune.

*Convention:* Conventions are established practices. Conventions are customs regulating significant social behaviours. These are common to all civilised cultures, e.g.

1. Breakfast after bath.
2. Westerners use knife, fork and spoon rather fingers for eating.

Parents generally do not leave such learning to chance; they instruct their children about their conventions. Conventions are violated less often than folkways or usage, and if violated, the sanctions are more severe; like ridicule, condemnation, strong disapproval, gossip, etc.

### Mores and taboos

*Mores:* Mores are the patterns of behaviour considered essential by society. The difference between folkways and mores is largely a matter of the degree to which they are enforced. Mores are rigidly enforced and if not followed, the individual incurs severe penalty from society. "Mores are those things which persons ought or ought not to do. Generally, the term 'mores' is used for the positive action things that ought to be done", e.g. (1) halal method of slaughter in Muslim society, (2) standing up during the playing of the National Anthem.

*Taboos:* Taboos are those things that persons ought not to do. The word 'taboo' in a strict sense refers to prohibitions of types of behaviour because of some magical, supernatural or religious sanction, e.g. prohibition against pork in Muslim society, prohibition against beef in Hindu religion.

The mores, because of their relationship to the ethical moral values, are slower to change than the folkways. Some mores have remained unchanged for centuries in our culture, e.g. Brahmin caste abstains from eating meat. Since mores are the customs that are held to be essential to the welfare of the people, they will remain stable.

*Ritual:* A pattern of behaviour or ceremony which has become the customary way of dealing with certain situations, or is the pattern that has been established by law, as in the case of governmental affairs or is a part of the rules of a particular organisation. In India, there are rituals that are identified with religious groups, colleges and universities, government, etc.

### Acculturation and ethnocentrism

*Acculturation:* It means contact between culture when people of different cultures come in contact with one another. They may influence each other in different ways. It depends on period of contact. If the contact is long and frequent, there is greater impact which may be one-sided or reciprocal.

*Ethnocentrism:* It is the tendency of man to consider his own culture superior to all others and to judge other cultures in terms of standards and values that exist in one's own culture, e.g. an arranged marriage, which is common in India may be looked at with curiosity, surprise and even horror in the United States. The American father may claim that he would never "sell his daughter in marriage to any man".

## Importance of Culture in Extension

An extension worker will be more efficient if he understands the social and cultural background of the farmers with whom he works. He will then be in a better position to offer advice that will be highly suitable to the existing culture of the society, and can use the structure and culture of the society to the benefit of his work. It is useful, therefore, to examine the main features of societies and cultures that are relevant to extension work. The more an extension agent learns about and comes to respect the culture of the people with whom he works, the more he will be accepted by them.

Hence, before starting his actual project in an area, the extension worker should be aware of the culture of particular society. If he gives respect to the local customs, people will consider him as one among them. This will help the extension worker to develop a good rapport with the farming community. Then people will readily accept his ideas. For example, in villages, before entering into the house, people remove their shoes. Without knowing this folkway if an extension worker makes farm and home visit and enters the farmer's house with shoes onto accept his tea he may not be liked by the farmer. If this sort of activities continue in his course, he will lose respect and confidence of the farmers of that area. Ultimately he will not succeed either in the transfer of technology or in implementation of his programme. Therefore, thorough understanding of the culture of the society is highly important for an effective extension work.

Each aspect of the culture of the society has a definite purpose and function. This is important to remember when planning the extension programmes. Changes in one aspect of culture are likely to produce unforeseen or unacceptable effect on other aspects. Then a programme may have a little chance of success. This is one of the reasons why local leaders and farmers should participate in planning an extension programme.

## Cultural Change

Social structure, cultures are never completely static, they can and do change. Cultural change in society has two major aspects:

a. Cultural change by discovery and invention.
b. Cultural change by diffusion and borrowing.

The first comes from within the society and culture, the second from another culture, outside of the society. The extension worker should help to bring about cultural change in farming. This may in turn contribute to wider social change, e.g. ox drawn plough to tractors.

## Important Local Cultures

There are five particular aspects of local culture that the extension agent should be aware of:

1. **Farming system:** Before he can offer any advice to farmers the extension worker must understand their present farming system. Once he is familiar with local farming systems, the extension worker can explore the possibilities for improvement. New farming practices will be more acceptable to farmers if they can be introduced into existing systems without drastic changes.

2. **Land tenure:** Land tenure consists of the ways in which people obtain the right to process and use land. Land tenure systems vary from one society to another.

3. **Inheritance:** The way in which land and other possessions pass from one generation to the next also affects extension work. For example, in some cultures, a man's possessions are inherited not by his children but by his mother's brothers and their children. Extension agents should understand the local inheritance rules, because they will affect the ability of young farmers to acquire land, and the interest of farmers to take their advice.

4. **Ceremonies and festivals:** Ceremonies are a central feature of culture. They include religious festivals, celebrations to mark important seasons. Elders start off the planting and the end of harvest and their presence is considered to be very important for events (marriage, birth and death) within the life of a family or community. An extension agent needs to know when these take place so that he can plan his activities around them. He should also take care to behave in the appropriate way on such occasions.

5. **Traditional means of communication:** All societies have ways of spreading information and sharing ideas, e.g. songs, proverbs, drama, dance, religious gathering and village meetings. The extension worker could make use of these traditional means of communication to pass information and ideas to the rural people.

## Jallikattu

Jallikattu, a bull taming game in Tamil Nadu acts as an evidence of social relation between human being and bull in ancient Tamil culture. The bull taming game in Tamil Nadu has been called in different names like erukol, eru thazhuval, eruthu kattu, kaalai anaiththal, maadu anaiththal and manju virattu. Eru thazhuval which means "bull embracing" is the oldest form of bull taming game in Tamil culture. Tamil literatures namely kalithogai and Silappatikaaram has references on importance of ancient bull taming game in Tamil culture. Historians stated that the bull taming game has its origin from pastoral community in Mullai landscape, which then got spread to other landscapes. Seal dated between 2500 BC and 1800 BC discovered at Mohenjodaro acts as an evidence of bull taming games in Indus valley civilisation. Ancient paintings of bullfight have been found in Kalloothu Mettupatti near Madurai and Karikkiyur in The Nilgiri (Annamalai, 2015).

Epigraphists state that bull taming game has its place in all ancient civilization. In ancient Tamil culture once a girl is nearing puberty age, the father decides to buy a cow with male calf. The calf is reared as ferocious bull along with that girl. Once the girl attains puberty, the man who tamed that bull in a jallikattu won the woman as bride. Though the game has its origin from pastoral community, it has defined rules. Tom-tom, a traditional audio aid used for drawing attention of the mass, was used to announce the rules to the public and injured were taken for treatment immediately from the spot. More importantly, it was always a one-on-one fight, unlike the modern day 'free-for-all. Jallikattu has been playing a crucial role till today on conservation of native breeds of cattle in Tamil Nadu. As on now the bull reared for jallikattu has been considered as a member of the family and it also fetches pride to the family rearing the bull.

## ▌SOCIAL VALUES OR VALUE SYSTEMS

Extension work per se is meant for amelioration of the rural society. Any rural welfare measure could be successfully implemented and carried on only if there is necessary co-operation and participation of the people concerned.

Hence, it is highly important to gather details about the attitude, behaviour of the villagers. Behaviour is seen, whereas attitude of the people is known by their nature of action or reaction to stimuli.

The fate of any welfare work done by any extension workers has a close connection to attitudes and tendencies of the people. And it is an individual's values that form or give shape to his/her attitudes or tendencies.

Value, according to S.C. Dodd, is "desiderata, i.e. anything desired or chosen by someone some time". They are attitude related attributes that are projected upon people, objects and situations.

In other words values are that relative worth, importance or preference that an individual attaches to a material, symbol, situation,or extra mundane aspects of life. The importance attached by an individual to a thing in comparison with the other, be it of same class or of a different class, has a direct bearing over the individual's value system. The thing that has been given importance in the case above may be overlooked or even ignored by another individual who might hail from a different school of thought or possess a value set-up different from the individual referred to in the former case.

For instance, villagers in general attach more importance to the finger ring than to their footwear. On the other hand, a city dweller attaches more importance to his footwear than to his finger ring.

## Importance of Values for an Extension Worker

Uniformity of values is seen in highly homogeneous communities for these communities more or less follow similar culture and pursue similar occupation.

Above all, homogeneous communities (rural) unlike heterogeneous communities (towns, cities) undergo socialisation that is effected by more or less similar agents, environment, situations and so on. In heterogeneous communities, socialisation is effected by a series of agents (college, clubs, factories, media, etc.). Hence, there are marked differences in values between rural and urban population.

Such being the case, an extension worker, to be successful, needs to be aware and knowledgeable about the values of the villagers that in all probabilities are similar at the same time, and indispensable.

In some societies honesty, loyalty, obedience, etc. might be the guiding values of the population. In some, unity, honour, self-respect, etc. might be the prime values. Hence, an extension worker needs to have a thorough understanding about the values rooted deep in the minds of the people.

This is because if the extension programme traces along the prescribed values besides achieving its actual purpose the efforts and task undertaken by the extension worker will receive due recognition, encouragement, participation, co-operation, so on and so forth. On the other hand, if the same extension worker ignores or sidelines the values of the villagers during the course of action then the programme or result would be counter productive besides jeopardizing the credibility of any further extension work in the village. Hence, for all the above said reasons the extension worker would do well to understand the values of the villagers that would be manifested in their behaviours, approached signs, symbols, etc.

## SOCIAL CHANGE

Human being is a dynamic creature that is ever prone to change. Human beings have never been static. Change in human society has been a continuous feature ever since the emergence of human society. However, change does not happen at all societies at the same time. Similarly, the pace at which things undergo a change in a particular society may not be the same in all societies. For example, change with respect to status of women in Western societies when compared to the change in status of women in Indian society has marked differences wherein change in this regard has been faster and more intensive in Western society than it has been in Indian society.

It needs to be said that change in a particular institution in a particular society does have its impact over other societies at varying degrees. For example, love marriage, though not totally unheard of in Indian societies, has become quite common due to the influence of the west. Constant variations are seen in the society and these variations are noticeable in (1) Social relationships, (2) social patterns, and (3) social interaction.

### Meaning and Definition

The word change denotes difference in anything observed over a period of time. Social change, therefore, means observable differences in any social phenomenon over a period of time.

Social change is meant to only such alterations that occur in social organisation vis-à-vis its structure and function.

H.T. Mazumdar defines social change as a new fashion or mode either modifying or replacing the old in the life of people in a society.

According to Johes, social change is a term used to describe variations or modifications of any aspect of social processes, social patterns, social interactions or social organisation.

According to MacIver and Page say, "Our direct concern as sociologist is with social relationships. It is the change in these relationships which alone we shall regard as social change.

### Forms of Social Change

The general way or patterns of social change may be classified into: (1) Unilinear, (2) Pendular, and (3) Evolutionary.

(1) In unilinear type of change, the society is following its onward march in a constant way towards an end which, the society believes, as predetermined by blind forces of nature, fate or divine province.

(2) In pendular or rthythmical change, the change implies a sequence of periodically recurring change similar to the movement of the pendulum.

(3) In evolutionary type change, everything, be it a living organism or an institution, is ever undergoing change but the change is mostly latent, gradual, slow, uniform, rather than being abrupt, radical and conspicuous. Though it is said change is ever happening it is only when the transformation brings in some remarkable difference that the change is vividly felt.

### Agencies of Social Change

There are quite a number of agencies that affect the process of social change. And if a change is brought about in an institution in a society, the change should not be seen as a result of any single agency instead it should be understood that change is brought about by a combined action of certain forces (agencies). For instance, if the change is felt with regard to the status of women it is necessarily the influence of educational, economic, political institutions. The following agencies play an important role in aiding or preventing social change in a society.

### Family

The principal member of the family, a lot depends on such a person for a change to happen, for the person is seen in the light of his socialisation, environment, occupation and so on. For instance, if the head of the family is going well in the surrounding then he/she is not likely to invite or ask for a change and impose change over his/her family members.

### Religion

Man, in general, is bound by his religious convictions hence one's religion plays an indispensable role in one embracing or resisting the change. If the society or an individual feels that the change may strengthen their religious institution then the individual or society invites the change. On the contrary, if the change posses a challenge to religious practices then the change is likely to be resisted by the society.

### Government

Political institution: A government is one of the most important influencing factors in the process of social process. For it is the political institution vis-à-vis legislation, norms, etc. that could thrust change if need be on its people for the political institution aids or prevents a change keeping in view the principle of greatest good for the greatest number.

### Education

Education is the sum total of experience that moulds the attitude and determines the conduct of both child and the adult. Education induces rational power in the minds of the human beings. Rational thinking enables the human beings to reflect on change in an objective way than preventing one from being carried away by one's blind, emotional subjective feelings and beliefs.

## Characteristics of Social Change

1. **Social change is a universal phenomenon:** No society can remain untouched by change permanently rather no society remains completely static. When the population changes, change does occur in technology, education, material production and so on.
2. **Social change is a community change:** Social change is not a change in the life of an individual or the life patterns of several individuals. It is a change that occurs in the life of the entire community.
3. **Speed of social change is not uniform:** Change in a society could be engineered by its members themselves or it could be brought about by nature. The pace at which manmade change is brought about varies from abrupt to gradual depending upon the consequence of change and people's interest in the change. But natural calamities such as floods, earthquake bring in drastic, even

overnight changes, in the lives of the people.
    A change in a society vis-à-vis its pace and direction varies between one society and another. Highly civilized societies welcome change that they feel is good for their posterity and themselves, on the other hand, primitive barbaric societies view every change with skepticism and a lot of apprehension.
4. **Change is a law of nature:** Man by nature desires change. Our needs keep changing and so changes are essential for our lives, e.g. automatic shaving kits, compact discs, dish washers, etc. are some of the changes that man finds very essential in today's world.
5. **Prediction of social change is difficult:** Prediction of social change is difficult for it is hard to discern as to what factors induce change and when the change is going to be brought about. It is already said in the evolutionary form of change, that change is ever occurring in the society but we are unable to see or feel the changes for they are latent and highly internal in their period of transition.

## Factors Affecting Social Change

The following are the factors influencing the social change: (a) Demographic factor, (b) Technological factor, (c) Economic factor, (d) Cultural factor, (e) Legislation, (f) Planning, (g) Education

(a) **Demographic factor:** Demography is defined as the study of quantitative and qualitative aspects of human population. Thus, the demographic factor denotes the size, structure and distribution of population. The size of the population is based mainly upon three factors—birth rate, death rate and migration. The composition of population depends upon variables like age, sex, marital status, literacy, etc.
    The social structure of a society is closely related to the size and composition of human population. Thus, the change in demographic factor can bring a social change in varying degrees. Changes in the demographic factors such as changes in birth rate and mortality rate have their consequences on the structure of family, kinship, politics and other institutions.
    The size and structure of population have their direct impact on the social relationships like age of marriage, value of education, ability to get job, family size and other factors. In animal husbandry point of view, the size and composition of population has its impact on demand and supply of livestock products, growth of livestock sector, entrepreneurship model, etc.

The demographic factor has an effective impact on nation's economy and poverty. As an extension agent, we have to plan a scheme or project for the farmers based on the demographic factors.

b. **Technological factor:** Technological invention is an important factor having impact on social and cultural change. The use of fire and invention of wheel played an important role in the human transformation. Likewise the invention of the pot, the compass, the printing press, the telephone, steam engine, motor car, radio, internet, atom bomb and weapons, cell phones, etc. played a major role in social and cultural changes in human society.

Technological invention not only had brought changes in attitudes, beliefs and tradition of human society, but it also had impact on the caste and class behaviour among human beings. For example, the technological developments like industries, railways, bus services, etc. had an impact on caste and class behaviour. People of different caste and class are working together in the same atmosphere without any differences due to technological invention and services. The milk producer organizations and poultry farmers organization consists of farmers of various caste and class without any differences among them.

Technological interventions helped India to achieve number one milk producer, third in egg production in the world. But at the same time, technological interventions also bring in negative consequences like pollution, introduction of exotic germ plasm leading to decrease in disease resistance.

c. **Economic factor:** Karl Marx, the famous historical economist, has given the best description on the economic interpretation of social change in his book "Das Capital". In his point of view, a classless society has to emerge in which no one owns anything and everyone owns everything. The core point is abolition of poverty.

According to Marx it is the economic factor which determines social, cultural, religious and political aspects of human life. He stressed the mode of production is the factor behind the social formation corresponding to feudalism. Capitalism and socialism.

The economy can be divided into five types, namely tribal economy, the peasant economy, the pre-industrial urban economy, industrial economy, and corporate economy. Even in the era of globalisation, still 65% of our population live in villages revolving around peasant economy.

Indian economy, where all five types of economy co-exist, the policy makers should focus on measures to increase employment especially in rural areas, inorder to alleviate poverty. White revolution coupled with abolition of traditional landlord system has brought a new level of social change led to the formation of cooperative farming giving equal opportunities to all sectors of livestock farmers.

d. **Cultural factors:** Cultural factors have an intimate relationship with social change. The cultural factors like values, ideologies, attitudes, ideas of great men have impacts on society. According to W.F. Ogburn, culture can be classified into two categories, namely material culture and non-material culture. Material culture comprises books, utensils, houses and such other forms of technology, while non-material culture includes beliefs, values, attitudes, norms, religion, education, etc.

The changes come first in material aspects of culture. But, the non-material culture takes more time to cope up with the material aspects of change. As a result, non-material culture falls behind material culture, which is known as 'cultural lag'. Thus, the changes in the conditions of life have influence over the values, attitudes, beliefs and habits of the society at different pace. For example, nowadays the status of a person in a society is not determined by his birth but by his power.

e. **Legislation as a factor of social change:** Law is a system of rules that are enforced through social institutions to govern behaviour (Wikipedia, 2016). The function of law is to ensure a certain degree of uniformity among the members of the society which has various cultural and behavioural patterns. It also influences the members of the society to bind with the group expectation. Law alone cannot bring a social change without the support of the people. For example, even if we have strong law against food adulteration, it still persists in the society. But, apart from these limitations, law is an instrument of social change.

f. **Planning as a factor of social change:** Planning is a process of thinking and organising activities to achieve a desired goal. The change in a society could occur in a planned or unplanned manner. The government plan and implement a scheme or project to bring a positive social change in the concerned society. Five-Year Plan is an example of planned social change. However, sometimes due to natural calamities like flood, drought, etc. unplanned changes may occur in a society.

g. **Education as a factor of social change:** Education is process of acquiring knowledge, skill and attitude. Education is the key element in the social change. Educating a society brings a positive change in the society towards economic and social welfare. Thus, the government focus on education through "Mid-day Meal Scheme" and "Right to Education Act" to bring a social change in the society. Education not only brings improvement in personal living, but also towards social living.

## SOCIAL TRANSFORMATION IN RELATION TO ANIMAL REARING

**Social transformation** is the process by which an individual *alters* the socially ascribed social status of their parents into a socially achieved status for themselves. However, another definition refers to large scale social change as in cultural reforms or transformations. The first occurs with the individual, the second with the social system.

Early human history can be divided into three ages namely **stone, bronze,** and **iron**. The dating of these ages is important to understand the social transformation of human being in relation to animal rearing.

| | Stone age | | | Bronze age | Iron age |
|---|---|---|---|---|---|
| Lower paleolithic | Middle paleolithic | Upper paleolithic | Mesolithic, neolithic | | |
| 2,500,000– 200,000BC | 200,000– 50,000BC | 50,000– 10,000BC | 10,000– 3000 BC | 3000– 1000 BC | 1000 BC– Present |

The evolution of first human species termed *Homo habilis* in sub-Saharan Africa was marked as the beginning of stone age, as *Homo habilis* was a maker of stone tools. The stone age is divided into the Paleolithic (old stone age), mesolithic (middle stone age) and Neolithic (new stone age) based on the social transformation in human species. In old stone age, humans were hunters while in middle stone age they were nomads and in new stone age they were peasants. In course of time the human species who dependant on wild food resources were transformed to domestication of animals and agriculture.

### Domestication of Animals

i. **Dogs from 12,000 years ago:** Man's best friend was the first animal species to be domesticated by the human around 12000 years ago. As the wolves were similar in hunting characters of human, dogs which evolved from wolves were easily domesticated by the human.

ii. **Sheep and goats, cattle and pigs: 9000–7000 BC:** The animal which was first domesticated for food purpose is sheep around 9000 BC followed by the goats later. The nomadic pastoralists life was depend on these animal species. Cattle were domesticated little later in Asia but probably not long after 7000 BC. Pigs were first domesticated in China.

iii. **Draught animals from 4000 BC:** The domestication of oxen around 4000 BC and discovery of wheel and plough increased agriculture production. In tropical regions of Asia water buffaloes were domesticated and used for draught purpose. Water buffaloes were used for dual purpose both as draught and milch animal in rice grown areas. The other animals domesticated were cats from before 3000 BC, horses and assess 3000 BC, poultry 2000 BC, etc. The domestication of animals played a major role in social transformation of human being into two different groups, namely pastoralist and peasants. The peasants settled in permanent settlement and their livelihood rely on agriculture while the pastoralists whose livelihood depend on livestock rearing, live as a community moving from one place to another.

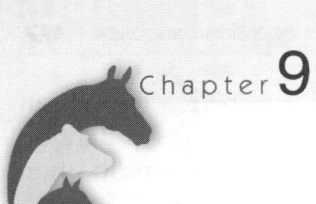

Chapter 9

# Communication of Innovation

Communication is a process by which two or more people exchange ideas, facts, feelings or impression, in ways that each gains a common understanding of the meaning, intent and use of message[1]. The word communication originates from the word 'communis', which means common/establishing commonness. In essence it is the act of getting a sender and a receiver tuned together for a particular message or series of messages.

Communication is the process of transferring meaning in the form of ideas or information from one person to another. A true interchange of meaning between people includes more than just the words used in their conversations. It includes shades of meaning and emphasism, and facial and involuntary gestures that suggest real meaning. An effective interchange requires more than just the transmission of data. It requires that the persons sending the message and receiving it rely on certain skills (speaking, writing, reading, listening, and the like) to make the exchange of meaning successful.

You can see, then, that communication is the chain of understanding that links the members of various units of an organisation at different levels and in different areas. This concept has the following elements: (1) An act of making oneself understood, (2) a means of passing information between people, and (3) a system for communicating between individuals. This tradi-tional view of communication, however, as occurring between two or more individuals, is being modified by the technological revolution to include communication between machines and other machines.

## TYPES OF COMMUNICATION

1. **Intrapersonal communication:** Communication within an individual, e.g. thinking, feeling.

2. **Interpersonal communication:** Interpersonal communication most commonly occurs in face to face situations, where we can see, hear, and even touch the other person or persons. It provides opportunity for immediate feedback, based on the result we can alter our communication style and structure.

3. **Mass communication:** It is a communication system in which an identical message is originated by an institutional organisation and sent to a large number of receivers through public channels (TV, radio, newspaper, magazines, film and computer, Internet).

4. **Non-verbal communication:** "Communication without language is known as non-verbal communication". It is also known as gestural communication.

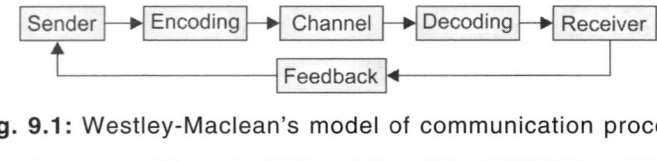

**Fig. 9.1:** Westley-Maclean's model of communication process[2]

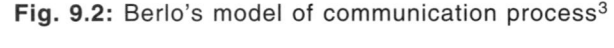

**Fig. 9.2:** Berlo's model of communication process[3]

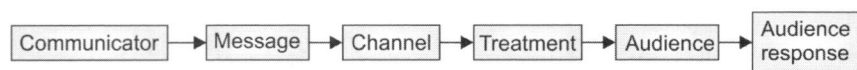

**Fig. 9.3:** Leagan's model of communication process[4]

1. Farquhar, R.N. Agricultural Liaison Officer, CSIRO—Australian Agricultural Extension Conference—Reviews, Papers and Reports, 1962.
2. Westley, B. H. & McLean, M. S., Jr. (1957). A conceptual model for communications research. Journalism Quarterly, 34, 31–38.
3. Berlo, D. K. (1960). The process of communication; an introduction to theory and practice. New York: Holt, Rinehart and Winston. Claude E Shannon, W. W.
4. Leagans, J. Paul, The Communication Process in Rural Development, (Ithaca, New York: Cornell University, International Agricultural Development Bulletin, No.1, 1963), p.5.

# COMMUNICATION MODELS

## The Communication Process

Communication is a process that involves inter-dependent and interrelated elements together to achieve a desired goal or outcome.

### Characteristics of Communication

1. Mutual presence of sender and receiver of messages is required.
2. Each person assumes roles as both sender and receiver of the message.
3. It involves mutual needs to communicate.
4. Both the sender and receiver of the messages are interdependent and interchangeable.

### Elements in the Process of Communication

1. Aristotle model: Speaker-speech-audience.
2. "SMCR" model given by Berlo: Communication source-encoder-message-channel-decoder-communication receiver.
3. Leagan's model: Communicator-message-channel-treatment-audience-response.

There are many different models of communication, depending on the context of communication involved. But we concentrate on the interpersonal communication model. The model illustrates the most important elements involved in communication between and among organisation members. Source has an idea, thought, or impression that is encoded or translated into words and symbols that are transmitted or sent as a message to the receiver, the receiver picks up the symbols and decodes or retranslates them back into an idea and sends some form of feedback to the sender.

### The Source

The source or originator of the message occupies the first place in the communication process. The source controls the type of message sent; the construction used, and frequently the channel through which the eventual message passes.

Let us place you in the source's predicament so that you are able to examine this first element. The intended communication is based on satisfying some internal need in which someone else (a receiver) plays some role. The first step is that something happens to stimulate the thought processes. You receive an order, or perhaps your boss enters the room, or you observe a slowdown in production. The event stimulates you to recognise the need for transmitting your feelings and ideas to someone else. The stimulation creates in you a desire to communicate and helps provide a need or purpose for your communication, whether it reflects your need to offer advice, to solicit an opinion, to create a given impression, to take a given action, or whatever.

### Encoding the Message

The second step, encoding the message involves transmission of some form of verbal or non-verbal symbol that is capable of transferring meaning, such as spoken or written words, gestures, or actions.

From among the available symbols, the person transmitting a message selects that will fulfil a specific need and arranges them in some sequence of significance. One must think not only of what is going to be said but also of how it will be presented to have the desired effect on the receiver. Thus, the message must be adapted to the level of understanding, interest, and needs of the receiver to achieve the desired consequences. It is also important, however, to consider possible unintended consequences and to present the message so that these are avoided.

The language of a given culture originates in people's interactions with each other. Pre-historic people used picture symbols; the American Indians used smoke signals; some Arab cultures used gestures. Spoken symbols were developed as a means of transmitting ideas, feelings, and attitudes as the need to communicate with others increased. These symbols were modified to meet particular needs at a given time.

A word symbolizes an event, idea or object. For example, the words, tool and machine represent particular objects.

Even in today's organisations, whenever managers write letters or memos, compile figures, issue orders, solve a problem orally, or answer employees' questions, they are using symbols to communicate. Symbols should be selected on the basis of the meaning they will have for the listeners or readers. That is, effective managers need to understand human nature and develop sensitivity not only to the meaning of words but also to the effects those words and symbols might have on others.

### Transmitting the Message

The third step, transmitting the message reflects the communicator's choice of medium or "distribution channel". Oral communication may be transmitted through many channels in person, by telephone, by dictating machine or by video-tape. It may take place privately or in a group meeting of many persons. In fact, one of the most important decisions the source has to make is in determining the appropriate channel for transmitting a given message.

In addition to its speed, a fundamental advantage of oral, person-to-person communication is the opportunity for interaction between source and receiver, commonly known as feedback, the final step.

Written communication may be transmitted through channels such as memos, letters, reports, notes, bulletin boards, company manuals, and newsletters. Written communication has the advantage of providing a record for future reference, but the major disadvantage is that it does not allow spontaneous, face-to-face feedback.

### Advantages of Written and Oral Messages

| Written | Oral |
| --- | --- |
| 1. Provides a record of questions, clarification. | 1. Lends itself to more immediate feedback. |
| 2. Allows greater attention to message's organisation and wording. | 2. Allows non-verbal communication—tone of voice, inflection, body language. |
| | 3. Transmitted rapidly. |

### Receiving the Message

The fourth step is the reception of the message by the receiver. How do people receive messages? Basically, people receive messages through their five senses—seeing, hearing, tasting, touching or being touched, and smelling. Full transmission has not occurred unless a receiver actually receives a message. Many important attempts at communication have failed because someone never received the message.

### Decoding the Message

The fifth step of the communication process is decoding. It involves giving meaning to the symbols the receiver receives. The receiver searches his or her memory bank for a translation of the symbols received. This, in turn, is the result of the receiver's heritage, culture, education, environment, prejudices, biases, and distractions in the surroundings. There is always the possibility that the source's message, when decoded by the receiver, will yield a meaning far different from the one the sender intended. The receiver thus shares a large responsibility for communication effectiveness, for communication is a two-way street. Managers and subordinates may occupy both source and receiver roles throughout an interaction. Moreover, they engage in a variety of interactions of different scope, importance, and duration.

### Feedback

After the message has been received and translated, the receiver may transmit a return message that stimulates the original communicator or someone else. Thus, communication is a continuous and never-ending process. A person communicates, the receiver responds by further communicating with the original sender or another person, and so forth. The response is called feedback.

Management might distribute a policy bulletin to a group of supervisors, but until there is a response in the form of questions, agreement, comment, or behaviour or until there has been a check to see whether the policy is being followed, the management does not know how effective the statement has been.

Communication is an exchange, and, if it is to be successful, information must flow back and forth from the originator to the receiver or at least the originator must have some knowledge of the receiver's reaction. Although the term feedback may be new, its importance is not.

## ORGANISATIONAL COMMUNICATION

Organisational communication is the process involving the transmitting and receiving instructions, orders, decisions, reports, and requests between the members of the organisation. Communication is important to managers, and it is needed by all employees. Organisational communication is a widely accepted important function of management. A large part of the typical manager's time is spent in some form of communication—writing, reading, speaking, or listening.

### Meaning

Organisational communication means exchange of ideas, opinions, facts and emotions between two individuals or group. It is the process of passing messages and understanding from one individual to another. It is also the process of acting on information.

### Scope

Without communication, administration cannot move even an inch in any organisation. It is the life-blood of the organisation as only through this the objectives of the organisation can be achieved. So, the scope is wide.

### Importance

1. To make the members of the organisation to understand the objectives, policies and problems.

2. To build up human relations and create working atmosphere.

3. It is essential to initiate action, understanding, co-operation and satisfaction.

4. To get opinion, ideas, and suggestions from sub-ordinates as feedback for an improvement. In organisational functioning, production and marketing.

5. It is important to save time, labour and money.

6. It is important to avoid wastage.

7. It is essential to solve problems and conflicts.

8. It is to satisfy basic human needs for recognition, self-improvement, a sense of belonging and sharing the feelings.

## Flow of Communication in an Organisation

You can better understand organisational communication if you examine the basic directions in which it moves. Formal communication channels are dictated by the organisation's structure or are prescribed by some other formal means. The basic channels are vertical (upward and downward), horizontal or lateral, diagonal and circular.

**i. Vertical communication:** Here the communication flows either upward or downward.

1. *Downward communication* (Fig. 9.4): Downward communication is generally thought of as following the organisation's formal chain of command from top to bottom. It tends to follow and reflect the authority, responsibility, relation-ships shown in the organisational chart. Some examples of downward communication are listed here:

   1. Information related to policies, rules, procedures, objectives and other types of plans.
   2. Work assignments and directives.
   3. Feedback about performance.
   4. General information about the organisation such as its progress or status.
   5. Specific requests for information from lower levels.

   Downward messages may be in either written or oral form. They are typically passed through bulletin boards, memos, reports or other documents, conferences, meetings, speeches and in person-to-person or small group interactions. Management traditionally concentrates most of its communication effort on downward communication. But the important point is that the results are usually alarmingly ineffective.

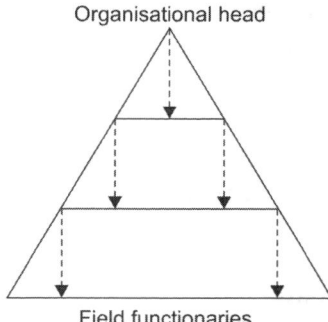

**Fig. 9.4:** Downward communication

2. **Upward communication** (Fig. 9.5): Upward communication usually takes the form of progress or performance reports and requests for resource. It may be viewed as a feedback of data or information from lower levels to upper management levels. But, whereas progress and performance reporting are perhaps the major forms of upward communication, other forms are also vital to management. These include the following:

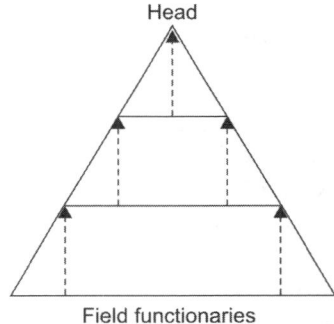

**Fig. 9.5:** Upward communication

1. Ideas and suggestions for improvements and problem solving.
2. Requests for assistance or information.
3. Expression of attitudes, feelings, and gripes that influence performance directly and also indirectly.

From an organisational standpoint, the "open door" policy, grievance system, attitude surveys, employee management councils, or the military's inspector general system are designed to provide upward communication to top management.

*Advantages of vertical communication*
- Authoritative.
- Binding.
- Most legitimate type.

*Disadvantages of vertical communication*
- Formal and impersonal.
- Slow moving.
- Conceal true motives.

**ii. Lateral or horizontal communication** (Fig. 9.6): Lateral or horizontal communication includes the following:

1. Communication among peers within the same work group.
2. Communication that occurs between and among departments of the same organisational level.

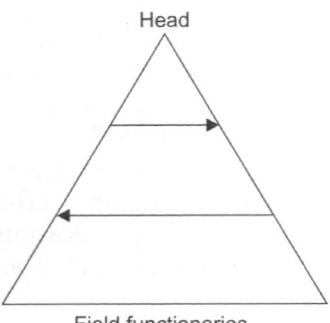

**Fig. 9.6:** Horizontal communication

This form of communication is essentially co-ordinative in nature and results from the concept of organisational specialisation. That is, if you are to function effectively in your own job, you will likely need to interact with, and be dependent on, other organisational units. Moreover, organisations today seek to use the abilities of specialists by creating special project teams, task forces, or committees that pull together representatives from various specialities. Communication helps co-ordinate these lateral activities. The contents are half formal and half informal—written or verbal middle management.

*Advantages*
- Co-ordinating in nature.
- Simpler than vertical.
- Time saving.
- Learning from each other.

*Disadvantages*
- Chief uninformed.
- Disuniting effect.
- Increase misunderstandings.

**iii. Diagonal communication** (Fig. 9.7): Diagonal communication includes that which cuts diagonally across an organisation's chain of command. It most frequently occurs as a result of line-and-staff department relationships. Several different relationships may exist between line-and-staff personnel. These may range from a purely advisory staff relationship to one in which staff exerts strong functional authority over line.

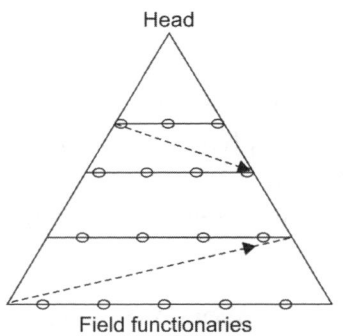

**Fig. 9.7:** Diagonal communication

*Contents:* Tactical situations, hostage situations, cases of civil unrest, and usually verbal.

*Advantages*
- Direct method.
- Hostage situations.
- Cases of civil unrest.
- Usually verbal.

*Disadvantages*
- Destroy lines of authority/command.
- Uninformed immediate superiors.
- Conflicting orders/confusion.
- Usually verbal, thus untractable.

**iv. Circular communication** (Fig. 9.8): In circular communication a chain of messages pass from one person to another person in circular manner among the members of the organisation.

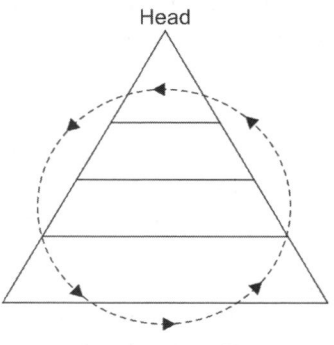

**Fig. 9.8:** Circular communication

*Contents:* Communication by conference, representatives from all ranks and controversial issues.

*Advantages*

- Most democratic.
- Produces instant feedback.
- Resolves issues quickly.

*Disadvantages*

- Too time-consuming.
- Status differences.
- Success based on verbal skills.

v. **Grapevine communication** (Fig. 9.9): It is also known as informal communication. Often information, exchanged in an informal way, i.e. not specified by the organisation's structure, is called grapevine communication. The term was first used during the Civil War, when intelligence telegraph lines were strung on tree branches in a manner resembling a grapevine.

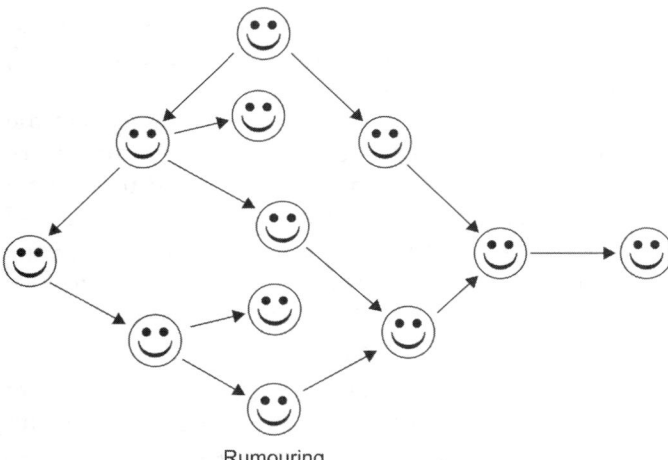

Rumouring

**Fig. 9.9:** Grapevine communication

*Serial transmission:* During serial transmission there will be a drastic difference between the original message and the one reported by the last person to receive it. Information will be lost from the message, facts distorted, importance changed, details added or reduced and totally the entire content and structure the information changed.

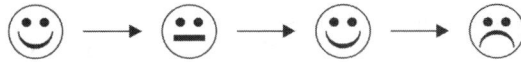

**Fig. 9.10:** Serial transmission

*Rumour:* Rumour emerges as a response to situations that are important to us, where there is ambiguity, and conditions that create anxiety.

Organisations contain such working atmosphere which makes rumours flourish in organisations. The secrecy and competition that typically exist in large organisations—around such issues as the appointments, transfer, etc. encourage and sustain rumour on the grapevine. The rumour will persist either until the needs and expectations creating the uncertainty underlying the rumour are fulfilled or until the anxiety is reduced. It is difficult to completely eliminate rumours. However, organisational management can minimise the adverse effect of rumour by announcing decisions, and open discussion.

## Barriers to Communication

- The use of jargon. Over-complicated, unfamiliar and/or technical terms.
- Emotional barriers and taboos. Some people may find it difficult to express their emotions and some topics may be completely 'off-limits' or taboo.
- Lack of attention, interest, distractions, or irrelevance to the receiver.
- Differences in perception and viewpoint.
- Physical disabilities such as hearing problems or speech difficulties.
- Physical barriers to non-verbal communication. Not being able to see the non-verbal cues, gestures, posture and general body language can make communication less effective.
- Language differences and the difficulty in understanding unfamiliar accents.
- Expectations and prejudices which may lead to false assumptions or stereotyping. People often hear what they expect to hear rather than what is actually said and jump to incorrect conclusions.
- Cultural differences. The norms of social interaction vary greatly in different cultures, as do the way in which emotions are expressed. For example, the concept of personal space varies between cultures and different social settings.

## DIFFUSION

Diffusion is the process by which an innovation is communicated through certain channels over time among the members of social system. It is a special type of communication in which the messages are compared with a new idea. It is the newness of the idea in the message content of communication that gives diffusion its special character.

Diffusion is a kind of social change, defined as the process by which alteration occurs in the structure and functions of a social system. When new ideas are formed, diffused and adopted or rejected, leading to certain consequences, social change occurs.

### Four Main Elements in the Diffusion of Innovations

An innovation is communicated through certain channels over time among the members of a social system.

i. **Innovation:** It is an idea or object which is perceived as new by an individual.

*Attributes of innovation:*[1] The characteristics of innovations, as perceived by individuals, help to explain their different rate of adoption. They are as follows:

*Relative advantage:* It is the degree to which an innovation is perceived as better than the idea it supersedes. The degree of relative advantage may be measured in economic terms, but social prestige factors, convenience and satisfaction are also often important components. The greater the perceived relative advantage of an innovation, the more rapid its rate of adoption is going to be.

*Compatibility:* It is the degree to which an innovation is perceived as being consistent with the existing values, past experience and needs of potential adopters. An idea that is not compatible with the prevalent values and norms of a social system will not be adopted as rapidly as an innovation that is compatible. An example of incompatible innovation is the use of contraceptives in countries where religious beliefs discourage use of birth-control measures, as in Muslim and Catholic nations.

*Complexity:* It is the degree to which an innovation is perceived as difficult to understand and use. Some innovations are readily understood by most members of a social system; others are more complicated and adopted more slowly. In general, new ideas that are simpler to understand will be adopted more rapidly than innovations that require the adopter to develop new skills and understandings.

*Trialability/divisibility:* It is the degree to which an innovation may be experimented with on a limited basis. New ideas that can be tried on the instalment plan will generally be adopted more quickly than

innovations that are not divisible. An innovation that is trialable represents less uncertainty to the individual who is considering it for adoption, as it is possible to learn by doing.

*Observability/communicability:* It is the degree to which the results of an innovation are visible to others. The easier it is for individuals to see the results of an innovation, the more likely they are to adopt. In general, innovation that is perceived by receivers as having greater relative advantage, compatibility, trialability, observability and less complexity will be adopted more rapidly than other innovations.

ii. **Communication channels:** Communication channels are the means by which messages get from one individual to another. For example, mass media channels are often the most rapid and efficient means to inform an audience or a potential adopter about the existence of an innovation, that is, to create awareness about it. Mass media channels are all those means of transmitting messages that involve a mass medium such as radio, TV, newspaper, etc. which enable a source of one/a few individuals to reach an audience of many. On the other hand, interpersonal channels are more effective in persuading an individual to adopt a new idea, especially if the interpersonal channel links two or more individuals who are near peers. Interpersonal communications involve face-to-face exchange between two or more individuals.

iii. **Time:** The time dimension is involved in diffusion:

- in the innovation-decision process by which an individual passes from first knowledge of an innovation to its adoption or rejection,
- in the innovativeness of an individual, i.e. the relative earliness/lateness with which an innovation is adopted compared with other members of a system, and
- an innovation's rate of adoption in a system, is usually measured as the number of members of the system that adopt the innovation in a given time period.

iv. **Social system:** A social system is defined as a set of interrelated units that are engaged in joint problem-solving to accomplish a common goal. The members or units of social system may be individuals, informal groups, and/or sub-systems.

The social system constitutes boundary within which an innovation diffuses. The social structure, norms, roles of opinion leaders and change agents affects the degree of diffusion process.

---

1. E.M. Rogers. "Communication of Innovation", The Free Press, New York, 1971.

# ADOPTION PROCESS

"Adoption process is the mental process through which an individual passes from hearing about an innovation to final adoption".

The adoption behaviour of an individual farmer has been conceptualised by researchers as a process composed of a number of successive stages. They are awareness, interest, evaluation, trial and adoption.

## Awareness

At this stage an individual becomes aware of some new ideas. He knows about the existence of the idea, but he lacks details about it. For instance, he may know only the name and may not know what the idea or product is, what it will do or how it will work. This stage has been observed by some authors as the stage is to initiate the sequence of later stages, which will lead to adoption or discontinuance or rejection. This stage otherwise known as stage of random or non-purposive occurrence.

## Interest

At this stage an individual wants more information about the idea or product. He wants to know what it is, how it works and what its potentialities are? The individual favours the information but he has not yet judged its utility in his work situation the main function of this stage is to increase the individual's information about the innovation. This stage is otherwise known as knowledge stage and interest information stage.

## Evaluation

At this stage the individual mentally applies the innovation to his present or future anticipated situation and then decides whether to try the innovation or not. He asks himself: "Can I do it? And if I do it, will it be better than what I am doing now, will it increase my income; or otherwise bring me satisfaction"? This stage has been described by some researchers as application, acceptance and conviction stage.

## Trial

At this stage the individual uses the innovation in a small scale in order to determine the utility of the innovation in his own situation. The purpose or main function of this stage is to demonstrate the new idea in the individual's own situation and determine its usefulness for possible complete adoption. This stage has been described by some authors as dry-run stage. Rejection of innovation may also occur at this stage.

## Adoption

At this stage the individual decides to continue the full use of the innovation. The main function of this stage is consideration of the trial results and decide to continue the innovation.

**Discontinuance:** It is a decision to cease use of an innovation after previously adopting it.

**Rejection:** It is a decision not to adopt an innovation.

## Factors Affecting Adoption

  i. Social factors
    1. Social values.
    2. Local leadership.
    3. Social contact:
       **a. Nature of social contact.**
       **b. Extent of social contact.**
    4. Social distance.
 ii. Personal factors
    1. Age.
    2. Education.
    3. Psychological characteristics.
iii. Situational factors
    1. The nature of the practice.
    2. Farm income.
    3. Size of farm.
    4. Tenure status.
    5. Sources of farm information used.
    6. Level of living.

# ADOPTER CATEGORIES

It is obvious that people do not adopt new ideas at the same time. Some people adopt ideas when they are first introduced, others wait a long time; while some never adopt an idea. The criterion for adopter categorisation is innovativeness, which is the degree to which an individual is relatively earlier to adopt new ideas than other members of his social system. The research shows significant differences in selected personal and social characteristics when people are classified into five categories according to time of adoption, as follows (Fig. 9.11).

## Innovators

They are venturesome and the first people to adopt new idea. They are very few in number:
- Have larger farms
- High net worth and risk capital
- Willing to take risk

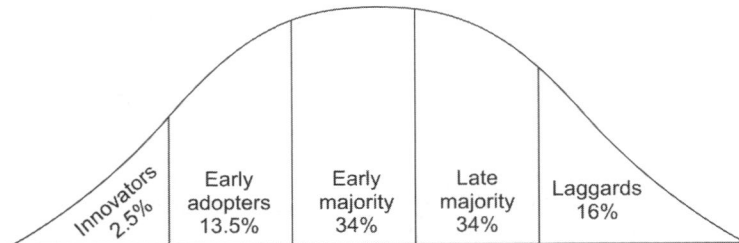

**Fig. 9.11:** Adopter categories

- Usually not aged
- Generally well educated
- Mentally alert and actively seeking new ideas.

They often bypass the local extension worker in getting information from the originating sources and may learn about new things even before he does. They subscribe too many farm magazines and specialised publications.

### Early Adopters

They are respectable. While innovators are cosmopolite, early adopters are localite. Younger than others but not necessarily younger than the innovators. They are quickest to use tried ideas in their own situation. Have large farms, higher education, high income. The early adopter category is generally sought by change agents as a local missionary for speeding the diffusion process. They read newspapers and farm journals and receive more bulletins than people who adopt later. They may be regarded as "Community adoption leaders".

### Early Majority

They are deliberate (local adoption leaders), and slightly above average in age, education and farming experience. They have medium high social and economic status. They adopt new ideas just before the average members of social system. They are most likely to be informal leaders, but not holders of elected positions. They associate mainly with people of their own community.

### Late Majority

They are skeptical. The late majority adopt new ideas just after the average member of a social system. Those in this group have less education and are older than the early majority. Pressure of peers is necessary to motivate them to adopt new ideas. They take fewer leadership roles than the earlier adopters, i.e. little opinion leadership. They read few newspapers and journals. They have little mass media exposure. They are below average in social status, have small farms, little specialisation and less income.

### Laggards

They are traditional. Laggards are the last in the social system to adopt an innovation. Decisions are often made in terms of what has been done in previous generations and these individuals' interests primarily with others who also have relatively traditional values. They have least education—old people → smallest farm → lowest income → little specialisation. They possess very little opinion leadership.

## CONSTRAINTS IN ADOPTION OF IMPROVED ANIMAL HUSBANDRY PRACTICES

### Labour

Non-availability of labour is a major constraint nowadays.

### Fodder and Feed

Inadequate land for fodder cultivation, non-availability of fodder throughout the year, non-availability of roughages, lack of grazing fields, high cost of feeds and fodder, lack of irrigation facilities, irregular supply of cattle feed, labour requirement for cross-bred animals is more as compared to desi animals, lack of clean water is the constraint which threatens the livestock farmers especially the farmers in small scale farming.

### Breeds

Poor adaptability of cross-bred cow in local climate condition, susceptibility of crossbred cow to disease, milk of cross-bred cow has poor consumer acceptability, low milk production by local breeds, poor quality of bulls at village, repeat breeding in cross-bred cows and buffaloes are the constraints faced by the farmers in adopting cross-bred animals.

### Lack of Knowledge

Lack of knowledge of fodder production, lack of knowledge about balanced feeding, ignorance about importance of deworming, lack of knowledge about feeding, breeding and management practice, ignorance of farmers about clean milk production, lack of knowledge about animals' treatments, lack of knowledge on keeping up to date management records, perception of AI as an unnatural process, inadequate knowledge of diseases through prevention and control, lack of knowledge about proper diagnosis of disease are the constraints which have direct impact on adoption of improved animal husbandry practices.

## Cost and Medication

Poor health coverage, lack of veterinary services in the village, high cost of treatment, location of artificial insemination centre at distance place, high charge for emergency service/feed, veterinary center/dispensary functioning without a veterinary assistant surgeon, high cost of high yielding breeds of animals, high cost of medicines, high cost of vaccine and treatment, high cost of improved breed and their maintenance, lack of space for isolation of sick animals, insufficient veterinary doctors or attendants, lack of capital are prime most constraints faced by farmers in livestock farming.

## Marketing

Lack of marketing infrastructure, middle man not exploitation, dairy co-operative society is far away from home, lack of guidance for available credit facilities, irregular and inadequate system of bonus distribution, less price of cow's/buffalo's milk offered by society, shortage of milk preservation facility, delay in milk payment, non-availability of timely veterinary services, lack of transport facilities and all weather road are the constraints faced by the farmers in marketing the livestock and livestock products.

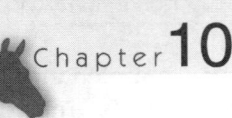

# Chapter 10

# Programme Planning and Evaluation

Extension programme planning is a continuous process. It is a blueprint or plan to an extension worker for effective execution. The purpose is to promote animal husbandry and agricultural production and elevate the quality of rural life through extension education. The changes produced must meet the peoples' needs. Therefore, the farmers' need is to be of importance to extension programme builders. "If we could but know where we are now, and where we ought to go, we could better judge what to do and how to do it". This statement by Abraham Lincoln stresses the importance of nature and role of planning for the people, by the people and of the people. So, a major emphasis in extension is given to active participation by clientele in decisions about both the immediate and the long range planning processes.

## PROGRAMME PLANNING TERMINOLOGY

There are certain terms related to extension programme management which have connotations that may vary with the context of their use. Therefore, their meaning, as employed here, is indicated below.

### Programme

Normally, this is a written statement which describes the extension activities proposed, the problems they address, the premises on which they are based, the objectives they seek to attain and the resources they require. This is an overall long range schedule of work containing a broad outline of things that need to be done and the methods of doing them. This serves as a basis for specific extension plans and projects. Extension programmes are formulated and publicised in order to promote understanding and generate interest among the client groups and others concerned.

### Plan

It is usually an annual schedule of extension work. It outlines the activities which are so arranged as to enable efficient implementation of the entire extension programme in stages. It answers the questions like what, why, how and when as well as by whom and where the work is to be done.

### Programme Planning

It is a process made up of sequential decisions and actions, the product of which is the extension plan. Working with the people, it seeks to identify the priority problems and needs, investigate the situations, assess the resources available and needed, define the possible solutions, determine the objectives, and indicate the causes of action.

### Extension Programme

According to Legans (1961), an extension programme is a set of clearly defined consciously conceived educational extension programme objectives derived from an adequate analysis of the situation, which are to be achieved through extension teaching. Situation is a brief statement of the more general factual information together with the needs and desires of the people.

According to Kelsey and Hearne (1949), an extension programme is a statement of situation, objectives, problems and solutions.

### Calendar of Work

It is a time schedule of work. It consists of activities arranged chronologically, according to a time period. It indicates, for any given point of time, the kind of activities to be pursued. It helps in avoiding lapses, and clumping of activities.

### Project

This pertains to one selected component of the extension programme. Thus, when extension programme is a composite plan of action, extending over a period of years, and extension plan is an annual plan of work, extension project refers to the plan of solving a single problem.

### Aim

Morris speaks of aims of programme as very generalised and broad statement of directions which life on the farm should be taking with respect to given activities. For example, improvement of the farmers' standard of living may be thought of as an aim. This may have more specific objectives such as better feeding practices, larger size of enterprise, improvement of soil fertility, more milk per cow, etc.

## Objective

The objective is defined as the direction of movement. For example, an objective in a extension programme may be to raise the average yield in a year from 280 eggs to 300 eggs per layer.

## Goal

The goal is defined as the distance in any given direction one expects to go during a given period of time. For example, the goal for the current year for the above objective of achieving 300 eggs per bird may be to achieve the yield of 290 eggs per layer.

## Problem

It is an unsatisfactory situation. One may know or may not know why it has occurred. All the same it is a situation that causes concern and its solution is not known. For example, a farmer may notice blood in cow's urine and may not know the reason. A farmer may notice low yields of milk due to mastitis but may not know how to control it.

## Need

It is a problem situation, the solution for which is also known. But the ability to make use of the solution is presently not there. For example, a farmer may want a milking machine to milk more animals but may not know how to apply it.

## IMPORTANCE OF PROGRAMME PLANNING

The benefits of programme planning can be stated as follows:

1. Avoid wastage of resources: Planning helps in minimising the wastage of time and money and provides general efficiency. Optimum results can be accomplished under the prevailing circumstances and conditions.
2. Provide guidance: Planning ensures establishment of objectives, gives direction for extension work and helps in evaluating the results.
3. Continuity: Because the plan is available in black and white, there will be continuity of the programme. Even when there are changes of personnel the tempo or direction of work and co-ordination among staff will be maintained.
4. Reliable information: The thorough analysis of the situation brings out all the information required for

programme, including the research findings. Thus, the plans are made based on the prevailing conditions.
5. Institutional support: For proper implementation the involved persons, including the affected, must be in agreement with the plan. The planning will help to justify the appropriations by public bodies and to obtain the support of the key personnel.
6. Leadership development: The study of groups and leadership indicates the necessity of leaders to plan and execute the programmes in a successful way in rural societies. The programme paves way for involvement of key persons in planning and execution of development programmes and thus it is one of the best methods of leadership development.
7. Minimise conflicts: Many conflicts like conflicts of resources, conflicts of personalities, etc. may arise while executing a programme. These can easily be removed at the planning stage. A good programme planning will avoid unnecessary conflicts.
8. Local support: A programme planned with the co-operation of the people and based on their need will get full support from them. The goal achievement will be difficult if local people do not support it. A good programme planning gets the co-operation of local people.
9. Future programmes: A good programme planning always identifies and monitors future development also.
10. Best use of innovations: The latest technologies and innovations are highlighted to the local people by the extension worker at the planning stage and included in the programme. Thus, the programme planning paves way for the best use of latest technologies.

## PRINCIPLES OF PROGRAMME PLANNING

These are certain essential principles based on which extension programmes are formulated:

1. Extension programme is built upon the needs and interests of the people.
2. It begins with a proper analysis of the existing situation to define problems, possible solutions and assess resources.
3. It starts where people are and with what they have.
4. People who benefit from the programme are made to participate in its formulation, implementation and evaluation.
5. Programme objectives and solutions offer satisfaction to the participants.
6. It provides educational benefit to the people in all its phases.

7. Programme evaluation provides insights for revisions and improvements.

8. It is comprehensive to cover the interests of all sections of the community but is based on priorities since all problems cannot be tackled at the same time, and it is flexible to meet the changing situations.

9. Extension programming is a continuous process which learns from past experience while taking into consideration the short-term and long-term objectives for the future.

## PHILOSOPHY OF PROGRAMME PLANNING

A well planned programme is broad-based, planned with the people and meets the urgent needs of a large number of people. It is also important to co-ordinate the programme with the programmes of other groups, organisations and agencies and those in the same or related problem areas.

## METHODS OF PROGRAMME PLANNING

1. **According to duration**
   a. Short-term plans.
   b. Medium-term plans.
   c. Long-term plans.
2. **According to extent of participation**
   a. Liberal participation.
   b. Restricted participation.
   c. No participation.
3. **According to place of planning**
   a. Centralised planning.
   b. Decentralised planning.
   c. Completely independent grassroot planning.
4. **According to the type of planning**
   a. Isolated planning.
   b. Integrated planning.
   c. Comprehensive planning.
5. **According to type of approaches**
   a. Democratic approach.
   b. Autocratic approach.
   c. Laissez-faire.

## ABILITIES NEEDED IN EXTENSION PERSONNEL

Management of extension programme is a skillful task. There are some particular abilities required in a good extension worker in this regard. These are:

1. Ability to sense and identify people's concerns in his contacts with them.

2. Ability to analyse local situations and draw sound conclusions.

3. Ability to derive pertinent lessons from past experience.

4. Ability to relate new technology to local situations.

5. Ability to work with people including identification and involvement of local leaders as well as mobilising people's participation.

6. Ability to develop a simple, written extension programme as an agreed basis of action.

7. Ability to guide participants step by step in formulating, implementing and evaluating the extension programme.

8. Ability to make educational use of the whole process.

9. Ability to harness both local and external resources and to draw upon the support of the supervisors, specialists and other resources.

10. Ability to evaluate the performance, draw lessons therefrom and invest them in the subsequent plans of action.

## NEEDS AND INTEREST

Needs is the difference between "What is" and " What ought to be". Interest may be defined as a feeling of curiosity or concern about something. A thing towards which one feels it. A farmer may have interest to learn and acquire information, knowledge and skill that he thinks is useful to him.

### Meaning of Need (Fig. 10.1)

Need means a circumstance in which a thing or course of action is required. It means a requirement, a thing necessary for life. It is a gap between two conditions.

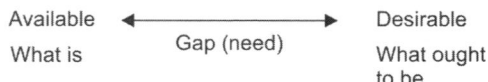

**Fig.10.1:** Meaning of need

What it is can be determined by observing and understanding the situation. What ought to be is determined by estimation (research). The estimation of needs will reveal the degree of the needs, i.e. the width of the gap. This indicates the significance of the existing problem. The wider the gap, the greater the need.

### Classification of Needs (Fig. 10.2)

Needs can be classified based on: (a) Hierarchy, (b) different forms, (c) general purpose, (d) psychology, and (e) desires.

## Felt Need

This can also be called recognised need. Felt need is one which is recognised by the individual group.

## Unfelt Need

It is also known as unrecognised need. Unfelt need is one which is not recognised by the individual or group.

## Security Need

Economic, social, psychological and spiritual security. Man wants protection for his physical being, food, clothing and shelter. It may also be satisfied by spiritual beliefs. In fact, in history whole cultures have put emphasis on security. The Great Wall of China, the innumerable forts and fortresses in several countries are striking example of social security.

## Affection or Response Need

Companionship, gregariousness and social minded-ness, the need for a feeling of belonging.

## Recognition Need

Status, prestige, achievement and being looked at the top. Each individual feels the need to be considered important by his fellowmen.

## New Experience Need

Adventure, new interests, new friends and new ways of doing things. Some people primarily want the thrill of something new, something different.

## Organic Needs

Organic needs like sex, hunger and thirst are also very important for human beings.

## Need to Study Need

Needs are the central concern in programme planning around which successful programmes are built. Once people believe that the programme is having something to meet their needs and solve their problems, they will immediately accept the programme. Hence, the degree of success of any programme depends upon the accurate identification and focus on the common needs and incorporation of suitable remedy to solve the problem and satisfy the needs of the people. To make the programme effective the people should understand and recognise the gap between what is and what ought to be. Once they recognise they will involve themselves.

Need is very important in any programme planning. Everyone has needs. Needs vary in nature, scope and significance. Needs are often individual in attainment

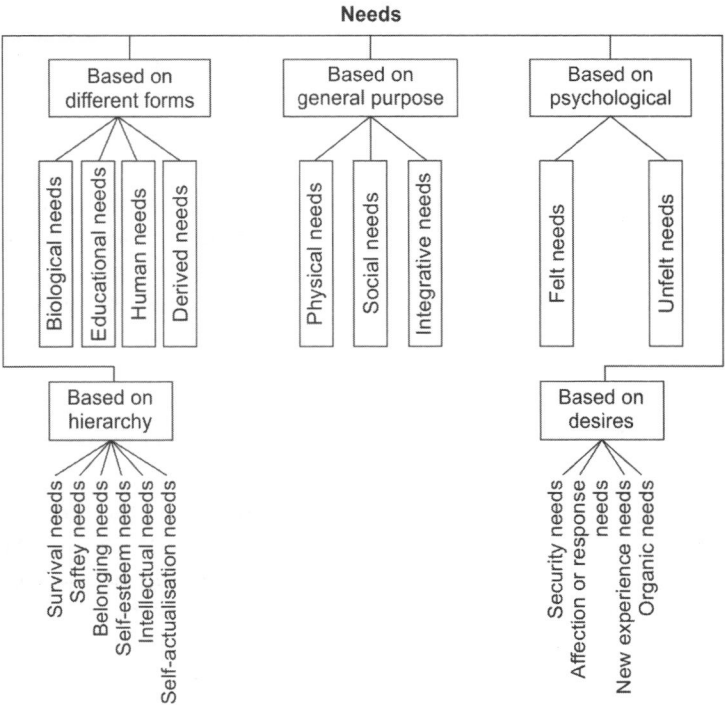

**Fig.10.2:** Classification of needs

but they also tend to be common among members of groups. As Karl Marx said, "Since everything, in this world change except the 'change' itself, needs also change with time and progress. The needs of people change with age, education, growth and with social, economic and family status situations".

Research on poultry farmers indicate that majority of the farmers are not aware of many of their most important needs.[1] It is true, because farmers have needs which are mostly unfelt. One of the difficulty in rural programming is helping people to identify their most important needs, they do not recognise.

In the programme planning process one has to list out the people's needs and decide whether to consider or ignore them from the programme. This step is very important because the needs accepted by the people and planners find place in the programme as the subject matter or content. Finally they are translated.

## Hierarchy of Needs (Fig. 10.3)

Human needs function as a hierarchy.[2] Lower order needs for survival and safety are the most essential. Everyone requires food, air, water and shelter and seeks freedom from danger. These needs determine the behaviour until they are met. But once we are physically comfortable and secure, we are stimulated to fulfil needs for belonging and love and esteem needs for recognition and approval. And when these needs are

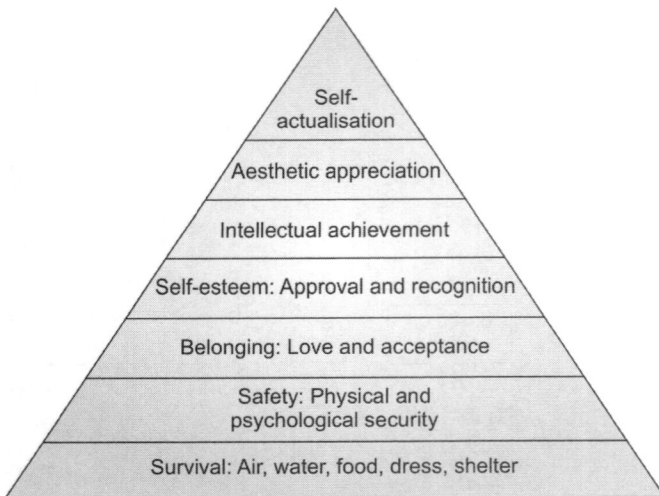

**Fig.10.3:** Hierarchy of needs

---

1. P. Mathialagan. "Training Needs of Poultry Farmers", Unpub. M.V.Sc., Thesis, Department of Extension, Madras Veterinary College, TANUVAS, Chennai, 1992.
2. A. Maslow. "Motivation and Personality". Harper and Row Publishers, Inc.

more or less satisfied, we turn to higher level needs for intellectual achievement, aesthetic appreciation and finally self-actualisation.

## Estimation of Needs

Needs can be assessed by three methods:

1. Participatory method.
2. Primary source method.
3. Secondary source method.

### Participatory Method

The most reliable method is applying Participatory Rural Appraisal techniques. This method involves 15 steps as suggested by Sabarathnam.[1]

1. Identification of key informants.
2. Listing and ranking the problems of rural people by key informants.
3. Estimation of economic importance of various problems.
4. Estimation of Rank-based Quotient (RBQ) for the problems.
5. Working out the average loss or extent of damage for the various problems.
6. Selection of farmers
7. Collection of technological problems as per the ranks of the farmers.
8. Estimation of RBQ for the problems as per the ranks of the farmers.
9. Estimation of loss or damage caused by the problem according to the farmers' experience.
10. Finding out the correlation between key informants value's and farmer's values for problem ranking and for loss or damage caused by the problems.
11. Assessing the magnitude of the problems.
12. Separation of research needs and extension problems.
13. Sending the technological research needs to concerned research institutes.
14. Sending the extension problems to the development departments for prioritisation. Selection and formulation of extension programmes.
15. Selection of the top-most extension problems. This methodology is applicable for identification of problems of rural people in any field of development which will go a long way in

---

1. V.E. Sabarathnam, S. Vennila. "Estimation of Technological Needs and Identification of Problems of Farmers for Formulation of Research and Extension Programmes in Agricultural Entomology". Expl Agri. 1996; 32:87–90.

formulation of need-based research and extension programmes.

### Primary Source Method

Discuss with the people and identify the needs during the course of conversation. While talking with the people for problem identification, see that your questions are open-ended. Meet as many people as possible for discussion. Make separate list for each discussion of what has been expressed directly or indirectly as a felt need. Set up a priority list of the above needs on the basis of the number of times the same need has been expressed by different group of individuals.

It is very difficult to arrive at actual felt needs by this method, because people are on their guard when asked questions. Answers are coloured by suspicion, and apprehension that the interviewer may be an inspector, tax collector, etc. and hence will be vague and meaningless.

### Secondary Source Method

Ask the various extension personnel working in that area, NGOs, other rural institutions like panchayat, youth club, co-operative, etc. about their perception of the needs of the people of that area. Then fix a priority. We can compare the needs perception of the people and the agencies. The area of unfelt needs of the farmers may be expressed by these agencies.

## ▌EXTENSION PROGRAMME MANAGEMENT

Extension programme management consists of three distinct phases. All these phases require close interaction with the people concerned. Also, all these interactions are essentially educational in purpose (Fig. 10.4).

1. Programme formulation.
2. Programme execution.
3. Programme evaluation.

### I. Programme Formulation

In this phase, decisions are made on what areas would receive extension work and why, as well as what goals would be pursued and in what manner. This involves, area appraisal, determining the objectives and formulating plan.

1. **Area appraisal:** Under this the problems and needs will be estimated, locally available resources will be assessed and promising solutions identified.

   a. *Estimation of problems and needs:* This is done by applying Participatory Rural Appraisal (PRA) techniques. First, the extension worker becomes aware of the local people and area, and develops good rapport with the people. He then identifies the key informants in the selected area, and adopts inter-disciplinary team approach to identify the needs and problems. For this, he makes a keen observation of the situation and becomes aware of the areas in which improvements are possible and new technology can make a contribution. The extension worker listens carefully to the people in order to know what their concerns are and to recognise the needs and problems as perceived by them. Next he interacts with the key informants and people regarding the scope for the alternative approaches to some of their practices and observes their responses. Based on these, he makes a tentative list of priority items to be investigated by preferential ranking technique.

   Generally, the problems can be classified as: (a) Problems which can be solved by the villagers with their own resources, (b) problems which need community co-operation without involving outside assistance, and (c) problems that require assistance from outside sources.

   b. *Assessing resources:* To make the people adopt new practice and to solve the identified problems often requires additional resources and efforts. The extension worker assesses the natural resources, indigenous technology and organisational resources available; advanced technical inputs material as well as financial resources, and socio-political resources required. For each of the priority problem, assess the resources needed like human resource, farm and home particulars, water, soil, pasture, forest, meteorological, etc.

   This is done by tapping the indigenous knowledge related to animal husbandry and agriculture, making an inventory of all groups and organisations that are available and exploring their complementary capacities and resources. This might include local NGOs already working with farmer groups of various memberships, religious centres, schools, etc.

   Technical resources like veterinary dispensaries, commercial companies, extension office, agricultural stations, research and training centres, field staff of nearby animal husbandry, agricultural projects, etc. are ascertained and financial resources like all infrastructural facilities, credit institutions (co-operative and

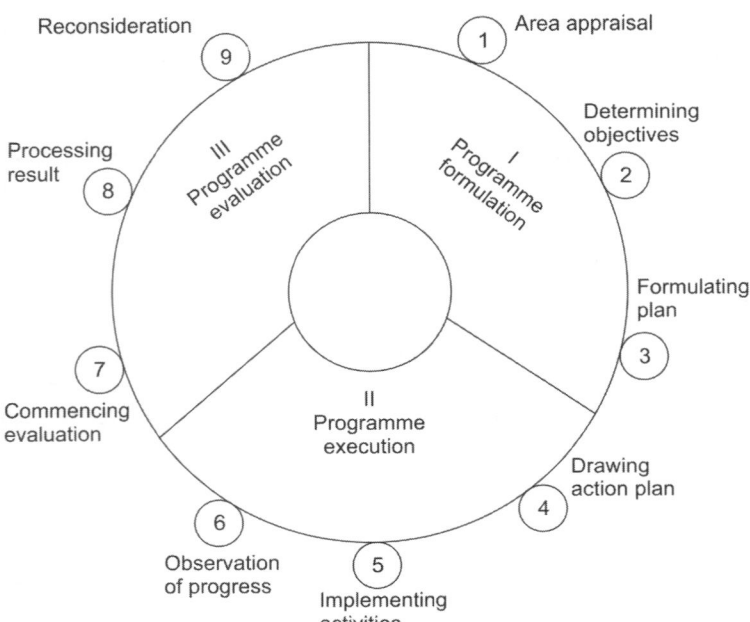

**Fig.10.4:** Extension programme management

nationalised banks), etc. are assessed. It is also important to be aware of socio-political resources like attitudes, behaviours, beliefs, social classes, groups, leadership, etc.

The extension worker, by conducting community walks (village transect) with the key informants, farmers and facilitators, identifies the resources available and efforts required to adopt the alternate approaches.

c. ***Identifying promising solutions:*** The extension worker, by conducting PRA, locates the specific constraints and also relates the new technology or alternate approaches suitable to deal with them. Once the range of problems is identified, the extension worker can organise group discussions, farmer–expert workshops with the concerned participants and opinion leaders and notes their responses and preferences. For each of the priority problems, identify some possible solutions and options. Then formulate tentative set of approaches to the problems.

2. **Determining objectives:** Objectives are the base of any programme. A good objective will provide possible directions for large number of people to move in some direction. Extension programmes must help people, define the directions in which they want and need to go. The level objectives are (a) fundamental, (b) general, and (c) working.

This step consists of selecting the solutions, setting the standards to be achieved and adopting

objectives. All these should be done only by participatory method (participation of local leaders and other people's representatives).

a. *Selecting the solutions*: Taking all factors into consideration, selecting the solutions best suitable under the circumstances.

b. *Setting standards*: Once the approach to deal with a particular problem is over then decision should also be made as to what level of achievement should be attempted and what quality of results should be worked for.

c. *Adopting objectives*: Specific objectives are then considered, stated in precise terms and adopted by all concerned. They identify what is to be achieved.

3. **Formulating plan:** Having finalised the programme objectives, the ways to achieve them should be spelled out in detail. The plan or strategy is a guide or blueprint for the persons responsible for the execution of the programme. It is the mechanics of achieving the objectives.

a. *Planning events*: The events that should be conducted in pursuit of the objectives have to be identified and arranged in a sequential order taking all other relevant factors into consideration. This should necessarily include programme evaluation.

b. *Planning resource mobilisation*: The financial, technical, material and manpower requirements needed at different stages should be estimated and their mobilisation should be arranged.

c. *Planning the time*: According to the availability of the resources and activity's proper steps should be taken to sort out the overall time requirement for completing the programme in order to finalise the plan.

## II. Programme Execution

This phase involves the decisions and actions related to the preparation of action plan, implementation of all specific activities and observation of the progress in order to avoid delays and lapses. This is a crucial phase wherein the co-ordinated time-bound, sequential efforts envisaged in the programme are put forth, adjustments being made only with regard to changes in the situation subsequent to planning decision.

4. **Drawing action plan:** It is important to put the planned extension programme into action. This should involve developing a detailed and complete calendar of action. In other words, this should specify what, when and where as well as by whom the necessary action is to be taken.

   a. *Activity planning*: After formulating the strategy, individual activities to be continued should be considered, listed and organised in a proper sequence.

   b. *Sharing responsibility*: The plan for sharing of programme action responsibilities at different time at different places in a co-ordinated way by the extension staff, other professionals, NGOs, lay leaders, and people should be followed. This lays down as to who should do what.

   c. *Designing calendar of action*: The dimension of 'when' and 'where' has to be added to 'what' and by 'whom' to form a comprehensive calendar of action. This is the key element in programme execution.

5. **Implementing activities:** Based on the calendar of action implementation of the events is the next step in programme execution.

   a. *Advance preparation*: For effective implementation advance preparation is essential to ensure that things happen without confusion and as per the plan. Make advance arrangement for all inputs and teaching aids.

   b. *Initiating action*: Persons involved have to join together for the action to be initiated. Explain the approved programme to the staff and local leaders.

c. *Guiding the process*: Carry out the planned programme, phase by phase, in a co-ordinated manner.

6. **Observation of progress:** This is essential to avoid lapses and to prevent slippages. When a number of activities are in progress, more or less at the same time due attention has to be given to each of them to ensure that the plan is executed properly and adequately.

   a. *Observing performance*: Having a great responsibility for different activities, it becomes necessary to watch the performance of each during the implementation state. This is to ensure that things are happening as designed, as far as practical, and deviations, if any are within the limits of tolerance.

   b. *Providing assistance*: If the performance is below the level of expectation, immediate effort is to be made to recognise the nature and effect of deficiency and provide assistance.

   c. *Ensuring correctives*: If there are lapses of some sort, either due to changed environment or due to human error, quick reckoning of the situation should be done to introduce appropriate correctives, wherever possible.

## III. Programme Evaluation

This is the last phase in extension programme management, but a very important phase. Evaluation is essential to measure the extent of achievement of the fixed objectives. It indicates the progress, and effective strong and week points if any. Evaluation helps to improve the skill of the extension worker in working with people and in determining the priorities in the plan of work.

Designing evaluation being a part of programme formulation phase, taking stock of evaluation efforts belongs to this phase. It covers several orderly steps including collection of relevant data, analysing, interpretating, getting conclusions, deriving implications and utilising the results (for further details refer to Chapter 10).

7. **Commencing evaluation:** There are two kinds of evaluation are formative and summative. (i) Concurrent evaluation, and (ii) terminal evaluation, generally two aspects are evaluated—the progress as well as the impact by the programme.

   a. *Ensuring data collection*: The required facts and figures should be collected at appropriate stages.

b. *Organising data*: The data collected should be organised and tabulated systematically so as to provide suitable basis for analysis.

c. *Analysis*: Should be systemically analysed to get meaningful results.

8. **Processing result:** It is important in order to benefit from the evaluation activity. This includes interpretation of the results for further use.

a. *Getting conclusions*: From the results of the analysis of the data, logical conclusions have to be drawn regarding the progress and impact of the extension programme.

b. *Deriving implications*: From the conclusions, relevant implications have to be derived.

c. *Drawing recommendation*: Based on the implications, appropriate recommendations have to be made to influence the current and future extension programmes.

9. **Reconsideration:** Nothing is more important for programme improvement in extension work than conducting the evaluation properly and using the results adequately.

a. *Reviewing the plan*: In the light of the recommendations, if they have immediate relevance, the ongoing action plans should be reviewed for possible changes and improvements.

b. *Reconstructing the programme*: If the extension programme is further going to continue, modifications and revisions may be considered if the recommendations so indicate.

c. *Preparing the report*: Extension reports are prepared periodically about the performance of the extension programme. Such reports should contain the findings of evaluation as well as the way they were utilised.

### Factors Affecting Programme Implementation

Though there are many obstacles in extension programme, the four important ones are discussed below:

i. **Village factions:** Many villages have factions which may be due to a variety of reasons such as social, domestic, religious, caste, etc. Extension workers accept the existence of factions as normal in a village, and help the members of both the factions to initiate programmes to fulfil their respective needs. They also use the competitive spirit of members of both the factions and change the villagers. Without proper realisation some extension workers encounter a number of diffi-

culties. They sometimes make the situation more difficult for further approach.

ii. **Emergencies:** In spite of the best efforts, emergencies may arise during the implementation of a programme like natural calamities. There need not be any serious disappointment or frustration over such emergencies. The extension worker's important responsibility is to analyse the reason for the emergency with the village leaders, apprise them of the emergency and stimulate them to think and plan for alternate action.

iii. **Administrative sanction:** In spite of a well thought out plan of work and definition of the roles of individual members, sometimes the one is disappointed by the delay in administrative sanction or in not getting necessary approvals for going ahead. Recurrence of such incidents can no doubt be minimised by proper advanced planning. However, when such delays occur the extension workers should try to ascertain their reason, and explain them to the villagers and plan alternate steps with them. In the programme planning such factors may block the programme. The extension worker has to analyse them, find out the reasons, apprise the planning group, and plan for alternate programme.

iv. **Changing market:** A change in market position also presses the extension workers and their plan.

### Participation in Planning Process

The participation of farming communities in programme formulation, execution and evaluation of extension programmes has been a long-standing fundamental guiding principle. But, throughout the world it not followed strictly.

### *People's Participation in Planning*

All people whose welfare is covered by the programme may be involved in this process. Representation of local lay leaders, farmers, panchayat president, co-operatives, non-officials, representatives of credit agencies and many others who have something to contribute need to be involved in this process. The purpose of involving people is that the programmes are meant for the people and hence it is better if the plans are prepared by the people who are to be benefited by the programme. It will help the people in fulfilling their responsibilities as citizens in a democratic way by preserving and strengthening values like freedom, progress and success.

Sometimes the rural clientele and extension officials are separated by variation in thinking and behaviour. Without adequate participation of the farmers and their family members in the planning process, it is not possible to integrate the programme's supply and services with the people's expectations and acceptance. The people's participation is essential to promise an appropriate balance of programme supplies, suitable timing or sequence of those supplies, and the closing of social, geographical and cognitive distance between extension agency and rural farmers.

Farmer will receive and utilise the services of extension agency only when he perceives that it will suit to his needs. So, highly centralised planning will not suit to local variations, indigenous experience and cognitive levels and their needs. People have every right to self-determination. The indigenous knowledge of our farming community is an ignored, unutilised resource of country. This imperfection in extension programme still continues, in spite of the growing number of well documented analyses of value and validity of indigenous knowledge. Absence of the participation of people and incorporation of their indigenous knowledge and experience restricts the success of extension programmes.

Collective involvement of farmers from all categories of farming community in programme planning, execution and evaluation is important because involving only the progressive farmers will widen the gap between the progressive farmer and other farmers and also the solution given by the extension agency which may be well suited to the big farmer and may not be compatible to the small farmers. So, collective participation is essential.

Reference group relationship on individual farmer behaviour is important to consider in planning process. People require time, and the confidence given by the presence of neighbours and accepted peers, in order to analyse and think of some prospective change in present behaviour patterns, whether the change be of a social or a technical nature. These factors should be recognised and related to by extension worker. The indigenous specialists (e.g. person having special knowledge or skill in treatment of cows) must be given due to importance by extension worker, as they play vital role in learning occurring within the local community and their advice is readily accepted.

### Village Leaders' Participation

These village leaders, who are identified for such purposes may be involved in performing the following works:

i. Help the extension worker in identification and analysis of problem and needs.

ii. When the extension worker finds solution for problems identified, the non-officials may provide him the indigenous technologies available to solve the problem. They can also indicate the local resources available to the extension worker.

iii. Assist in fixing the priorities and objectives.

iv. Assist in execution or carrying out the programme.

v. They strive hard to convince local people for large participation.

The success of the programme planning depends to what extent the local people, particularly the local leaders, are involved in this process.

Programme planning is an excellent means of developing leadership qualities of people. Developing skills in various steps in programme planning, i.e. fact collection, decision making, execution, etc. will lead to the development of competent leadership.

### Participation of Institution

Youths are much more energetic, enthusiastic and receptive to new ideas and to work on new programmes. They have great influence on their parents and therefore play a major role in acceptance of a practice at their own farm. So, the youth resource should be utilised properly by the extension agency in programme planning and management.

1. Voluntary organisations like youth clubs, women clubs—can prepare the people mentally to accept extension programmes. They also play crucial role in implementation of the programmes and its evaluation.

2. Village co-operatives help in preplanning, planning and execution stages, by providing data, assembling the people, involving their members and leaders in identifying problems and need, prioritising the problems, and fixing the objectives. Further, they may provide financial assistance to extension programmes and other physical facilities required for the extension worker.

3. Schools also help by providing data, giving place for organising training programmes and other meetings regarding the programmes.

4. Panchayats organisation and revenue division help in providing relevant facts and also in all the stages of programme planning and execution.

Farmers' associations can work to prepare and articulate collective demands to officials so that better decisions can be made about relevant and timely programme inputs. Extension personnel should involve farmers' associations in all the phases of programme planning process.

### Extension Workers' Participation

The following roles are to be performed by the extension workers at all levels in connection with programme planning:

a. To collect, organise and analyse facts.
b. To help in fixing objectives.
c. To identify problems and needs of the people.
d. To decide upon suitable solutions to problems or answers to wants and needs.
e. To help in fixing the priorities.
f. To develop complete procedures and train staff.
g. To teach and strive for larger participation by the people.
h. To co-ordinate all efforts and resources of other agencies and groups.
i. To evaluate results.
j. To publish and distribute programmes.

In addition to each of these works the extension worker has the full responsibility of successfully executing the programme.

### Assumptions in Extension Programming

1. Planning and development is a continuous process.
2. Improving the quality of life of rural farming community could be possible by solving their problems.
3. The indigenous knowledge and skill of the people and knowledge of the scientists can be added together to find suitable solutions to the emerging problems.
4. Everything keeps changing except change. Therefore change is often desirable and essential, but change for the sake of change is not always desirable. Any change should not be taken lightly, but rather it should be considered carefully. By creating conducive atmosphere and opportunities we can increase the rate of change in behaviour.
5. Quality of the life of rural community can be improved by proper planning and utilisation of certain resources of knowledge, technology, personnel, the physical environment and teaching methods and aids.
6. If innovations are better than the existing practice people will readily accept them.

7. Education has got great influence over the prosperity of people and their lives.

## EVALUATION IN EXTENSION

Evaluation is to ascertain whether an extension programme has achieved its objectives and whether these objectives could have been achieved more effectively in some other way. Data gathered in this process is analysed so that the relevance, effect and consequences of activities are determined as systematically and objectively as possible. This will be utilised to improve present and future activities such as planning, decision-making and programme implementation to achieve extension objectives more effectively. The evaluation can be done by the organisation concerned internally or with the help of an outside agency.

### Meaning of Evaluation

Evaluation its derived from the Latin word 'vale' which means, to value. Its dictionary meaning is: The determination of the value; an appraisal, the strength or worth of something; an estimate of the force of or the making of a judgement of something.

### Definition of Evaluation

Evaluation in extension can be defined as an endless or continuous and systematic process of appraising the value of extension programmes. According to Kelsey and Hearne (1955), evaluation is a process by which the values of an enterprise are ascertained or analysed by which one is able to understand and appreciate the relative merits or deficiencies of persons, groups, programmes, situations, methods and process.

### Objectives of Evaluation

1. Assessment of progress and impact.
2. Ascertain the merits and demerits.
3. Measuring the success or failure in implementation.
4. Analysing the reasons for success or failure.
5. Finding out the people's reactions.
6. Deriving lessons for improvement in the formulation and execution of programmes.

### Scope of Evaluation

After the birth of Community Development Programme and Panchayati Raj, the Central and State Governments are continuously launching programmes for rural uplift. So, the scope is wide. In future, there is a scope for internal evaluation of the impact of programmes like IRDP, SCAP, ITDP family planning and health education, etc. Such internal evaluations should be the department's responsibility and the evaluation organisations in the state can extend advice and guidance regarding this matter.

## Use of Evaluation

1. Evaluation gives a clear picture of progress and impact of the programme.
2. It directs and guides future action.
3. It can help to modify and improve ongoing programmes.
4. Evaluation of a completed programme provides no useful information for improving that programme, but the experience gained in this way is valuable for planning future programmes.
5. It helps in judging the effectiveness of methods or devices used.
6. It serves to appraise the effectiveness of programme management procedures.
7. It gives assurance and confidence to the persons involved.
8. It can serve important public relations functions.
9. Evaluation makes one take a systematic approach to decision-making. It can contribute to the development of professional attitudes of the extension personnel.
10. It provides clear information about the people in the programme operation area.
11. Evaluation provides a report to the people.
12. Under present economic conditions government increasingly requires evidence for the money spent on agriculture and animal husbandry. Evaluation can provide some of the information required for this accountability.

## Elements of Evaluation

1. Survey.
2. Applying some criteria or standard to information collection.
3. Getting conclusions, deriving implications and drawing recommendation.

## Types of Evaluation

Extension evaluation is an endless process. Every extension work involves and conscious and unconscious appraisal of progress and effectiveness. It is difficult to use systematic approach at every stage and on all the times. Therefore various methods are employed to conduct evaluation.

i. **Formal and informal evaluation:** According to Bym Darcle et al (1959) as quoted by Reddy (1993) informal and formal types of evaluations are a five-point continuum of degrees of evaluation.

*Casual everyday evaluation:* We make value judgements everyday (a good meal, best show I ever saw; one of the worst speeches I ever heard). Simple observations are important, but have their limitations. We must be careful to distinguish what is actually present from what we think, we see.

The following are some of the limitations of this type of evaluation: (i) Personal ideas used instead of standard measurements; (ii) institution and personal bias cannot be eliminated; (iii) no systematic plan for arriving at conclusions; (iv) may have only part of the information.

*Self-checking evaluations:* It makes conscious attempt to apply principles of evaluation, e.g. checking on ordinary observations, talking with others, getting other people's judgements.

*Do it yourself evaluation:* These involve more careful planning, and applying principles of evaluation more systematically. They usually require surveys, or score cards.

*Extension studies:* More complex, use more scientific approach. Scientific research: Experimental studies, scientifically carried out to determine cause and effect relationships. Must be:

- Factual or valid: Measure what you think you are measuring.
- Analytical: Analyse the relationship of various factors.
- Reliable: Sample representative of population consistency of results.
- Objective: Free of bias, others get similar results.
- Impartial: Approach with an open mind and spirit of enquiry.

ii. **Formative and summative evaluation:** The terms formative and summative are associated with two important roles of evaluation. Formative evaluation attempts to assess the demerits of the programmes during the implementation stage. Summative evaluation assesses the worth of the final results of a programme.

Previously the importance was given to summative evaluations that were conducted after the completion of the programme to estimate the accomplishments and whether selected objectives were achieved. Nowadays, more and more attention is being given to formative evaluation that is conducted during the implementation stage. Such evaluations provide early feedback of programme's demerits, which can be used to modify and improve the remaining phase of a programme.

iii. **Ongoing and ex-post facto evaluation:** Cernea and Tepping (1977) distinguished between ongoing evaluation and ex-post facto evaluation as quoted by Annamalai et al (1994) are as follows:

On going evaluation is an action-oriented analysis of a project's effects and impacts, compared to anticipations, to be carried out during implementations.

Ex-post facto evaluation would resume the effect several years after completion of the investment. It involves reviewing comprehensively the experience and impact of a project as a basis for future policy formulation and project design.

## Steps in Evaluation

According to the nature, scope and complexity of the programme and the availability of resources the procedure used in evaluation may vary. However, a series of steps can be followed which are basic to all formal evaluations:

1. Plan for evaluation.
2. Purpose of evaluation.
3. Reasons for evaluation.
4. Respondents for evaluation.
5. Standards for evaluation.
6. Levels of evaluation.
7. Evidence for evaluation.
8. Designs for evaluation.
9. Conducting evaluation.

### Plan for Evaluation

The evaluation plan must indicate what will be done, why it needs to be done, and how it will be done. In addition it should indicate who should evaluate and what. It is essential because, availability of resources are always limited. Planning will help to complete the evaluation within the limitations. An evaluation plan will also give the relevant respondent to be involved so that evaluation can address their quotations and

concerns. Planning will guide to identify which evidence would be considered 'credible' by such respondents. Further it will facilitate in getting useful input from all related persons.

### Purpose of Evaluation

"The major purpose of evaluation is to assist in programme decisions. Formal evaluations are worth doing only if they have a chance of affecting such decisions". The purpose of the evaluation will determine which data have to be collected for evaluating an extension programme. We can distinguish formative evaluation which gathers information for development of an effective extension programme, and summative evaluation which tries to measure the end results of a programme in order to decide whether or not it should be continued, expanded or diminished.

### Reasons for Evaluation

The reasons were already listed in the chapter under the sub-heading 'use of evaluation'.

But the evaluator should fix the priority and focus the evaluation accordingly.

### Respondents for Evaluation

Respondents are the audience for the evaluation. They may consist of farmers and their families, members of youth clubs, public, local leaders, members of rural institutions, NGOs, the evaluator, other extension staff, supervisors, and advisory councils. The evaluator should select the primary respondents according to the reasons for evaluation, because various respondents will have various concerns about the programme.

### Standards for Evaluation

Standards are the criteria or yardsticks applied to measure the impact of a programme. For example, a standard fixed for an extension programme may be the number of marginal farmers who adopt a particular practice. If an evaluation reveals that the specified number adopted then the programme can be considered as success as far as this standard is concerned. The objective of a programme is a major source of standards but sometimes, the programme emphasis may alter during the course of implementation, or the objectives may not be clear or precise. However, during evaluation objectives of special concern may be identified; also standards for assessing the impact of programme may be raised or lowered based on experience.

## Levels of Evaluation (Table 10.1)

We can evaluate extension programme at various levels. In the early stage we can evaluate how the extension programme was planned, and after completion of the programme, the impact on the farming community. We can also evaluate at one of the intermediate levels as follows:

**Table 10.1:** Levels of evaluation

| Sl. No. | Levels of evaluation | Levels |
|---|---|---|
| 1. | Changes in the society | 8 |
| 2. | Economic changes for the beneficiaries | 7 |
| 3. | Consequences for the beneficiaries | 6 |
| 4. | Behavioural changes of the beneficiaries | 5 |
| 5. | People's opinion about the programme | 4 |
| 6. | Beneficiaries' involvement in extension activities | 3 |
| 7. | Implementation of the programme by extension agents | 2 |
| 8. | Planning of the extension activities | 1 |

The higher levels in this table are generally the result of the lower levels. The higher the level that the extension worker is observing, the more accurately he will be able to state how far the ultimate goals of the programme have been reached. However, it is difficult to find suitable measurement standards for changes at higher levels. It is also more difficult to prove that changes at these levels are due to extension programme and not other factors. It is easy to demonstrate that this is the case if attention is also paid to the lower levels during evaluation, although the manpower and means may not always be available.

## Evidence for Evaluation

Evidence means information about a standard or criterion. To finalise which type of evidence to use, adjustments must be made between what is the best to use and what it is possible to obtain.

Evidence can be classified into two main types: (a) Changes in the behaviour of the people, e.g. change in level of knowledge, skill and attitude, extent of adoption, etc. (b) Opportunity and change may be difficult to measure so it is worth measuring work in terms of the learning situation we have set up. Learning situation means demonstrations, group meetings, reading materials, etc. There are several levels of evidence for programme evaluation. At each level what was expected can be compared to what was achieved.

## Designs for Evaluation

The survey is the most commonly used design on conducting extension evaluations. In this design, sampling is done first, i.e. list sampling, block or area sampling by stratified sampling, quota sampling, and purposive or judgement sampling. Questionnaire, interviews and observation techniques are applied to collect data. It gives information on people's perceptions and opinions about programme and the results of programme. It can also bring out facts on the status of participants prior to their participation in a programme.

The other designs like case study design, experimental design, matched set design and before and after study design are rarely used in programme evaluation. Case study results cannot be generalised but they can supplement other evaluation designs. The before and after study observations are made before and after participation in an extension programme. The other two designs are rarely used because they are expensive and difficult to conduct.

## Conducting Evaluation

a. **Analysing:** After collecting the data, it should be properly measured by using the devices like value scales, attitude scales, opinion polls, knowledge and comprehension tests, interest checks, skill or performance rating, etc. The data may be tabulated and analysed. Different kinds of data analysis can be applied ranging in complexity from percentages to statistical techniques. Good data analysis relies on emphasis on those aspects that are related to the particular issues addressed by the evaluation.

b. **Reporting:** The findings of evaluation need to be presented either by talk or written form. Different kinds of reporting procedures may be used like written reports, audio-visual reports, question–answer reports, etc. In the report, the evaluator should clearly state the reasons behind any implications and recommendations made.

c. **Applying:** The implications and recommendation drawn from evaluation should be used to improve the ongoing programme and/or in the planning of future programmes. The evaluation process has not served its purpose unless the results drawn are utilised. If it is found that the present activities of the extension worker has failed in certain objectives then he has to attempt to modify his methods and means so that they might reach the people.

The way in which results are presented for re-consideration is determined by the audience or the reader. In many cases, the results of evaluation have to be reported in more than one way to meet the needs of different categories of people.

## Six Keys of Evaluation

1. **Statement of objectives:** State the objectives of a programme to be evaluated in terms of behaviour changes in the participants. If a programme is developed in response to a particular need, a major concern of the evaluation should be whether the programme is meeting the need, or to what extent it meets the needs. Many times, the objectives may be vague, consisting of very general statements of expected outcomes. Much difficulty will be encountered in attempting to translate such objectives in evaluation criteria.

2. **Source of evidence:** Evidence consists of information related to a particular criterion or standard fixed for evaluation. This information we can get only from people involved in that particular programme, e.g. men, women, farm families, members of youth club, other support groups.

3. **Representative sample:** Sampling means selecting a small number from the whole group concerned, from which an estimate can then be made for the whole group. The opinion of the selected a few should represent the typical of universe (whole people participating in the programme). The sample size and method of sampling also should be relevant.

4. **Suitable methods:** The methods of obtaining evidence must be appropriate to the kind of information being collected. Evaluator can collect information by questions and interview, and some evidences by direct observation. Therefore, depending upon the purpose of evaluation suitable methods must be employed, e.g. information about change in attitude and skill imparted can be collected by direct observation method.

5. **Reliable question:** The question should be to the point. It must be carefully constructed so as to obtain relevant, unbiased data, e.g. when asking question about District Livestock Farm visit, relevant question should be as below:
   - Did you observe any new breed of sheep in District Livestock Farm?
   - If yes, what were they?

The irrelevant question may be as follows:
- What new breeds of sheep did you see during the farm visit?
- Did you think the farm visit was helpful? (yes or no)

6. **Plan to apply findings:** The evaluation should not be regarded as complete until the findings have been applied to improve the ongoing programme and/or in the planning of future programmes. It should be remembered that evaluation should never be conducted for just its own sake. Decide how you will analyse and use the evaluation findings before evaluation is conducted.

## Problems of Evaluation

Basically, the purpose of evaluation is to estimate the impact of a programme usually in terms of how well it has achieved its objective. Evaluation must be properly conducted. However, many problems are faced at different stages of evaluation. Some of the important problems as quoted by Annamalai et al (1994) are: (a) Error of observation, (b) error of measuring instrument, (c) error of measurement, (d) error of quantification, (e) error due to lack of control, and (f) error of true response.

a. **Error of observation:** Evaluations observe various phenomena and give opinion. Difference is observed in the description of the phenomenon between two evaluators. Sometimes it is also noticed that the same observer gives different opinions about the same programme at different occasions.

b. **Error of measuring instrument:** It is difficult to design a perfect instrument for evaluation. There is chance of error in social sciences because no instrument can judge the human behaviour with absolute correctness. However, proper care will help in reducing error in data collection.

c. **Error of measurement:** It is generally impossible to measure all of an individual's behaviour or knowledge in a social environment. Therefore, an attempt is always made to measure a representative or a typical sample of the behaviour or knowledge. The information based on a sample is likely to contain errors.

d. **Error of quantification:** In order to assess the achievements and to know the significance of achievements, data have to be quantified. There are chances of error during the process of transfer of data from qualitative form to quantitative form. Moreover, few absolutely constant units of measurement are available in social research.

e. **Error due to lack of control:** Most of the time evaluation deals with human beings. The human beings are constantly changing and difficult to control. A poultry scientist or a pharmacologist is able to handle his material in any way he chooses, but it is difficult to do the same with the human beings.

f. **Error of true responses:** Most of the information obtained are based on the expressed opinion of respondents. They may not be giving the true responses. It is very difficult to check the truthfulness of the information.

g. **Error of operational difficulties:** A researcher has to face many operational difficulties while collecting data. Respondents of the baseline may drop out at the terminal stage. The selected respondents may or may not be present at the time of researcher's visit. The availability of instruments of evaluation by their very nature is limited.

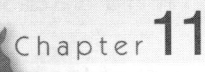

# Chapter 11

# Livestock Marketing Extension

## THE ROLE OF LIVESTOCK

Since the pre-historic time, livestock has been part of human life. Bulls have been worshipped both in India and in the Mediterranean areas, two of the most advanced cradles of human civilisation. There are plenty of references of the pre-Christian worship of calves in the Bible (Exodus:32), by way of deprecating idol worship. The term cattle have been used as synonym of wealth of a man. The unmatched wealth of man is good learning, and nothing else (Kural). The oldest pre-Aryan civilisation of India was the one discovered in the Mohenjodadro and Harappa. In these excavations, we find an advanced city civilisation and worship of Shiva with the bull as his vehicle. Bulls have also been used as seals of authority.

The wars in ancient India were started by seizing the cattle of the invaded country (as oil wells are seized by Americans now) as the prime wealth of the country. The cattle had great economic value to man and that is why hospitals for cattle were in vogue in India even in the pre-Christian era of Ashoka (300 BC).

### Animal Husbandry—The Earliest Avocation of Mankind

Man, as the descendant of ape, living in the caves and tree tops, has been hunting and eating animals, and the fish he caught or angled, from time immemorial, and he started domesticating animals even before taking to agriculture. Since man was quadruped, before standing up erect, and using his forelimbs as hands, he must have fought the animals with all four limbs to subdue the animals; or its young ones should have been subjugated and domesticated by him. In fact, he was a nomad, taking his cattle, sheep, goat and his friend, the dog, from pasture to pasture, as he took to cultivation. Until cultivation was extensive, animal flesh was the prime food apart from roots and fruits available in the wild. The idea of agriculture sprouted from early, mans brain only by constant observation of naturally occurring fruit-bearing trees and cereals dropping their seeds on earth, the seeds germinating and coming to yield on maturity. This process requires the development of reasoning capacity and thinking. Hence, that animal rearing preceded agriculture.

Earlier, man lived in the protected cattle pen along with animals. In fact, most of our villages are named the cattle pen of X or Y such as Kondmanaickenpatty, Erumapatty (meaning buffalo pen), a block headquarters in Namakkal Taluk, Kondichettipatty, Pattyveeranpatty, Mattupatty (in Kerala) and Mysore (meaning village of buffaloes), etc. Those places should have been cattle pens, which later on grew into bigger habitations with village artisans, etc. settled together, based on other needs. The cattle pen has been the nucleus of later habitations. The importance of livestock is prominent, leaving alone the master, if you consider the names Mysore, Erumapatty, Mattuppatty, etc. You can see even now the practice of herdsmen going out grazing the animals in rough out the day, sleeping with the animals during the nights, and visiting their own homestead once in a bluemoon, particularly at festival time. They either get food from home, if nearer home, or cook for themselves, when they go out to far off places grazing and camping on agricultural fields.

### Economic Role

#### Livestock as Human Food

Until the advent of vegetarianism as propounded by Buddha and Mahaveera, the whole of mankind ate meat. Nowhere vegetarianism is mentioned in Bible or other holy literatures except in India, that too, after advent of the above spiritual heads and animal lovers. Worldwide, the protein need of man is mainly met by meat. The deficiency of protein in India leads to malnutrition and poorer health of Indian men and women, who lack in average stamina compared to their counterparts in other countries, particularly the white world. Milk is the wholesome food, balanced in protein, fat, carbohydrates, vitamins and minerals. It is virtually an elixir nourishing the young and old alike, including the sick. Milk is the second largest agricultural commodity next to rice. The monetary value of milk is about ₹ 4,95,841 crores annually. Milk, meat, egg, wool, etc. contribute about 4.1% of GDP of the country.

Egg is another produce of livestock. It is produced in poultry farms by the rural folk, and is a complete and unadulterated food, at affordabe price.

Meat: The meat from sheep, goat, cattle and broiler birds, and fish forms the major supply of meat needs. The poorest Dalit population survive on beef, buffalo meat and pork.

### Livestock as Draught Animals

Animal rearing and agriculture went hand in hand. In fact, cattle are useful in many ways to agriculture, particularly as draught animals, drawing the ploughs and carts, taking loads. The bullock power provides the motive power to the Indian agriculture and allied activities. About 80 million of working animals provide about 40 million MW of electrical energy equivalent power to the rural sector for agricultural activity. About 20 million people are engaged in bullock cart transportation system which provides self employment opportunity. In the hill tracts, animals like mules, yalks, elephants and horses are the only means of transport. To the present day, the animals are used for threshing the corn ears, by driving them over. They are used for baling out water, though with the advent of its diesel and electricity has become a rare phenomenon now. Man has been riding both horses and bullocks, and had also laden goods on the backs of bullocks, horses, mules, elephants and asses. The great Indian God, Lord Shiva or Mahadev is glorified as the only rider on the bulls.

### Manure

The cow dung and urine have been used as valuable manure in the farms from times immemorial. There are people who keep sheep and goat in large flocks as a whole time occupation. Their pens are used by farmers, on payment, for fertilizing the vacant lands during the off season, the droppings and urine of the animals forming rich manure. The advent of chemical fertilisers has however, overshadowed its use for some time. Now, with a renewed interact in it, which is equivalent to ₹ 43.47 billion the world is going for dung of animals as manure, i.e. organic farming, considering the harmful effects of chemical fertilisers.

### Energy Source

The dung is a source of energy which is equivalent to ₹ 43.47 billion annually. It is used for extracting biogas and well digested manure at the same time, and also killing all the seeds of weeds. Biogas is a renewable and non-polluting fuel. Often, the dung of animals is converted into cakes and used for household cooking, and often for burning dead bodies, particularly in the towns. With the rising prices of petroleum gases, gobar gas has again gained importance.

### Ready and Steady Money for Farmers

The milk and its products, the calves, the goats, sheep, (mostly the male ones) and the fowls and their eggs are ready money for farmers whenever they need to buy inputs for the farming or for paying the physician or buying other household ariticles. Sometimes, certain animals are set apart for preplanned items of expenditures. The agricultural income is seasonal and only at the time of harvest, provided there is no drought or flood unseasonal rains, or other epidemics of plant diseases, whereas the milch income and income from sale of animals, fowls, eggs, etc. is continuous, spread over the year. Even if the animals die, the carcasses are eaten as food, and the skin/hide is sold. Establishment of the milk co-operatives has led to an assured income to the milch animal rearers.

The author knows of an instance of a destitute widow, working as daily labours, educating her son and finally marrying of her daughter with a dowry of 20 sovereigns of gold jewels and ₹ 20,000 in cash all earned from the milk of a buffalo, which was stall fed with the leaves of sugarcane, from the sugarcane fields in which she worked during the day.

Most women in agricultural families jealously save the money from the milk sales, and sale of fowls, etc. and go for jewellery for their daughters, without bothering the men, except when the men are drunkards and take away such savings. They also meet out the petty household expenditure from such savings. Hence, the livestock has been rightly called wealth in most languages such as 'maadu' in Tamil, 'sommulu' in Telugu, and 'dhanagalu' in Kannada.

### Alternate Source of Living

It is a fact of life, that when agriculture fails due to vagaries of nature, particularly in dry tracts, livestock comes in handy for the farmers to tide over the adversity. Often it so happens that landless labourers take up the job of rearing calves or sheep/goat bought for them by those with money, particularly elderly rural people with money who cannot look after the cattle and cannot otherwise invest. They both share the difference in value after rearing and calving, at the marketing stage. The livestock is often pledged for loan taken from money lenders.

### Employment

Animal husbandry is a great source of employment to the rural folk, both to the labourers and small landowners. One can see a labourer leading his/her single cow or single goat to his workplace, which is also the spot where fodder is available for his animal. The weed of groundnut field, or leaf sheddings from sugarcane, tapiacco, etc. is often the feed for the animals, whereas in countries with sparse populations, such vegetable matter is be treated as waste and often burnt.

They also keep fowls at the backyard, to breed and serve as food for themselves or for sale in the market. The livestock and fowl rearing is mostly done by women, for whom it is a great source of self-employment and income. It is estimated that on an average, farmers spend three to five hours a day on animal husbandry activities.

Whereas agriculture can provide employment for 180 days in a year, and mere 100 days in dry tracts, animal husbandry keeps the people employed all through the year.

### Used by Police and Army

Dogs are used both by army and police for tracing hidden bombs, stolen articles and the thieves, who had handled the articles. Horses again are used both by police and army, the police for crowd control, the army for transport and physical fitness. Camels are valuable means of transport for both army and police in deserts.

### Use in Research

Dogs, cows and horses, besides rabbits and guinea pigs, have been frequently used for preparing vaccines, testing drugs, etc.

## Social and Cultural Role

### Mark of Social Status

The ownership of animals, particularly of good pedigree breed, is a sambol of social status, and financial status too. The famous Kangeyam breed is the handiwork of the prestigious family of Palayakottai pattagars (the zamindars of Palayakottai in Erode district of Tamil Nadu). It brought them both fame and money.

### Animal Recreations

The bulls, horses rams and fowls are often reared and brought up for racing and gaming (fighting) purposes during festivals, fairs, etc. Bull fight during Govardhan Puja in Madhya Pradesh and other Nothern Indian states. In the field of modern entertaining society race course and cock fight is another typical socio-psychological ventrue. Amongst these, cock fighting is a matter of heritage enjoyed by mainly the tribes of many parts of the country and race courses is a tradition of urban rich people. So, it is said that not only the companion or sports animals but the animals as a whole plays a significant role in the sociopsychological upliftment of our society. The trained animals, perform on commands and are a source of joy in the circuses.

### Great Cultural Sport of Bull Taming

Bull taming is a great sport of Tamils of ancient and present times too. The farmers used to groom well fed bulls for challenge and whichever young hero subdued the bull took the hand of the young maid, as per the ancient Tamil lores. The equivalent of the sport is the Spanish or South American sport of almost the same type, the only difference being the riding on the angry bull's back or drawing the animal with a red rag and killing it with a sword, a cruel practice by our vegetarian philosophy. The famous Alanganllur (in Madurai district of Tamil Nadu) bull taming sport draws ever-increasing local and foreign crowds.

### Cow as Dowry to the Beloved Daughter

The milch animals are valued dowry taken by daughters to their husband's place. It is part of our ancient culture.

### Thanks Giving to the Animals on Pongal Days

The great Pongal festival of Tamils is a unique harvest festival with great cultural significance and emotional impact. It is an occasion for man to thank his animals, which are his revered wealth. He washes and decorates the animals and feeds them with his own food, cooked in fresh pots with all sanctimony, using only the firewood. The Pongal rice is mixed with the sweet jaggery and fruits, before being served to guests. His gratitude is such that he eats after they are fed. Beating or using the animal for labour is forbidden on that sacred day.

### Legends and Religions

Man's imagination with regard to animals has taken various shapes. He has created winged horses, men with horse bodies in Greek mythologies, a thousand horses drawing the chariot of the sun, the gods choosing and riding animals such as Durga riding tiger, the Mahadev the bull, the Vigneshwar the bandicoot, the taker of life, Yama, the buffalo, and Lord Muruga, the Indian national bird peacock, etc. Even the dog is held to be the incarnation of a god, Bhairava Moorthy.

Lord Vishnu flies the eagle. Our gods had incarnated as pigs, fish, tortoise, etc.

**Animal sacrifice to propitiate Gods**: The animals are given in worship to the gods as sacrifice, both in the Biblical and Koranic faith, and in other faiths, notwithstanding the alien vegetarian philosophy grafted onto Hindu religion by the enterprising Brahman, under attack from Buddhists and Jains. The Bible (Exodus 13:2) states: "Then the Lord said: Dedicate to me ... every first born male animal. They are mine." The Aadhi Hindus, unlike the migrant non-Hindu Brahmins coming from Central Asia, still worship their ancestors, such as Karuppanar, Ayyanar, the Kali, etc. and offer as sacrifies anything from the first born cock to bucks, buffalo calves, and boars, and eat them too. The first milk and first ghee are offered to gods to keep them well pleased! Recently, Nepal's King came to India and offered all these types of animal sacrifies at the Kali temple in Bengal, and ate their meat.

**Astrological reading by animal chart:** Man's flight of imagination has gone to such an extent that his astrological readings go in the name of various signs of Zodiac named after animals.

**Even the dung and urine are sacred in India:** The Indian farmers' ready stuff to make idols is cow dung. To spray the house with cow's urine is to cure one of pollution! God help this country! To smear the ground and the floor of rooms with cow dung is an age-old practice. The first thing a rural Indian does, after getting out of the bed, is to spray dung solution on the courtyard. The release of ammonia from dung incidentally can act as killer of germs, and hence this practice can be given an air of scientific wisdom of ancient Indians.

**Sacred milk bath of idols:** The practice of bathing the idols of Hindu gods with milk is held sacred in among the Hindus.

**Tonsuring of heads and buck slaughter:** The Hindu believers take their children to temple and have their heads tonsured and ear pierced. Even the elders have their heads tonsured in the presence of god and offer the hair to the deity. During these occasions, the deities, mostly meat eating ancestors, have to be pleased by sacrificing a buck or cock, or even pigs and male-buffaloes, and every one eats after serving the God first with unpolluted sacrificial food!

**Gratitude towards the cow:** The Indian is grateful to the cow with which he is associated. Nor would he eat beef. Only the landless destitute eat beef or buffalo meat. His religious faith holds the cow in reverence. The Hindu mythology holds the cow capable of granting anything one needs, particularly food for any number of men. It is said that the great army of King Viswamitra was fed by the sage Vashishtha with the help of his holy cow, the Kamadhenu (the giver of whatever one wanted). The King wanted to have the cow for himself. This request was declined by the sage. Viswamitra took it by force, but the divine cow defeated him and his troops and returned to its owner. Such was its prowess! Flight of great fanciful imagination! The fortune tellers take the decorated bulls to doorsteps and cater to man's wish to know answers to his problems. The nodding of the bull is either affirmative or negative, and the fortune teller interprets accordingly, as the divine answer!

**Grieving the death of animals:** Since the livestock is the wealth of the farmer, whenever a big animal like a cow, bullock, or buffalo or a flock of sheep or goat die, the relatives of the owner, and others are bound by social custom to go and express condolence at death/deaths. The death of cow or bullock is considered inauspicious for the future of the family.

**Superstitious beliefs:** The birth of a male calf on a Friday, and laying of eggs by birds after nightfall or are considered inauspicious, and the bird is eaten the next morning! The animal, even if a good milker, will be sold off promptly. The sheep delivering twins or more, are unwelcome, and are got rid off.

## Psychological Role

From time immemorial, domesticated animals have been the companions of men, often deeply entrenched in his beliefs and psychology. Men were very much attached to animals such as cow, which is a surrogate mother for many children whose mothers do not lactate sufficiently.

### Cow and House Warming

Indians have gone to the extent of treating the cow as holy and give it the status of a mother god and worship it. During house warming ceremony of a newly-built house, a cow is a must, and it is made to walk across the house. Its urinating in the house is held auspicious.

### Cow in Mother's Status

Even if the cow goes dry in its old age, the diehard Sanatanist insists upon keeping it just like a mother, and feeds it till its death. It is not given to be eaten, but buried with ceremony.

### Human Bond Toward Animals

The relationship of a farmer with a milch or draught animal or a dog is almost human in nature. The farmer knows the moods of his animal. He would apologise to his animal in so many words for not feeding it in time, in case he had to rush out in an emergency or some such thing. The animal would show its love to its master or mistress by its body language, by licking or brushing against his/her body, and the man would pat, groom, and wash the animals to express his love to them. The animals whine, or moo to express their needs, such as need to piss (in the case of a dog in leash), and quench their hunger or thirst. Once, they are obliged they lick the master express their gratitude. They almost speak to you.

### Animal's Human-like Intelligence

The author heard of a recent incident of a dog. On witnessing a ghastly accident in which several people were killed on the spot, ran to the village and whined and cried, and drew the people to the scene of accident. What a sense nature has given the creature!

### Rescuer of the Distressed

The reader could well have read of a dog, caught in the attack on the twin towers of World Trade Centre in New York, leading his blind master rapidly down the stairs and out of danger!

### Near Human Companion

There is a real time story of a boy, starved of parental society and love, going hysterical and suffering from mental derangement, being cured by the suggestion of a veterinarian to buy a pup to give company to the boy and the boy regaining his normal mental equilibrium by sharing his love with the pet animal. The stories are legion where men and animals have shared their mutual love in myriad ways.

A campanion animals like dog, cat, often develops an emotional and social attachment with the community. They can give a mental relief and reduce mental tension of our daily life. These animals can be acquinted the sympathy of his masters by showing their obedience, patience, friendship and company. They can guide of handicapped or blind persons by their natural instinct. Nowadays these pet or companion animals designed as one of the most important family members of our society. Man is deeply attached to his animals, and has given it an important place in his religion and sacrifices to his gods.

## TYPES OF FARMING AND SYSTEMS OF FARMING

The type of farming refers to the nature and degree of products or combination of products being produced in a farm and the methods and practices used in the farm. The system of farming is concerned with the organisational set up under which the farm is being run. The system mainly involves the question like who is the owner of the land, whether resources are public or owned individually and who makes the managerial decisions.

### Factors Determining the Types of Farming

The nature of the farm business is such that once resources are put under some use, it becomes difficult to shift them easily to some other enterprise. For example, if a farmer owning a dairy enterprise is being attracted by the profit of poultry and wants to replace dairy by poultry, he will have to sell the cows or buffaloes in order to purchase poultry birds and has to modify the dairy buildings.

The factors affecting the types of farming can be broadly classified into two types, viz. (i) physical factor and (ii) economic factor.

| Physical factor | Economic factor |
|---|---|
| 1. Climate | 1. Comparative advantage but not absolute advantage |
| 2. Soil | 2. Market facilities |
| 3. Topography | 3. Location of processing unit |
| | 4. Availability of capital |
| | 5. Availability of labour |
| | 6. Profitability |

a. **Physical factors:** These are the factors due to which the type of farming differs from place to place.
   1. *Climate:* Climate plays an important role in different types of farming. This factor differs from place to place.
   2. *Soil:* Generally deep soils are the best suited for most of the agricultural crops. Loose and shallow soils will have less water holding capacity and hence major crops cannot be grown.
   3. *Topography:* Refers to slope and height of the place. For example, different crops may be cultivated at different elevations. Similarly, livestock enterprises also depends upon the topography.

b. **Economic factors:** These factors are mainly concerned with the profit of the farm.
   1. *Comparative but not the absolute advantage:* It is a comparative advantage which is considered in the yield of farm management.

2. *Marketing:* Marketing is an important factor deciding the type of farming. The market cost is a function of distance of the farm to the consumers and the nature of the product.

3. *Location of processing unit/plant:* For example, the presence of egg powder plant of Erode influenced the poultry farmers, besides the natural condition. Thus, the location of processing units affects the type of farming.

4. *Availability of capital:* Technologies in modern times are changing very quickly and adoption of these technologies need more and more capital. Therefore, the availability of capital affects the selection of enterprises and ultimately the types of farming.

5. *Availability of labour:* Some enterprises are more labour intensive than others and these enterprises can be taken up only when the availability of labour is assured, e.g. poultry farming.

6. *Profitability of the enterprises:* Change in the profitability may occur due to change in the price and yield of different livestock products out of new research finding. For example, in 1980, the price of the egg increased significantly whereas the price of other farm products remained constant. This resulted in increased poultry area in the very next few years. Hence, this factor mainly influences the type of farming to a great extent.

## Types of Farming

1. **Specialised farming:** When income is derived from a single enterprise, the farming system is known as specialised farming. Under this type of farming, the major enterprise contributes more than 50% of the total farming income, e.g. dairy farming, sheep farming, poultry farming, piggery, etc.

2. **Diversified farming:** In this system a number of enterprises are taken up in the farm, and no single enterprise is relatively more important than other enterprises. In other words, no source of income is equal in terms of percentage of total income of the farm. Thus, the difference between diversified farming and specialised farming is the extent to which different enterprises are undertaken, e.g. crop + livestock + fishery.

3. **Mixed farming:** The type of farming under which crop production is combined with livestock, e.g. crop with cattle or sheep or poultry. This is the definition given by Tondon and Dhon Dayal.

According to Chauhan, the term mixed farming is used for the type of farming in which growing of crop is combined with some type of livestock rearing. The principles of agricultural economics dictate that a farm gets at least 10% income from livestock and the upper limit 49% would be it to be described as mixed farm. It provides employment and better income throughout the year. It ensures more efficient utilisation of land, labour, equipment and other resources. Crop residues are better utilized for livestock. It satisfies the family food needs.

4. **Dry farming:** It refers to the area which receives less than 500 mm of annual rainfall, where mostly mixed farming is taken up. Areas where the rainfall is up to 750 mm along with high temperature and greater velocity wind, witness heavy loss of water. This type of area also comes under dry farming, e.g. agro-forestry/sylviculture.

5. **Irrigated/garden land farming:** It refers to artificial resources of water for raising a crop in areas where rainfall is insufficient or not well distributed over a period of time. This type of cultivation is called garden land cultivation or wet land cultivation, e.g. sericulture.

6. **Small-scale farming:** Here the flock or herd size is very small. It is easy to manage interfamily labour. Loss due to natural calamities is minimum. Per unit output may be high as compared to large-scale farming. But mechanisation is not possible and farmers do not get employment round the year.

7. **Large-scale farming:** Here the flock or herd size is large. It needs more capital and labour and the risk is also high. When the factors of production are large in quantity, such farming is called large-scale farming. Since the production is in large-scale, the cost of production per unit will be less. Feeding and watering can be mechanised. Better marketing of products is possible because processing, packaging and transportation of the produce will be economical. But natural calamities, labour strike, price fluctuation will result in more loss.

8. **Extensive farming:** When more area is brought under operation to increase the output, it is termed extensive farming, e.g. deep litter system of poultry farming.

9. **Intensive farming:** When more capital is used in a small area. In other words, land remains fixed in size while other factors are increased, e.g. raised platform multi-tier cage system of poultry farming.

10. **Ranching or pastoral farming:** It is a type of farming practised in which livestock is reared on pasture. It is a common practice in cooler regions with sparse populations like Australia, New Zealand and North America where wool production is a common feature.

It refers to an area that is not under the control of any owner nor is it enclosed by any boundary (government wasteland, panchayat wasteland). Ranching means grazing animals on public land. Sometimes such a land is also utilised for rearing dairy stock; then, it is called dairy ranch.

**Pastures:** Pastures are grassland where grasses are grown and animals are allowed to graze. In pasturing the animals, there is no expenditure involved for raising fodder, harvesting and distribution as in the case of stall feeding and therefore the cost of production of the livestock product is minimised or reduced.

Pastures are of two types. These are: (a) Natural pasture and (b) artificial pasture.

a. *Natural pasture:* Grasses are grown on wastelands which offer this facility in natural pasture. In this method, grasses get established spontaneously, e.g. Hariyali, Denanath grasses grow without sowing and they provide excellent grass cover under good management. Some of the pastures are closed for grazing and grasses are used for hay making, after allowing the grasses to grow to the full height. These pastures are called meadows. The grasses that are established after the main harvest are called the aftermath, which in the later stage can be used for the animals to graze.

b. *Artificial pasture:* The inclusion of grasses in crop rotation is a common feature in foreign countries. Grasses are kept in the field for 3 to 10 years, then the field is ploughed and brought under other crops. These grasslands are otherwise called temporary pastures or leys and the pratice is known as lay farming. The land is prepared similar to other crops. In this method, grass seed and legume seeds are mixed together and sown as a mixed crop. The inclusion of legume is advantageous in many ways. They are rich in protein content. They enrich soil by fixing atmospheric nitrogen and consequently, the grasses that are associated with legumes make a better growth than the grasses which are grown alone. The selected grasses and legumes should be rich in foliage growth which in turn have rich protein and minerals.

Rotational grazing or compartment grazing: In this the pasture is divided into different blocks or compartments which are grazed one after another in regular rotation. The extent of land available for grazing at a given time is thereby limited to the use of animals and they graze the grasses completely. After grasses are grazed thoroughly, the animals are not let into that particular compartment. In turn the other block is opened for grazing. By this ways, the animals are let into the compartments in rotation, i.e. from one block to another. The type of grazing is called rotational grazing or compartment grazing.

Advantages of rotational grazing: In this method, pastures are uniformly grazed by the animals without any break and ensure the availability of grasses for grazing throughout the year.

Carrying capacity: It is the capacity of the field or the pasture land to allow a number of animals for natural grazing. This is called the carrying capacity of pasture.

11. **Landless livestock farming:** Majority of the agricultural labourers always maintain one or two dairy cattles or one or two sheep and goats or a few fowls or both in their backyard. They generally have to graze their animals on the roadside, or in the government lands or forest. They also collect the weeds and grass from the agricultural farms in which they are working and from roadside. They normally buy dry fodder and concentrates to feed their animals. Also, some labourers have a contract with the landowners for making a specified quantity of green fodder available to them, while a few also purchase standing fodder crops for their animals. Only a few landless farmers, who adopt dairying as their main profession, purchase compound cattle feed manufactured by public and private feed companies.

## Systems of Farming

1. **Peasant farming:** This refers to an organisational set up in which individual cultivator is the owner, manager and organiser of the farm. He makes the decision and formulates the plans for farm depending upon the available resources. The advantage is that the farmer himself is the owner. Therefore, he is free to take all types of decisions. The disadvantage is that the resources are limited.

2. **State farming:** The operation and management is done by Government officials or university. Such a farm is either attached to institutions or they themselves are institutions. Supervision is done by

the farm manager and labourers are hired on daily or monthly basis. The farm may be mechanised or non-mechanised depending upon the size of the farm. There is no limitation for resource. Because of the lack of personal interest and personal stake of the individual, this type of farming is not profitable.

3. **Capitalistic farming:** The management and the ownership of this farm are under rich person or capitalist. The size of such farm is sufficiently large and the management is very efficient. These farms are owned by individual or a group of individuals or shareholders. The resources are plenty and the latest technology know-how are used and hence they are very efficient. These types of farms or farmings are very common in Western countries like USA and Canada and on hills of India, i.e. tea/coffee estates.

4. **Collective farming:** It refers to the collective management of resources, wherein large number of families live in the same village. The members surrender their land, livestock and machineries to the society. The members work together under a management committee elected by themselves. The committee maintains or manages the farm activities by proper allocation of work. Then, the resources do not belong to any of the farmer or the member but to the entire society and the individual farmer has only a limited voice. The payment to workers are in terms of workday units, i.e. a standard quota for each kind of farm operation is fixed in relation to one working day and the amount of work done by each farmer in a day is calculated accordingly, both in respect of quality and quantity. An unskilled worker has to work more hours than the skilled worker to complete the quota of his workday. This type of farming is very common in Communist countries.

5. **Co-operative farming:** A co-operative farming is one in which members pool their lands or resources voluntarily and manage it jointly under a democratic set-up. Each farmer retains right on his own land, but the land is treated as one unit and cultivated primarily under the direction of an elected management. A part of the profit is divided in proportion to the land contributors and the rest is distributed in proportion to the labour contributed by each farmer.

6. **Contract farming:** The farmers look after the maintenance of the birds on contract while the enterpreneur takes care of the investments in terms of chicks, feeds and cost towards health measures and general maintenance. This system has been adopted in broiler farming in India. Such an approach has been successfully tried in some places for production of baffalo meat from male buffalo calves.

## LIVESTOCK PRODUCTS' MARKETING EXTENSION

As animal husbandry, agriculture and society develops, marketing becomes more important. Livestock occupies an important place in agricultural economy of India. It is recognised as an important source for generating equitable income and employment in rural areas. The contribution of livestock to total gross domestic product (GDP) was 4.0% in 2000–2001. The farmer, therefore, has to take on commercial and marketing skills. The extension agent at the grassroot level has high responsibility in developing these among them.

### Livestock and Livestock Products

India's livestock sector is one of the largest sectors in the world with a holding of 11.6% of world livestock population. Total livestock population in India is 512 million (annual report, 2016–17). Of the total global buffalo population, India accounts for 57.83%. Similarly, 17.93% of the world's goat and 15.06% of cattle are in India. The poultry population has shown manifold increase.

### *Products*

The products may differ according to the states, lifestyle and culture of the people. The value of output of livestock and fisheries sector was estimated to be ₹ 5,91,691 crore during (2015-2016) which was 28.5% of the total value of output from agriculture and allied areas. However, the major products through which the livestock contributes to the income are milk and milk products, meat draught power eggs, chicken, bones, hides, etc. depending on the major demands of the people.

### *Milk*

Milk production of India reached 155.5 million tonnes (2016-17) and accounted for about 65 per cent (Rs 3,49,672 crore) of the total value and the output from livestock and was higher than wheat and sugarcane.

### *Meat and Beef*

In India, meat production is largely a byproduct of livestock production, utilising spent animals at the end the production life.

The second largest production of livestock origin is meat and beef. Total meat production including poultry meat was 7.0 million tonnes in 2015–16.

### Egg and Chicken

The egg production in India was about 82.93 billion from 2015 to 2016 out of which 21% eggs were produced by desi layers. Also 3.26 MT of meat is also produced by poultry.

### Other Products

Apart from meat, the other products derived from animals like eggs, wool, hide, fur, etc. also contribute a similar percentage of the market share.

### Consumption

The per capita availability of milk is about 322 g per day in 2014-15. It is more than the world average of 294 g per day, while in the advanced countries the per capita availability of milk is about 700 g.

The meat and beef consumption is common in daily diet of the people of the developed countries. However, it is an occasional or ceremonial recipe in the diet of a large segment and Indian population. The per capita consumption of meat in India is only 14 g per day, whereas the ICMR recommendation is 34 g per day.

Though India is the world's third largest egg producer, its per capita availability is poor, being about 66 eggs per year, and poultry meat about 3.1 kg. However, 70% of this poultry product is consumed in urban and sub-urban areas, which account for about 25% of the country's population.

### Export

India's total export value of milk products was ₹ 4,274.1 crore during 2013-14. Export value of beef and meat fetched ₹ 27,212.9 crore and the export value of poultry product was estimated to be 0.6 billion. The total value of export of livestock and livestock products during 2013-14 was 58,910.9 crores. India has a bright future in exporting and livestock products.

### Throes and Woes of Indian Livestock Farmer

Before understanding the concept of livestock marketing extension and its importance it is important to understand the status of farmers in India.

1. Small fragmented holdings.
2. Poor per animal/flock yield as compared to international standards.
3. Inferior quality produce.
4. Market competitiveness and vacuum in the market.
5. Poor post-harvest and seasonal dependence.
6. Multiple products in small qualities with heavy wastages.
7. Selling everything wholesale and buying everything in retail (no storage facility).
8. Distress sale of produce.
9. Poor bargaining power.
10. Weak market intelligence.
11. Everything exploited by commission agents.

### Marketing

Marketing involves finding out what customers want and supplying it to them at a profit. This description stresses two crucial points of marketing, i.e. firstly, the whole marketing process depends on what the customers want or need, and secondly, the marketing is a commercial process and is only sustainable if it provides all the participants with a profit.

Marketing can also be defined as 'the series of activities involved in making available services and information, which influence the desired level of production relative to market requirements and the movement of the product (commodity) from the point of production to the point of consumption.

This definition covers the services, which should be covered by the extension officer, such as providing information and advice. This role includes: (1) Finding out what the customer wants, and (2) supplying it to him at a profit.

The key activity of an extension officer or any public servant concerned with improving livestock agricultural marketing is the commercialization of the rural economy.

### Marketing Process

There are three stages in the marketing process:

1. **Concentrating or assembling:** This is the collection of the marketable surpluses from the producers and pooling them into huge size lots, generally on the basis of grades, quality, uniformity, etc.
2. **Equalisation:** This is the adjustment of the supply (market arrivals, stocks) to the demand (market disposals), and is an important function of holding (stocking) commodities with seasonal production.
3. **Dispersion:** This is the distribution of commodity to other market functionaries like wholesalers, retailers, agents, etc. according to demand.

In the process of marketing the marketing cast forms the dominant factor. This can be studied in three different ways:

1. **Functional approach:** The marketing functions are exchange functions, physical functions and facilitating functions.
   - Exchange function involves the transfer of title of commodity like buying (assembling) and selling. Selling involves the merchandising activities like packaging promotional activities, etc.
   - The physical functions are storage and transportation.
   - Facilitating functions are standardisation, financing, risk bearing and market information.

2. **Institutional approach:** That is market institutions. These are agencies involved in the marketing process. The institutional approaches to understand the marketing functions are as follows:
   a. Merchant, middlemen, retailers and wholesalers. They take title and own the commodity.
   b. Agent, middlemen, brokers and commission agents. They act as representatives of sellers and buyers.
   c. Speculative middlemen. They take title to the commodity as well as the risk involved in marketing.
   d. Facilitating organisations. They aid the middlemen by providing facilities for physical functions and exchange functions, including credit facilities.

3. **Commodity approaches:** This approach is combination of the functional and institutional approaches by specially taking a commodity.

## Problems in Marketing of Livestock Products

### i. Milk

a. *Problems of producers*
   1. In India, marketing of milk is sizeably in the unorganised sector which provides for ample scope for malpractices like use of false measurements in buying and selling milk and adulteration by vendors.
   2. Milk is bulky and perishable. Hence, it has to be disposed of within a short period which results in limited bargaining power of producers. Milk supply is characterised by a vertical supply curve.
   3. Procurement price is based on fat content which gives lower price for cow milk and higher price for buffalo milk.
   4. Intermediaries dictate the price by advancing loan to the milk producers.
   5. Producer finds it difficult to adjust supply with the demand within a short period.
   6. Seasonal variation in production. During winter, milk production will be more and price will be more. Because of this, the producer is not in a position to enjoy the maximum benefit.
   7. The absolute gap between the procurement price and retail price is increasing. Retail price is increasing at a faster rate, whereas procurement price is not increasing at the same rate.
   8. Cost of inputs like dry fodder, green fodder, concentrates, medicines and labour had shown greater increase over the years.

b. *Problems of processors and producers*
   1. High cost of collection and transportation. Since the milk production units are scattered over a large area.
   2. Pronounced seasonal fluctuation in milk production makes the collection costlier and adds to overhead charges.
   3. Since collection is lower, it leads to underutilization of capacities.
   4. High capital investment in buildings and equipment.
   5. Handling losses at various stages have not been standardised.
   6. Lack of adequate maintenance, which results in increased inefficiency.
   7. Widespread adulteration leads to quality control problems and expenses.
   8. Studies on consumer preference are not available.

c. *Problems of consumers*
   1. Irregular supply
   2. High retail price
   3. Sanitary laws are not enforced strictly
   4. Milk is not available in different grades to suit the preferences of consumer.

### ii. Egg and broiler

a. *Problems:* Presently, the poultry traders and commission agents operating in various metropolitan cities, fix wholesale prices of eggs and table birds on day-to-day basis, taking into account the supply and demand. The prices so fixed have a little effect on the cost of production. The rural producers find it extremely difficult to get reasonable returns from the small poultry units because prices offered to them are not remunerative.

The state poultry corporations/federations have been providing marketing support but their impact has been very limited due to financial constraint. The Government of India has entrusted the responsibility for marketing of eggs and poultry at regional and national level to National Agricultural Co-operative Marketing Federation of India Ltd. (NAFED) by providing financial support. However, efforts of NAFED have not had the desired impact on the overall egg marketing situation in the country.

b. *National Egg Co-ordination Committee (NECC):* In 1982, a private sector agency was created under the name of National Egg Co-ordination Committee (NECC) to declare prices after monitoring the supply and demand position in different parts of the country. This organisation, however, is not able to administer the declared prices due to scarcity of funds and cold storage facilities for bulk procurement and storage. Two important constraints in poultry products' marketing are: (a) Unproductive, and often unremuneraive, wholesale price of eggs and broilers, and (b) lack of marketing infrastructure in terms of collection, processing and storage.

There is an urgent need for an agency at the national level like National Poultry Marketing Board to understand marketing operations and ensure prices based on the cost of production and to co-ordinate the marketing activity with various existing organisations in the public and private sector.

iii. **Meat:** Marketing of meat covers all the activities involved from the point of producer, who sells the meat animals to the first buyer, and extends up to the stage where the meat and other byproducts reach the consumer. In India, marketing of meat involves several intermediate operators or groups of them and it is difficult to assess how many hands it has to change before it reaches the consumers. At present, various functions, such as assembling of animals, slaughter, processing, storage, transportation and merchandising, are performed by groups of individuals, each taking undue margins of profit

for the services rendered. Though the retail prices of meat have gone up considerably, proportionate benefits have not reached the primary producers.

It is important to establish an organised marketing service for meat animals in the government or co-operative sector. Livestock markets can be operated as terminal markets owned by the State Government or co-operative and should provide facilities for yarding, feeding and watering of meat animals. Though in some states meat corporations facilitate marketing of meat animals, most of the state meat corporations are not promoting meat animal marketing activities. So the State Government should take adequate steps to establish a better marketing system and meat products.

### Defects in Present System of Livestock Products' Marketing in India

1. **Perishability:** In relation to other products, livestock and poultry products by nature are perishable. These perishable products require speedy handling and often special refrigeration which raise the cost of marketing.

2. **Forced sales:** Average Indian farmer is so poor and indebted that he cannot afford to wait till he gets higher price. In order to meet his commitments and pay his debt, he is forced to sell the produce just after the production at whatever prices are offered to him.

3. **Inadequate and expensive facilities of transport:** Forced and distress sales by the farmers are further compounded by the fact that the means of transport available to the farmers are inadequate and expensive. Most of the rural villages are not well connected by main roads or with marketing centres.

4. **Seasonality in production:** The production varies from one season of the year to another. Hence, storage facilities must be made available to preserve the products until they are consumed. This seasonality in production, thus, raises cost of marketing in terms of storage cost. The seasonal variability in production of items like milk, egg, butter, etc. is not as acute as it used to be years ago. The widespread use of rapid transportation and refrigeration has tended to reduce the seasonality.

5. **Superfluous middlemen and malpractice:** In-between farmers and consumers, there is a large army of middlemen who function at various stages in the process of assembling and distribution of farm produce. Many market surveys in India have

revealed that middlemen take away major share of consumer's price that varies for different commodities.

6. **Absence of grading and standardisation and inadequate storage:** Grades and standards for many livestock products have not so far been prescribed by many State Governments. A good number of farmers have a little knowledge of grading their produce and usually mix up good and bad quality products in a single lot which secures them a lower price in the market. There is general inadequacy of good storage facilities both in urban as well as rural areas. The indigenous methods of storage adopted in village do not adequately protect the produce. As a result, physical losses go on increasing if the period of storage is lengthened.

7. **Multiplicity of charges:** The sale proceeds of the farmer is subjected to many unauthorised deductions. Besides these, a number of other charges, legitimate or illegitimate, claimed by the middlemen lead to lesser share being received by the producer out of consumer's money.

8. **Substitutability:** There is always the possibility of substitution of one product by another. Mutton can be substituted by pork, beef or chicken and vice versa. Substitution is more effective in terms of shortages of meat and price rise. Abnormally rising price of meat may make the consumers switch over to another, completely affecting marketing of the farmer.

9. **Lack of communication and marketing information:** Most of the Indian farmers do not get the necessary information regarding prices of different farm goods, in different markets. Only the middlemen provide some information which is more biased in favour of the traders and hence the farmers are not able to realize reasonable returns for their produce. Though different communication media are available, due to lack of associated amenities, the farmer fails to get fuller advantages in this regard.

Among these problems, communication plays a vital role in determining the success or failure of commercialisation/marketing of the livestock produce in rural India. The extension system in the rural areas should be reoriented to meet the challenges in 21st century due to globalisation. The following systemic approach will help the extension officers to a greater extent in increasing the profits of small and marginal farmers in the rural India.

## Promoting Marketing Extension

The following are the stages involved in promoting marketing extension in rural India:

1. **Audit of local resources and facilities:** This involves carrying out an investigation of the area/region/country. The objective is for the extension officer to thoroughly familiarise himself with both the problems or constraints as well as the opportunities (main selling points of the area) through interaction. The extension officer's role is to listen and learn. He/she should try to understand how farmers might react to new ideas and which farmers are likely to be most positive so that. At the end of this stage, the extension officer will have a clear idea of the livestock, the marketing system, the individuals and the problems of the area. He/she will also have some idea of the possible solutions, which are worth investigating. The break-even price of delivering produce to the markets should have been calculated.

2. **Determining what the market wants in terms of product now and in future:** This is finding out from the market what product or products are wanted and in what form, i.e. customer wants. At this stage one need to know: Who currently supplies the market? At what times? At what prices? What volumes are sold? How the produce is packed and presented?

   All these will help the extension officer in understanding either to increase/start supply to the market. Answering all these questions is again a process of information gathering. Opinions of knowledgeable individuals, who are commercially involved with trading, valuable statistics, such as price data/information on the volumes of produce delivered to the market and the self-experience of the extension officer helps in getting fruitful information.

3. **The marketing system:** The previous stage deals with what the customer wants in terms of product, while this stage deals with determining what the customer wants in terms of service. In other words, finding the best way to work within the existing marketing system. It involves building up an understanding of how produce is distributed and sold and binds the relationships between different sales points in the marketing chain.

   In this stage, the extension worker needs to understand:

   i. *Produce distribution system:* The product distribution systems not only vary from country to country but also sometimes from product to product. The extension officer will need to fully understand the marketing system if he wants to make it work for the benefit of farmers.

ii. *Understanding how the marketing system works:* In this system it is the contractor who is taking the most risk. Risk and profit are very closely linked. About 30 per cent of the produce, normally that of the larger growers, is marketed direct to the wholesale markets. These wealthier farmers are in a better position to absorb the risks involved with marketing the produce themselves. It is completely different in the case of small and marginal farmers who mostly depend on local commission agents for marketing their produce.

iii. *Marketing margins at various levels:* The proportion of the final retail price that is reaches to the grower arouses much emotion and discussion. Calculating the marketing chain is a very difficult task as it varies depending on the retail price of the product, its perishability, marketing costs (for transport, packaging). For example, it is often assumed that the difference between the retail price and wholesale price is the retailer's profit. This is wrong because it fails to take into account the fact that the produce is often sold at different prices and that some produce is downgraded or even wasted entirely. To do this properly the extension officer will need to retrace each step in the marketing chain and establish from each middleman his buying and selling price. Typically, margins are greatest when the middleman pays a firm price and actually takes ownership of the produce.

iv. *Wholesaler and middlemen's selection as trade partners:* An important part of the extension officer's work is to identify suitable and reputable middlemen as trading partners. This involves finding out which companies are best equipped and most prepared to trade in the produce from his area. Secondly, he should find out whether these companies have a reputation for integrity and honesty. Discovering this information involves not only meetings with possible trading partners but also in effect, taking references about their reputation from other traders.

v. *Information services:* The producer requires rapid feedback on the state of different markets for knowing information on prices and on the demand of the market in terms of quality and quantity. This information can be used to maximise sales when the market is short and quality demands are not as stringent.

4. **Decision-making and agreeing on an action plan:** This involves deciding on what to do by choosing the best course of action. The challenge to the extension worker with special responsibility for marketing is firstly to decide how the marketing problems of the area can be solved. Secondly, he or she needs to think of the best way to get advice or plans across to the maximum number of farmers.

The two chief functions of an extension officer are: (i) To reduce the learning time of an individual farmer to accept a new idea/technique, (ii) to increase the number of farmers, who understand the new ideas.

The extension officer can better perform these functions by working with the farmers' groups and by helping farmers indirectly by providing guidance and advice to private sector companies and by adopting a project approach. The following four potential activities can help the extension officer to achieve the desired goals.

- Giving advice to an individual farmer.
- Providing market advice to farmers through mass extension methods.
- Providing advice/information to critical individuals, organizations or private sector companies in the marketing chain whose actions can have a beneficial effect on marketing.
- Adopting a project approach by co-ordinating the activities of a number of different intermediaries in a marketing chain.

5. **Implementation of action plans:** To improve the rural incomes and profitability of small and marginal farmers, the extension officer must understand and work for what is required for them. The suggestions are not comprehensive. As each individual situation is different for achieving the goals of improving rural economy and profitability of the farmers, the extension officer must advise the farmers at various stages of livestock production besides making him aware of marketing aspects like pre-production. (Input supply finance and credit and production planning.)

6. **Review stage:** In this stage the progress will be compared with the action plan drawn. The deviations will be identified and analysed for further modification of the action plan. Based on the deviations, the new action plan will be prepared

and analysed through SWOT analysis. Lesser the deviations from action plan more will be the rate of success and vice versa.

# E-COMMERCE

Electronic commerce or e-commerce is a popular business model where the buying and selling of products occurs over the electronic network, viz. internet and other computer networks. Through e-commerce, trade can be done from doorstep. Almost any product or service can be offered via e-commerce, from books and music to financial services. For example, a poultry farmer can purchase, poultry implements for his poultry farm through e-commerce. At the same, the farmer can also find market and sell his products through e-commerce. Thus, e-commerce helps both the traders and consumers towards easier mode of transactions from the doorstep. Since the internet usage is widespread all over the world, the amount of trade conducted via e-commerce has increased tremendously. Modern e-commerce uses wider range of technologies such as World Wide Web, email, mobile devices, etc.

The e-commerce has its scope in the wide areas, viz. online marketing, supply chain management, online transaction processing, electronic data interchange, inventory management systems, automated data collection systems, spurring and drawing on innovations in electronic funds transfer.

## Applications of E-Commerce in Agriculture and Animal Husbandry Sectors

Some common applications related to the electronic commerce are enlisted below:

- This helps farmers in documenting automation in supply chain and logistics
- The farmers do online trading using domestic and international payment systems via e-commerce.
- The farmers or the traders can popularise their products through enterprise content management.
- E-commerce favours the farmers in group buying of inputs needed for their farm at low cost.
- The farmers get automated online assistants through e-commerce.
- E-commerce keeps the farmers updated with the trades and fund transfer instant messaging.

- The farmers can form or join newsgroups related to their trade through e-commerce.
- The farmer can track the product purchased through online shopping
- Online banking helps the farmers towards banking services at their doorstep.
- Teleconferencing
- The farmers can buy electronic tickets for exhibitions, Agri mela organised anywhere in the country through e-commerce.

## E-commerce Law

Online sellers should abide Federal Trade Commission (FTC) laws which regulate most e-commerce activities, including the use of commercial emails, online advertising and consumer privacy. Online sellers, particularly those selling internationally or across state lines, face different legal and financial considerations, especially in regard to privacy, security, copyright and taxation. Over the past decade, federal and state governments have passed new online advertising laws.

The Digital Millennium Copyright Act (DMCA) protects digital works on the internet. The farmers or entrepreneurs who want to involve in e-commerce business need to be aware of, including copyright infringement liability and a service provider's responsibilities.

### Advantages

- **Convenience and door step service:** E-commerce can be done all over the day without any time constrain.
- **Selection:** E-commerce favours the consumers to select wider range of products based on their interest and budget through online marketing.

### Disadvantages

- **Limited customer service:** The customer cannot contact the sales person to seek advice on the product which he intends to buy.
- **No instant gratification:** When you buy something online, you have to wait for it to be shipped to your home or office.
- **No ability to touch and see a prodsuct:** Customer can sometime be dissatisfied with e-commerce when the purchased product is not up to the quality what he expected on seeing the images on the internet.

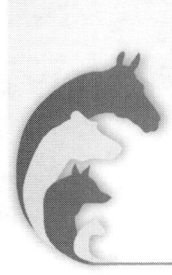

# Bibliography

1. Annamalai H, Manoharan RM, Netaji Seetharaman R. and Somasundaram S. "Rural Sociology and Psychology as Applied to Extension Education", Palaniappa Printers, Tirunelveli Jn., 1993.

2. Annamalai H, Manoharan RM, Netajiseetharaman R, Somasundaram S. "Rural Development and Programme Planning", Palaniappa Printers, Tirunelveli Jn., 1994.

3. Annamalai S. Part and parcel of the Tamil tradition, The Hindu. January 26, 2015.

4. Anonymous. "White Revolution by Co-operatives in Tamil Nadu", The Tamil Nadu. J. of Co-operation, 1994; 86: 4.

5. Anonymous. Introduction to Agricultural Extension Management, Post Graduate Diploma in Agricultural Extension Management, National Institute of Agricultural Extension Management, 2016.

6. Baskaram K, Somasundaram T. "Techniques of Extension Training", EEI, APAU, Hyderabad, 175.

7. Bhatia HR. "General Psychology", Oxford and IBH Publishers, New Delhi, 1981. Balister and R. Singh. Price spread in the marketing of eggs in Delhi. Agricultural Marketing, 1982; 25 (2) : 9–12.

8. Bell ML. Marketing Concepts and Strategy. New York: Macmillan Company, 1966.

9. Bhusan I, Sachdeva DR. An Introduction to Sociology, Kitab Mahal, Allahabad, 1980.

10. Brown, Ovor. "Mind your language." Capricon Books, New York, 1962.

11. Busset GM. "A Teaching Manual for Educational Psychology", Osmania University, Hyderabad, 1961.

12. Chandrakandan K, Palaniswamy S. Decentralised and Participatory Extension System: A need of the 21st Century. International Extension Forum Newsletter 1999; 142:(3): 5.

13. Chauhan SS. "Advanced Educational Psychology", Vikas Publishing House Pvt. Ltd., New Delhi, 1982.

14. Child D. " Psychology and the Teacher". Holt, Rivebart and Winston, Great Britain, 1975.

15. Clark Robert, C. Administration in Extension. University of Wisconsin, Madison, 1960.

16. Collinson MP. Farming Systems Research: Procedures for Technology Development. Expl. Agri. 1987; 23: 365–86.

17. Commissioner of Rural Development Training. "Training Rural Youth for Self-employment, Guidelines for Implementation". Govt. of Tamil Nadu, Chennai, 1995.

18. Crow LD, Crow A. "Educational Psychology", Urasia Publishing House (P) Ltd., Ram Nagar, New Delhi, 1979.

19. Dahama OP, Bhatnagar OP. Education and Communication for Development, Oxford & IBH Publishing Co., New Delhi, 1985.

20. Dass SS. "General Psychology", Asia Publishing House, Delhi. 1964; 455.

21. Deh PC. 'Rural Sociology: An Introduction", Kalyani Publishers, Delhi, 1981.

22. Department of Animal Husbandry and Dairying, Forty-first All India Livestock and Poultry Show Souvenier.

23. Ministry of Agriculture, Government of India, New Delhi, 1993.

24. Department of Rural Development. "IRDP and Allied Programmes of TRYSEM and DWCRA: A Manual", Ministry of Agriculture, Government of India, New Delhi, 1988.

25. Desai AR. "Rural Sociology in India". Popular Prakashan, Bombay, 1961.

26. Dillon JL, Plucknett DL, and Vallaeys GJ. Farming Systems Research at the International Agricultural Research Centres, TAC of the CGIAR, Rome, Italy, 1978.

27. Directorate of Extension. "Extension Education and Community Development", Govt. of India, New Delhi, 1961.

28. Draft of Five-Year Plan. "Planning Commission of India", New Delhi, 1980.

29. Draft Report on EEC Sheep Development Programme. Dept. of Animal Husbandry, Govt. of Tamil Nadu, Chennai, 1990.

30. Draft of Five-Year Plan. "Planning Commission of India", New Delhi, 2002.

31. Dull R, Sundaram KPM. "Indian Economy", S. Chand and Company Limited, New Delhi, 1995.

32. Ensminger D. "A Guide to Community Development, Government of India, New Delhi, 1962.

33. Ernst B, Peter R, Tonino Z. Agricultural Extension, Guidelines for extension worker in rural areas, International Book Distributing CO, Lucknow, 1995, pp 4.3, 4.7, 4.12.

34. Franco JD. "Extension Education and Community Development", Cornell University, New York, 1958.

35. Gangrade, KD. "Community Organisation in India", Popular Prakashan, Bombay, 1975.

36. Gelenn J Cook,"The Art of Making People Listen to You" Vikas Pub. House P. Ltd., New Delhi, 1976.

37. Hass Kenneth B, O Packer Harry. "Preparation of Audio-Visual Aids", Prentice-Hall, London, 1955.

38. Hergehahn BR. "An Introduction to Theories of Learning", Prentice-Hall, London, 1966.

39. Hough EM. The Co-operative Movement in India. Oxford University Press, London, 1966.

40. Hulton JH. Caste in India: Its Nature, Function and Origins, Oxford University Press, New Delhi, 1986.

41. Indian Poultry Industry Year Book, 1994.

42. Jagdish Prasad and Arbind Prasad, Indian Agriculture Marketing: Emerging Trends and Perspectives. New Delhi: Mittal Publications, 1955.

43. Jeelani R, Khandi SA, Kumar P, Bhadwal MS, Beig MY. Constraints Perceived by the Gujjars regarding Adoption of Improved Animal Husbandry Practices. Journal of Animal Research, 2015(5); 2:269–75.

44. Kelsey LD, Hearne GC. "Co-operative Extension Work", Comstock Publishing Associates, New York, 1963.

45. Kieffer RE and Lochran LW. "Manual of Audio-Visual Techniques", Prentice-Hall, 1966.

46. Kotler P. Marketing Management. New Delhi: Prentice-Hall of India Pvt. Ltd, 1989.

47. Kurien V. "White Revolution: After Anand what?", Survey of Indian Agriculture, 1988;179–83.

48. Kuryenson, "Rural Reconstruction Principles and Methods". Madras, 1950.

49. Misra DC. "Defining Agricultural Extension for 1990s". Occasional paper 1 Directorate of Extension, Ministry of Agriculture, New Delhi, 1990.

50. Misra DC. "New directions in extension training : A conceptual framework". Occasional paper 3 Directorate of Extension, Ministry of Agriculture, New Delhi, 1990.

51. MacIver RM, Page CM. "Society", Rinehart and Co., New York, 1949.

52. Mahesh Chand, VK Puti. "Regional Planning in India", New Delhi, 1983.

53. Mamoria CB, Joshi RL. Principles and Practices of Marketing in India. New Delhi : Prentice-Hall of India Pvt. Ltd, 1978.

54. Manivannan C. Principles and Techniques of veterinary and AH Extension, 2015.

55. Mathialagan P. "Animal Husbandry Extension and Rural Development: Seminar Paper, Dept.of Extension, Madras Veterinary College, Chennai, 1992.

56. Mathialagan P. "Priniciples & Extension Education Manual", Department of Extension Education, VC & RI TANUVAS, Namakkal, 1993.

57. Mathialagan P. "Seminar Paper: Partcipatory Technology Development" Department of Extension, VC & Rl, TANUVAS, Namakkal, 1996.

58. Mathialagan P. "Personality Development", Self-Confidence, 1995; 6(10): 3–10.

59. Minu Singh, Ritu Chakravarty, Adhiti Bhanotra and Sajad Ahmed Wani Constraints perceived by the tribal dairy farmers of Ranchi, Jharkhand in animal health care and management practices Indian J. Dairy Sci. 2015; 68(5).

60. Minjauw B.Training of trainers manual for livestock farmer field schools. participartory workshop held on the 17th to 29th September 2001, Mabanga FTC, Bungoma, 2001.

61. Morgan CT."A Brief Introduction to Psychology", Tata McGraw-Hill Publishing Company Ltd., New Delhi, 1977.

62. Mosher AT. "An Introduction to Agricultural Extension", Agricultural Development Council, Inc., New York, 1978.

63. Mukerji B. Objectives and Methods of Community Development, Extension Education in Community Development. Directorate of Extension, Government of India, New Delhi, 1961.

64. Narasimha Reddy CV. "How to be a good PRO"? Sharada Publications, Punjagutta, Hyderabed, 1976.

65. Newman WH. Administrative Action. Prentice-Hall, Inc., England, 1960.

66. Noxman DW. The Farming System Approach to Research. Farming Systems Research Paper No.3. Kansas State University, Manhattan, Kansas, USA, 1982.

67. Operation Flood: A Progress Report, NDDB, Anand, 1989.

68. Patil AP, Gawande SH, Nande MP and Gobade MR. Constraints Faced by the Dairy Farmers in Nagpur District while Adopting Animal Managenment Practices Veterinary World, 2019; 2(3):111–112.

69. Pilot Project: On Technology Assessment and Refinement Through Institution—Village Linkage Programme (IVLP) Action, KVK, IVRI, Izatnagar, Bareilly, April–September, 1997.

70. Prasad C. Extension Education System of the ICAR -A First Line Mechanism. Souvenir on the Occasion of Sixth National Seminar-cum-Workshop on KVK, 9–13 September, Divyayan KVK, Ranchi, Bihar, 1989.

71. Progress Report of NDDB. 1990.

72. Ramasamy C, R Prabaharan, A study of Marketing of Eggs in Madras City. Animal Husbandry Economics, Research Report No.1 Madras Veterinary College, Chennai, 1981.

73. Ray GL."Extension Communication and Management" Naya Prokash, 206, Bidhan Sarani, Calcutta,1996

74. Reddy AA. "Extension Education", Sree Lakshmi Press, Bapatla, 1993.

75. Report on Annual Plans. Planning Commission, Govt. of India, New Delhi, 1975.

76. Report on Livestock Census. Dept. of Animal Husbandry, Govt. of Tamil Nadu, Chennai, 1990.

77. Richard L Kohls and Joseph M. Uhl (1980). Marketing of Agricultural Products. New York : Macmillan Co., Inc.

78. Rogers EM. "Social Change in Rural Society", Appleton Century Crofts, New York, 1960.

79. Rural Development Department, "Workshop on Implementation of IRDP in Tamil Nadu, Report", Govt. of Tamil Nadu, Chennai, 1986.

80. Sabarathnam VE. R/R/PRA (PLA) for Agriculture, Rapid, Relaxed and Participatory Rural Appraisal Participatory, Learning and Action for Research and Extension in Agriculture (for crops and livestock), Vamsaravath Publishers, Hyderabad, 2002.

81. Samanta RK. "Women in Agriculture, Perspective, Issues and Experiences", MD Publications Pvt. Ltd., New Delhi, 1995.

82. Sanderson D. "Rural Sociology and Rural Social Organisation", John Wiley and Sons, New York, 1948.

83. Sanders HC. "The Co-operative Extension Service", Prentice-Hall, London, 1966.

84. Sathiadhas R, Noble D, Sheela I, Jyan KN, Sindhu S. Adoption Level of Scientific Dairy Farming Practices By IVLP Farmers in the Coastal Agro Ecosystem of Kerala. Indian Journal of Social Research Vol. 44(3) (243–250).

85. Shan PJ. "How to Develop Effective Public Speaking", Sultan Chand and Sons, New Delhi, 1988.

86. Shanmugasundaram S, Mathialagan P. "Sheep Development Programmes: A Few Constraints", Milcow. 17(1). Chennai, 1995.

87. Sharma RN and Sharma RK. Social Anthropology and Indian Tribal Media Promoters and Publishers, Mumbai, 1983.

88. Sharma RN. "Social Psychology", Kedaranath Ramnath, Meerut, 1973.

89. Sharma OP. "Practical Photography", Hind Pocket Books Private Ltd., Delhi, 1977.

90. Simmonds NW. A Short Review of Farming Systems Research in the Tropics. Experimental Agriculture, 1986; 22: 1–14.

91. Singh AK. Agricultural Extension: Impact and assessment, communication the tool for extension, Agrobios Publisher, Jodhpur, 2012; 218–19.

92. Singh J. Indian Social System, Prakashan Kendra, Lucknow.

93. Singh CB, De Boer AJ, Patil BR, Rai SN. Farming Systems Research and Extension for Livestock and Crop Residue Research and Development: Some Experiences, NDRI, Karnal, India, 1995.

94. Singh JP. Strategy for effective agricultural marketing extension to meet the challenges in 21st century, Manage Extension Research Review, July–Dec: 2001; 1–8.

95. Skinner CE. "Educational Psychology", Prentice-Hall, Metra, New Delhi, 1974.

96. Somasundaram T, Warren L Prawl. "Audio-Visuals: Their Role in Agriculture", APAU, Division of Extension, Hyderabad.

97. Supe SV. "An Introduction to Extension Education", Oxford & IBH Publishing Co. Pvt. Ltd., New Delhi, 1994.

98. Swanson Burton E. ed. "Agricultural Extension: A Reference Manual", Food and Agricultural Organization of the United Nations, 1989.

99. Tanwar PS. Constraints Perceived by Goat Keepers in Adoption of Goat Husbandry Practices in Semi-Arid. Rajasthan Journal of Community Mobilization and Sustainable Development, January-June 2011; 6(1): 108–111.

100. Taylor C Call. "A Critical Analysis of India's Community Development Programme", 1956.

101. Van den Ban AW, Hawkins HS. Agricultural Extension, CBS Publisher, and Distributers, New Delhi, 1998.

102. Veeramani K. "Why Reservation"? The Diravidar Kazhagam Publication, Chennai, 1983.

103. Waghmare SK, Waghmare VS. "Teaching Extension Education", Metropolitan, New Delhi, 1989.

104. Yella Reddy M. "Audio-Visual Aids in Teaching, Training and Extension", EEI, APAU, Hyderabad.

105. Dubey YK, Sharma ML, Yadav KN. Problems faced in adoption of improved dairy farming practices by the dairy farmers of Raipur City Research Journal of Animal Husbandry and Dairy Science 2012; 3(1): 30–3.

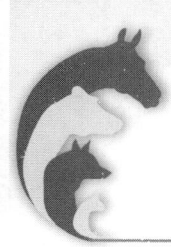

# Index